5 86   RE $ 2875

D0597447

NURSING INTERVENTIONS
Treatments for Nursing Diagnoses

GLORIA M. BULECHEK, R.N., Ph.D.
Assistant Professor, College of Nursing
University of Iowa, Iowa City, Iowa

JOANNE C. McCLOSKEY, R.N., Ph.D.
Associate Professor, College of Nursing
University of Iowa, Iowa City, Iowa

With a Foreword by
MYRTLE K. AYDELOTTE, Ph.D., F.A.A.N.
Professor of Nursing
University of Iowa, Iowa City, Iowa

W. B. SAUNDERS COMPANY   1985
Philadelphia □ London □ Toronto □
Mexico City □ Rio de Janeiro □
Sydney □ Tokyo

W. B. Saunders Company: West Washington Square
Philadelphia, PA   19105

1 St. Anne's Road
Eastbourne, East Sussex BN21 3UN, England

1 Goldthorne Avenue
Toronto, Ontario M8Z 5T9, Canada

Apartado 26370—Cedro 512
Mexico 4, D.F., Mexico

Rua Coronel Cabrita, 8
Sao Cristovao Caixa Postal 21176
Rio de Janeiro, Brazil

9 Waltham Street
Artarmon, N.S.W. 2064, Australia

Ichibancho, Central Bldg., 22-1 Ichibancho
Chiyoda-Ku, Tokyo 102, Japan

Library of Congress Cataloging in Publication Data

Main entry under title:

Nursing interventions.

1. Nurse and patient.   I. Bulechek, Gloria M. II. McCloskey, Joanne Comi. [DNLM: 1.
   Behavior Therapy— nurses' instruction.   2. Critical Care—nurses' instruction.   3.
   Nurse-Patient Relations.   4. Stress, Psychological—prevention & control—nurses' in-
   struction. WY 87 N9755]

RT86.3.N87   1985   610.73   84–14056

ISBN 0–7216–1310–1

Nursing Interventions: Treatments for Nursing Diagnoses   ISBN   0-7216-1310-1

© 1985 by W. B. Saunders Company. Copyright under the Uniform Copyright Conven-
tion. Simultaneously published in Canada. All rights reserved. This book is protected by
copyright.   No part of it may be reproduced, stored in a retrieval system, or transmitted in any
form or by any means, electronic, mechanical, photocopying, recording, or otherwise, without
written permission from the publisher. Made in the United States of America. Press of W. B.
Saunders Company. Library of Congress catalog card number 84-14056.

Last digit is the print number: 9   8   7   6   5   4   3   2   1

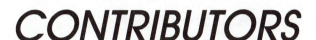

CONTRIBUTORS

Janet Davidson Allan, R.N., M.S.
Adult Health Nurse Practitioner, University of California, Berkeley, California
Exercise Program

Linda Jo Banks, R.N., M.S., M.A.
Surgical Nurse Clinician, Mercy Hospital Medical Center, Des Moines, Iowa
Counseling

Pamela J. Brink, R.N., Ph.D., F.A.A.N.
Professor, College of Nursing, University of Iowa, Iowa City, Iowa
Culture Brokerage

Kathleen C. Buckwalter, R.N., Ph.D.
Associate Professor, College of Nursing, University of Iowa, Iowa City, Iowa
Music Therapy; Sexual Counseling

Gloria M. Bulechek, R.N., Ph.D.
Assistant Professor, College of Nursing, University of Iowa, Iowa City, Iowa
Nursing Diagnosis and Intervention; Future Directions

Geraldine Busse, R.N., M.P.H.
Adjunct Associate Professor and Emeritus Associate Professor, College of Nursing, University of Iowa, Iowa City, Iowa
Nutritional Counseling

Martha A. Carpenter, R.N., M.A., M.S.
Assistant in Instruction, College of Nursing, University of Iowa, Iowa City, Iowa
Support Groups

Norma J. Christman, R.N., Ph.D.
Assistant Professor, College of Nursing, University of Illinois at Chicago, Chicago, Illinois
Preparatory Sensory Information

Sandra Cummings, R.N., M.S.
Psychotherapist, Mid-Eastern Iowa Community Mental Health Center, Iowa City, Iowa
Group Psychotherapy

M. Patricia Donahue, R.N., Ph.D.
Associate Professor, College of Nursing, University of Iowa, Iowa City, Iowa
Patient Advocacy

Cynthia M. Dougherty, R.N., M.A.
Instructor, College of Nursing, University of Iowa, Iowa City, Iowa; Staff nurse in SICU and Cardiac Catheterization Lab; The University of Iowa Hospitals and Clinics, Iowa City, Iowa
Surveillance

Geraldene Felton, R.N., Ed.D, F.A.A.N.
Professor and Dean, College of Nursing, University of Iowa, Iowa City, Iowa
Preoperative Teaching

Jill Gaffney, R.N., M.A.
Quality Circles Facilitator, VA Medical Center, Knoxville, Iowa
Music Therapy

Diane L. Gardner, R.N., M.A.
Instructor, College of Nursing, University of Iowa, Iowa City, Iowa; Nursing Coordinator—Maternal/Child Health, Mercy Hospital, Cedar Rapids, Iowa
Presence

Diane Bronkema Hamilton, R.N., M.A.
Doctoral candidate, University of Virginia, Charlottesville, Virginia
Reminiscence Therapy

Jane W. Hartsock, R.N., M.A.
Instructor, Medical Surgical Nursing, Moline Public Hospital School of Nursing, Moline, Illinois
Music Therapy

Janet Helms, R.N., M.A.
Instructor in Nursing, Moline Public Hospital School of Nursing, Moline, Illinois
Active Listening

Deborah Perry Jensen, R.N., M.A.
Instructor, College of Nursing, University of Iowa, Iowa City, Iowa
Patient Contracting

Kathleen Kelly, R.N., M.A.
Assistant Professor, College of Nursing, University of Iowa, Iowa City, Iowa
Discharge Planning

Karlene M. Kerfoot, R.N., Ph.D.

Senior Associate Director, Department of Nursing, University of Iowa Hospitals and Clinics, Iowa City, Iowa
Sexual Counseling

Carolyn K. Dreessen Kinney, R.N., Ph.D.

Assistant Professor and Coordinator of the R.N. Studies Program, University of Michigan School of Nursing, Ann Arbor, Michigan
Support Groups

Karin T. Kirchhoff, R.N., Ph.D.

Associate Professor, University of Illinois at Chicago College of Nursing, Chicago, Illinois; Clinical Nursing Research Coordinator, University of Illinois Hospital, Chicago, Illinois
Preparatory Sensory Information

Robert J. Kus, R.N., Ph.D.

Assistant Professor, College of Nursing, University of Iowa, Iowa City, Iowa
Crisis Intervention

Debra Livingston, R.N., M.S.

Psychiatric-Mental Health Clinical Nurse Specialist, University of Iowa Hospitals and Clinics, Iowa City, Iowa
Truth Telling

Rebecca Mannetter, R.N., M.A.

Clinical Nursing Specialist, Psychiatric Nursing Division, University of Iowa Hospitals and Clinics, Iowa City, Iowa
Support Groups

Eleanor McClelland, R.N., Ph.D.

Associate Professor, College of Nursing, University of Iowa, Iowa City, Iowa
Discharge Planning

Joanne Comi McCloskey, R.N., Ph.D.

Associate Professor and Chairperson, Organizations and Systems, College of Nursing, University of Iowa, Iowa City, Iowa
Nursing Diagnosis and Intervention; Future Directions

Marilyn T. Molen, R.N., Ph.D.

Associate Professor and Assistant Dean, Graduate Program, College of Nursing, University of Iowa, Iowa City, Iowa
Surveillance

Sue Ann Moorhead, R.N., M.A.

Assistant in Instruction, College of Nursing, University of Iowa, Iowa City, Iowa
Role Supplementation

Nola J. Pender, R.N., Ph.D.
Professor, Community Health Nursing, School of Nursing, Northern Illinois University, DeKalb, Illinois
Self Modification

Barbara K. Redman, R.N., Ph.D.
Executive Director, American Association of Colleges of Nursing, Washington, D.C.; Adjunct Professor, University of Maryland School of Nursing, Baltimore, Maryland
Patient Teaching

Anne G. Sadler, R.N., M.S.
Psychiatric Clinical Nurse Specialist, University of Iowa Hospitals and Clinics, Iowa City, Iowa
Assertiveness Training

Sharon Scandrett, R.N., Ph.D.
Associate Professor, University of Tennessee Center for the Health Sciences, Memphis, Tennessee
Relaxation Training; Cognitive Reappraisal

Sue Ann Thomas, R.N. Ph.D.
Associate Professor of Nursing, Clinical Director, Psychophysiological Clinics, University of Maryland, Baltimore, Maryland
Patient Teaching

Toni Tripp-Reimer, R.N., Ph.D.
Associate Professor and Chair, Theory and Methods, College of Nursing, University of Iowa, Iowa City, Iowa
Culture Brokerage

Susan Uecker, R.N., M.A., C.S.
Adjunct Instructor, College of Nursing, University of Iowa, Iowa City, Iowa; Clinical Specialist, Psychiatric Clinic, University of Iowa, Iowa City, Iowa
Relaxation Training

Veronica Wieland, R.N., M.A.C.S.
Psychotherapist, Mid-Eastern Iowa Community Mental Health Center, Iowa City, Iowa; Adjunct Appointment, University of Iowa, Iowa City, Iowa
Group Psychotherapy

James Z. Wilberding, R.N., M.A.
Clinical Instructor, Department of Nursing Service Education, V.A. Medical Center, Iowa City, Iowa
Values Clarification

Cassandra Williamson, R.N., M.A., C.S.
Psychiatric-Mental Health Clinical Nurse Specialist, University of Iowa, Hospitals and Clinics, Iowa City, Iowa
Truth Telling

FOREWORD

Within the last twenty-five years, major attention of nurse scholars has been directed toward the development of the intellectual base of nursing practice. A number of concepts underlying clinical nursing practice and drawn from the physical and social services have been well described by nursing authors, and descriptions of these concepts now appear in the nursing literature. What has not received the same attention is the systematic organization of that knowledge as it relates to specific decisions made by practicing nurses, decisions concerning the phenomena they observe in caring for patients and clients and the actions they undertake in dealing with those phenomena. Bulechek and McCloskey, the editors of this volume, have chosen to confront that task. They are congratulated upon their effort.

The early efforts to study nursing practice made use of task analysis, time and motion studies of nursing procedures, and bacteriological studies. Gradually, other kinds of methodologies and knowledge from other disciplines were introduced in nursing practice research. But in spite of the growth of nursing research, we are still lacking a system of standardized nomenclature describing the kinds of patient and client problems nurses treat and a set of standard treatments that apply to the task of resolving those problems. The lack of standardized nomenclature has been recognized and is being addressed, but the unavailability of standardized programs of treatment, designed within a framework of research and science, is not being remedied.

In this book, which is a major pioneering effort, Bulechek and McCloskey have brought together a set of nursing interventions for practicing nurses to use in their work. They point out that although controversy and lack of agreement surround the terms *nursing diagnosis* and *nursing intervention*, this nomenclature is both valid and useful. As a form of logical clinical inquiry, the use of the *nursing process* leads to junctures at which the nurse makes decisions about the nature of the phenomena with which he or she is dealing and about the selection and execution of specific nursing interventions to modify, interrupt, alter, or eliminate forces or factors giving rise to those phenomena. This is, in essence, the nurse's task, and the effect of that intervention is the outcome of the client problem. The editors have selected contributors, who, through review of research and literature and through their own experience, are attempting to standardize the treatment program (the intervention) for specific nursing diagnoses. These interventions are generalizations derived from studies of groups of patients or clients and from analyses of case studies. The generalizations can be modified to meet the nursing diagnoses of patients or clients in particular situations. The variety of interventions described and the diagnosis for which they can be used are representative of the independent actions nurses perform. In the introduction to each section of the book, the editors make a specific connection between the nursing diagnoses and the interventions.

Bulechek and McCloskey state that the book is primarily a text for undergraduate and graduate students. They believe it also serves as a reference and stimulus for clinical nursing research and as a basis for curriculum change. These are legitimate claims, but the value of the book's content far surpasses these modest assertions. The book offers to practicing nurses a basis for viewing their practice as requiring knowledge of intellectual depth. It reflects a domain of practice which is theirs and theirs alone, independent of physician prescription and hospital policy, procedures, and rules. It is a domain of practice that exacts from the nurse clinical nursing knowledge, clinical judgment, and evaluation of results. The stimulus to the nurse's own professional growth is great. Nursing administrators will do well to take advantage of this book's potential and encourage professional nursing staffs to make use of its content for self-development. Novice nurses, instead of methodologically and tediously designing their own interventions, can draw upon the experience of these experts and use this conceptual framework, which is so well synthesized.

The editors recognize the need for further study of the effectiveness of the intervention selected for each particular nursing diagnosis. Clinical testing of both diagnoses and interventions is also indicated. This would lead to increased reliability of the labeling of the diagnoses and standardization of the interventions. The recognition of the need for further studies in no way reduces the value of the book. This pioneer work will initiate a much needed re-examination of how nursing practice is taught, perceived, and organized. The intellectual activity it can generate and the satisfaction it will produce among practicing nurses are exciting to contemplate. The value of the work reaches far into the future. The editors and their contributors have made a rich gift to the nursing field.

MYRTLE K. AYDELOTTE
PROFESSOR OF NURSING
UNIVERSITY OF IOWA

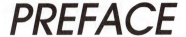

PREFACE

We are seeing today the evolution of nursing into an autonomous profession. Many factors in the past decade have contributed to this change: women's liberation, university education for nurses, political assertiveness, primary care, collective bargaining, change in licensure laws, and increased specialization. One measure of nursing's autonomy is the growing body of nursing knowledge. Knowledge of nursing practice has increased through the identification, categorization, and testing of nursing diagnoses and interventions. As the knowledge is defined, nursing curricula are changing to reflect the expanded scope of nursing practice.

The chapters in this book identify and define twenty-six nursing interventions. The idea for the book was born when we were unable to find adequate teaching materials for a course in adult health nursing at The University of Iowa that focused on nursing intervention. As part of our teaching assignments in the graduate program we cotaught two clinical courses on care of the adult client.

The first course dealt with nursing assessment and nursing diagnosis. Several books, many of them new in 1981, were available for use in this course, including the works of the National Conferences on Nursing Diagnoses. In addition, several "concept books" served as useful reference material for the course: the concepts in these books were almost unanimously diagnostic concepts.

The second course focused on nursing interventions. We were dismayed to find only a meager amount of literature in this area. The CURN project (1982) was one of the few works available. While it is a monumental piece of work in nursing—bridging the gap between research and practice—this series of monographs is difficult to use in a course because of the high cost to students. We found a handful of other books, each dealing with a single intervention concept, such as therapeutic touch, patient contracting, patient teaching, crisis intervention, and advocacy. But what we needed for the course was one textbook that discussed the various definitions of the intervention phase of the nursing process and presented a collection of nursing interventions. Since no such textbook is available, we have developed this book to fulfill the need.

In the summer of 1982 we began contacting prospective authors. We decided at the outset that the chapters should be written by nurses with graduate preparation because we wanted to emphasize the research base and the theoretical framework underlying the interventions. To assure an integrated book, each author was asked to use the following chapter outline:

A. Description or definition of the intervention.
B. Literature related to the intervention, both general and research.
C. Identification of any available intervention tools.
D. Identification of associated nursing diagnoses and appropriate client groups.
E. Recommendations for practice and research.
F. Case study examples.
G. References.

Occasionally a chapter varies from this outline when the content requires a slightly different organization. Because definitions of the intervention concepts and the associated research base are quite variable, the chapters differ in practice implications. Most include a case study but a few do not. Although some interventions have clear protocols that could be easily implemented, most do not. No one individual professional nurse can be adequately prepared to carry out all of the described interventions. Caution is recommended on the unsupervised use of unfamiliar interventions.

An introductory chapter on nursing diagnosis and intervention sets the stage for the remaining chapters, each on a separate intervention. The introductory chapter defines nursing intervention as a step of the nursing process, reviews the nursing process and nursing diagnosis movement, and then demonstrates how interventions relate to diagnoses. We recommend that all users of the book read Chapter 1 and then choose intervention chapters of interest to them.

Each intervention discussed here is linked to appropriate nursing diagnoses. The authors have used the list of established nursing diagnoses from the 5th National Conference on Nursing Diagnosis as well as diagnoses from their own expertise, as the Conference list is not all-inclusive.

Although the authors have identified nursing diagnoses that relate to the intervention, there has been *no research* that tests the effectiveness of an intervention in relationship to a particular diagnosis. We have made an index of interventions for particular diagnoses based upon the authors' ideas (see Future Directions), but we caution readers to use this only as a guide. Eventually research will provide clear indicators for practicing nurses concerning which intervention to choose for their patients according to the patient's nursing diagnosis. At present, however, this book is more correctly viewed as a useful guide to possibilities for clinical research into preferable interventions for nursing diagnoses. Each intervention is a broad, complex concept which has been operationally defined. Each chapter has been written by a nurse or nurses with graduate preparation drawing upon their practice experience. Each chapter concludes with comments and questions developed by the editors to facilitate discussion. The chapters are organized in four sections according to their central focus: stress management, life style alteration, acute care management, and communication. Each of the sections has an introduction that summarizes the material in the section. The sections and their titles evolved from the collection of interventions. In the beginning, we had planned to have an alphabetical listing of intervention chapters, but as chapters came in, we noticed that they grouped themselves in four areas. The four areas (stress management, lifestyle alteration, acute care management, and communication) can be viewed as one level of a taxonomy of interventions. A second, more concrete level would be the twenty-six interventions. Nursing orders, several of which would result from each intervention listed here, could be a third, even more concrete level of intervention. Like any emerging taxonomy, this beginning organization of interventions will be subject to many revisions in the future.

Selection of an intervention to be included depended mostly on our ability to find a knowledgeable and willing author. No attempt was made to include an exhaustive or inclusive list of nursing interventions. In fact there is one area that is noticeably lacking—that is the group of interventions to treat the self-care deficit diagnoses. Interventions such as Hygiene, Positioning, Mouth Care, and Bowel and Bladder Training would be included in this section. The reason for this limitation is that the research base on these interventions is very scanty and we were not able to locate clinicians who could write from their experience within a reasonable time frame. Being aware of this omission, we are already planning to cover this area if there are future editions of this book.

While the book was written with graduate students in mind, it should be useful in both undergraduate and graduate programs. The book can be used as a graduate course textbook in a clinical specialization course that focuses on interventions. It also can be used as a supplement to undergraduate clinical textbooks. These textbooks are often very global in their discussion of nursing interventions, frequently lumping them together in short sections entitled "Nursing management of the patient with . . . ." As the role of the nurse becomes more independent, we may see nursing intervention books, such as this one, replacing the traditional medical-surgical nursing, obstetrical nursing, and psychiatric nursing texts. We welcome that day; we welcome the day when nursing is able to fully articulate its independent role. This is our attempt to hasten the process.

Reference

Conduct and Utilization of Research in Nursing (CURN) Project. *Using research to improve nursing practice.* New York: Grune and Stratton, Inc., 1982, 11 volumes, 1548 pp.

ACKNOWLEDGMENTS

The cooperation and support of many people made this book possible. Our graduate students in adult health nursing responded enthusiastically to a new course devoted to interventions. Our contributors wrote and revised their manuscripts with fine professionalism. Our publisher decided to take the risk.

The book was written in a spirit of innovation, with the knowledge that we are extending the boundaries of nursing. The contributors made enormous efforts to define and clarify the interventions. Synthesizing the literature and their practical experience, they have made explicit what has previously been implicit. The best acknowledgment they could have is that other nurses use their ideas.

The College of Nursing at The University of Iowa provided typing and photocopying service. Steven Warner, our data processor, provided secretarial assistance. Our colleagues and students at Iowa have been most enthusiastic and encouraging.

CONTENTS

1

NURSING DIAGNOSIS AND INTERVENTION

GLORIA M. BULECHEK
JOANNE C. McCLOSKEY

For the first time in a century of organized nursing, nurses are defining an autonomous role. To this end we have seen in the past decade more specialization, changes in licensure laws, and the movement for nursing diagnosis. The key to an autonomous profession is a clearly defined base of knowledge. While nursing will continue to use knowledge from other disciplines, it must define what it is that nurses do and whether what they do makes a difference. This book is a beginning.

The focus of the book is nursing intervention. Diagnosis and intervention are two steps in the nursing process— a systematic problem-solving methodology which the nurse uses to deliver patient care.

THE NURSING PROCESS MOVEMENT

The nursing process can be conceived of as a description of the nurse thinking. In a sense, the nursing process was an offshoot of earlier attempts to define nursing. Although nurses have been licensed in the United States since 1903, it was not until 1938, when the first mandatory nursing practice act was passed in New York, that there was a recognized need to define nursing. Until 1938 all acts were "permissive," allowing unlicensed persons to practice as long as they did not use the title Registered Nurse. Although the laws were called nursing practice acts, none of those written before 1938 included a definition of nursing in terms of practice. Rather, a Registered Nurse was someone who had completed an acceptable nursing program and passed an examination, with the emphasis placed on the educational process. With a mandatory act that made it illegal for an unlicensed person to practice nursing, it became necessary in 1938 to define nursing. Attempts to define nursing, however, have been frustrated by the sheer size of the profession, its diversity in educational preparation, and its work demands. While we are closer to a definition of nursing today, the task is still before us.

If we cannot say what nursing is, we can at least describe what a nurse does. Nursing, then, is what a nurse does. Lydia Hall's attempt in 1955 to clarify the nurse's role was important; she suggested that we judge the quality of nursing care on a continuum from bad to good by whether the nurse did nursing at the patient, to the patient, for the patient, or with the patient. Another valuable contribution was that of Ida Jean Orlando in 1960, who addressed the interpersonal aspects of the client-nurse relationships. In 1966 Lois Knowles stated that a nurse's success as a practitioner depended upon her mastery of the five D's (Discover, Delve, Decide, Do, and Discriminate). The attempts of these and other nurses to describe nursing were important because they put into words the intellectual activity of the nurse, previously labeled as intuitive.

In 1967, the faculty at the school of nursing at The Catholic University of America in Washington, D.C., identified four phases of the nursing process: assessment, planning, implementation, and evaluation (Yura and Walsh, 1978). These four phases or steps of the nursing process are still the ones most often listed today, partly because they were the ones popularized in Yura and Walsh's book, *The Nursing Process: Assessing, Planning, Implementation and Evaluating* (1983; originally published in 1967). According to these authors,

> The nursing process is an orderly, systematic manner of determining the client's problems, making plans to solve them, initiating the plan or assigning others to implement it, and evaluating the extent to which the plan was effective in resolving the problems identified. (Yura and Walsh, 1978, p. 20)

In Yura and Walsh's steps, assessment begins with the nursing history and ends with the nursing diagnosis, planning includes goal setting and writing the care plan, implementation is the carrying out of the nursing actions called for in the care plan, and evaluation is a rethinking of the diagnosis and treatment in terms of the patient's response.

The popularity of these steps has overshadowed many other available alternatives. A comparison of steps proposed by different authors (see Table 1–1) reveals several interesting points:

1. The four-step model of assessment, planning, implementation, and evaluation is best known because Yura and Walsh popularized it in the first text on nursing process. Had they chosen to popularize the steps of perception, communication, interpretation, intervention, and evaluation proposed in the same year by the Western States Committee, the majority of nurses would probably label the steps of the nursing process differently.

2. All authors agree that the process is continuous. Evaluation leads in a circular process to reassessment.

3. Before 1973, nursing diagnosis was not listed as a step of the nursing process.

4. Although there are various alternatives, it appears that the four step model is being replaced by a five step model. The most popular five step model includes the steps of assessment, diagnosis, planning, intervention, evaluation.

What, then, is the nursing process? It is a problem-solving, systematic approach to care delivery which describes the intellectual activity of the nurse. It connects what a nurse does with why he or she does it; the nursing process requires actions based on judgment (Gordon, 1982).

The nursing process standardizes nursing care while providing individual service. Most nurses do not understand this. They continue to advocate "individual care planning" while using a process which encourages "group care planning modified for an individual when necessary." Mintzberg (1979), in an excellent chapter on the professional bureaucracy, explains the situation:

> The professional has two basic tasks: 1. to categorize the client's need in terms of a contingency, which indicates which standard program to use, a task known as diagnosis and 2. to apply or execute that program. [This categorization] allows the professional to move through the world without making continuing decisions at every moment. (Mintzberg, 1979, p. 352)

As examples of the professional, Mintzberg cites (1) the psychiatrist who examines a patient, declares him to be manic-depressive and thus initiates psychotherapy and (2) the professor who finds 100 students registered in a course and executes a lecture program but would run the class as a seminar if only 20 students registered. Similarly, a professional nurse using the nursing process would recognize such problems as anxiety, pain, knowledge deficit, and so on, and would have a precise and tested repertoire of skills designed to treat each of these problems. "A professional nurse, while cognizant of individual differences, seeks to identify nursing interventions and patient outcomes that are applicable to identifiable groups of patients" (CURN Project, 1981, p. xiv).

Table 1–1. STEPS OF THE NURSING PROCESS ACCORDING TO DIFFERENT AUTHORS

Yura and Walsh (1967, 1978)
  Assessment
  Planning
  Implementation
  Evaluation
	Western States Committee (1967)*
	  Perception
	  Communication
	  Interpretation
	  Intervention
	  Evaluation

Zimmerman and Gohrke (1970)
  Assessment
  Goal Setting
  Planning
  Action
  Evaluation
	Carrieri and Sitzman (1971)
	  Observation
	  Inference
	  Interaction
	  Assessment
	  Evaluation

ANA's Standards of Nursing Practice (1973)
  Collection of Data
  Nursing Diagnosis
  Goal Setting
  Planning of Nursing Care
  Nursing Action
  Reassessment
  Revision of Plan
	Mundinger and Jauron (1975)
	  Data-Gathering
	  Diagnosing
	  Planning
	  Implementing
	  Evaluation

McCloskey (1978)
  Assessment
  Diagnosis
  Goal Setting
  Intervention
  Evaluation
	Carlson, Craft, and McGuire (1982)
	  Assessment
	  Diagnosis
	  Plan
	  Intervention
	  Evaluation

Gordon (1982)
  Assessment
  Diagnosis
  Outcome Projection
  Planning
  Intervention
  Outcome Evaluation	

*See Yura and Walsh, 1978, pp. 24–25.

The nursing process is, then, professional nursing practice—the diagnosis and treatment of health problems within the scope of nursing. But just what is the scope of nursing? What problems do or should nurses diagnose? What treatments do or should nurses use? What treatments work for what diagnoses? The chapters in this book are a beginning attempt to outline nursing treatments and to relate them to nursing diagnoses. The term intervention is used to denote these nursing treatments.

NURSING DIAGNOSIS

Nursing diagnosis has made enormous strides in the past decade. After much debate in the early 1970s about what it is and whether nurses should do it, it is now generally accepted that a nursing diagnosis is

> a clinical diagnosis made by a professional nurse that describes actual or potential health problems which the nurse, by virtue of her education and experience is capable and licensed to treat. (Gordon, 1976, p. 1299)

Some users of nursing diagnosis have difficulty accepting the problem focus of Gordon's definition. Indeed, one criticism frequently leveled at nursing diagnosis is that it focuses on illness (problems) and not wellness. In an attempt to respond to this concern, Carlson, Craft, and McGuire (1982) in their textbook define nursing diagnosis as

> A statement of a potential or an actual altered health status of a client(s), which is derived from nursing assessment and which requires intervention from the domain of nursing. (p. ix)

The profession's acceptance of nursing diagnosis came (at least at the organizational level, if not at the individual level) in 1980 when the American Nurses' Association (ANA) published Nursing: A Social Policy Statement. According to this document, "Nursing is the diagnosis and treatment of human responses to actual or potential health problems" (p. 9). The definition is based on the 1972 Nurse Practice Act of New York State. The language, which has been incorporated in the nursing practice acts of many other states, defines both the independent and the dependent roles of today's nurses:

> The practice of the profession of nursing as a registered professional nurse is defined as diagnosing and treating human responses to actual or potential health problems through such services as case finding, health teaching, health counseling, and provision of care supportive to or restorative of life and well being, and executing medical regimens as prescribed by a licensed or otherwise legally authorized physician or dentist. A nursing regimen shall be consistent with and shall not vary any existing medical regime. (Kelly, 1974, p. 1315)

In the ANA document, human responses are viewed as

> (1) reactions of individuals and groups to actual health problems (health-restoring responses), such as the impact of illness effects upon the self and family, and related self-care needs; and (2) concerns of individuals and groups about potential health problems (health-supporting responses), such as monitoring and teaching in populations or communities at risk in which educative needs for information, skill development, health-oriented attitudes, and related behavioral changes arise. (American Nurses' Association, 1980, pp. 9, 10)

Gordon (1982) adds further clarification by noting that health-restoring responses are problems secondary to illness, medical therapy, developmental changes, or life situations, whereas health-supporting responses are problems in health management.

A comparison of the ANA model practice acts of 1955 and 1980 (see Table 1–2) demonstrates the profession's acceptance of diagnosis as an integral part of the nurse's role. In 1955, the act specifically precluded acts of diagnosis, whereas in 1980 the act acknowledged that nurses diagnose and treat.

Although the profession has accepted diagnosis as part of a nurse's role, there is as yet no fully acceptable definition of what a nursing diagnosis is. The ANA's "human responses to health problems" is cumbersome and unclear; Carlson and associates' "altered health status" is equally unclear. Our preference is with the guidelines provided by Gordon and the North American Nursing Diagnosis Association. In our own words, nursing diagnosis is the identification of a patient's problem that the nurse can treat. Thus, pain, decubitus ulcer, fear, and difficult adaptation to altered body image are nursing diagnoses, whereas organic heart disease, cancer, and bowel obstruction are medical diagnoses. Diabetes is a medical diagnosis, whereas knowledge deficit related to diabetes is a nursing diagnosis. However, it is not always this simple. For example, what is weight loss? Wound infection? Hypertension?

Some diagnoses are both nursing and medical. Some patients require many nursing diagnoses, some only one or two, and some none at all. Nursing diagnoses change more frequently than medical diagnoses, and some patients with no nursing diagnoses one day may require several a few days later as a result of medical intervention. Nursing diagnoses are more fluid, varying, and episodic than medical diagnoses (ANA, 1980).

In order to classify and standardize nursing diagnoses and treatments it is necessary that a diagnosis be accompanied by a noting of the signs, symptoms, and etiological factors that led to the making of the diagnosis. Several formats exist for stating a nursing diagnosis: PES (Problem–Etiology–Signs and Symptoms) format, "related to" format, supporting data format, and POR (Problem-Oriented Record) format. Examples of diagnoses made in each format are supplied in Table 1–3. The basic elements of each format are the diagnosis (problem), its etiology (cause) and its characteristics (signs and symptoms). Whatever the format, supporting data (etiology and characteristics) are important because they give clues concerning how to treat the problem. This will not always be necessary, however; at some point in the future a nursing diagnosis will mean, just as a medical diagnosis now does, a precise set of signs and symptoms and etiology which will call for certain treatments.

Although others have made important contributions to the identification and classification of nursing diagnoses (Campbell, 1978; Lunney, 1982; U.S.

Table 1–2. ANA'S MODEL PRACTICE ACTS, 1955 AND 1980

1955 Act:
  "The practice of professional nursing means the performance for compensation of any act in the observation, care and counsel of the ill, injured, or infirm, or in the maintenance of health or prevention of illness of others, or in the supervision and teaching of other personnel, or the administration of medications and treatments prescribed by a licensed physician or dentist; requiring substantial specialized judgment and skill and based on knowledge and application of the principles of biological, physical and social sciences. The foregoing shall NOT (emphasis added) be deemed to include acts of diagnosis or prescription of therapeutic or corrective measures." (Kelly, 1974, p. 1314)

1980 Act:
  "The practice of nursing means the performance for compensation of professional services requiring substantial knowledge of the biological, physical, behavioral, psychological, and sociological sciences and nursing theory as the basis for assessment, diagnosis, planning, intervention, and evaluation in the promotion and maintenance of health; the case finding and management of illness, injury or infirmity; the restoration of optimum function; or the achievement of a dignified death." (ANA, 1980b)

Table 1–3. NURSING DIAGNOSIS EXPRESSED IN FOUR DIFFERENT FORMATS

PES format
  Problem: ***Impaired Reality Testing (Acute)***
  Etiology; Psychosis
  Signs and Symptoms:
    1. Impaired perception
    2. Impaired attention span
    3. Impaired decision making (Bruce, 1979)

Related to format
  Anxiety related to impending surgery as characterized by verbalization.
  Knowledge deficit related to diabetes as characterized by inability to give self insulin,
    inadequate diet, and poor hygiene.

Supporting data format
  Knowledge deficit
    Supporting data: Newly diagnosed diabetic, Does not know how to give daily insulin
      injections. Daily intake list for past week reveals diet not followed, although instructed
      by dietitian 7/1. Overweight. Poor hygiene practices. Believes diabetes will go away in a
      few years.

POR format (Problem-Oriented Record)
  S. Believes diabetes will go away in few years. Says does not know how to give daily insulin.
  O. Newly diagnosed diabetic. Daily intake for past week reveals does not follow diet although
    was instructed by dietitian 7/1.
  Weight 180. Ht./wt. chart puts desirable weight at 155.
  Nails dirty and large toenails ingrown.
  A. ***Knowledge deficit*** related to diabetes.
  P. List above diagnosis as problem #3 on patient's problem list.
  Teach patient and wife about diabetes, complications and insulin.
  Stress need for foot care, diet and urine testing. Referral to visiting nurse for post-discharge
    evaluation.

Department of Health and Human Services, 1980), one group has taken national
leadership for the arduous task. In 1973 the National Conference Group for
Classification of Nursing Diagnoses was formed. Six national conferences have
been held since that time, and five books (Gebbie and Lavin, 1975; Gebbie,
1976; Kim and Moritz, 1982; Kim, McFarland, and McLane, 1984a and b) have
been published. In 1982, the National Conference Group became the North
American Nursing Diagnosis Association.

The purpose of all six conferences has been the development of a
diagnostic taxonomy for nurses: "the definition of a standard nomenclature
for describing health problems amenable to treatment by nurses" (Kim and
Moritz, 1982, p. xvii). At each conference approximately 150 nurse practitioners, educators, administrators, researchers, theorists, and graduate students
from the United States and Canada who have expertise and interest in the
development of nursing diagnoses have worked together to refine and expand
previous work. The methodology used by the conference group to define and
classify diagnoses is inductive—the identification of diagnoses by observing
and reflecting upon what it is that nurses do. Using a factor-isolating theoretical
approach (Dickoff, James, and Wiedenbach, 1968a, 1968b), the group is "doing
nothing less than describing the entire domain of nursing" (Kim and Moritz,
1982, p. 24).

To date, a list of 50 nursing diagnoses have been "approved" by the
National Conference Group (see Table 1–4). These have been identified by the
group for clinical testing by the nursing profession. The list is by no means
exhaustive, and most diagnoses need to be developed further to be clinically
useful. Additional research is needed on the diagnostic process; the validation
of the nursing diagnoses, their etiologies, and characteristics; the identification
of critical defining characteristics; and the identification of treatments that
work for each diagnosis.

Table 1–4. LIST OF 50 NURSING DIAGNOSES ACCEPTED FOR CLINICAL TESTING
   BY THE NORTH AMERICAN NURSING DIAGNOSIS ASSOCIATION, (1982)

*Activity Intolerance
 Airway Clearance, Ineffective
*Anxiety
 Bowel Elimination, Alterations in: Constipation
 Bowel Elimination, Alterations in: Diarrhea
 Bowel Elimination, Alterations in: Incontinence
 Breathing Patterns, Ineffective
 Cardiac Output, Alterations in: Decreased
 Comfort, Alterations in: Pain
 Communication, Impaired Verbal
 Coping, Ineffective Individual
 Coping, Ineffective Family: Compromised
 Coping, Ineffective Family: Disabling
 Coping, Family: Potential for Growth
 Diversional Activity, Deficit
*Family Processes, Alteration in
 Fear
*Fluid Volume, Alteration in: Excess
 Fluid Volume Deficit, Actual
 Fluid Volume Deficit, Potential
 Gas Exchange, Impaired
 Grieving, Anticipatory
 Grieving, Dysfunctional
*Health Maintenance Alteration
 Home Maintenance Management, Impaired
 Injury, Potential for
 Knowledge Deficit (specify)
 Mobility, Impaired Physical
 Noncompliance (specify)
 Nutrition, Alterations in: Less than Body Requirements
 Nutrition, Alterations in: More than Body Requirements
 Nutrition, Alterations in: Potential for More than Body Requirements
*Oral Mucous Membrane, Alterations in
 Parenting, Alterations in: Actual
 Parenting, Alterations in: Potential
*Powerlessness
 Rape-Trauma Syndrome
 Self-Care Deficit (specify level; Feeding, Bathing/hygiene, Dressing/grooming, Toileting)
 Self-concept, Disturbance in
 Sensory Perceptual Alterations
 Sexual Dysfunction
 Skin Integrity, Impairment of: Actual
 Skin Integrity, Impairment of: Potential
 Sleep Pattern Disturbance
*Social Isolation
 Spiritual Distress (Distress of the Human Spirit)
 Thought Processes, Alterations in
 Tissue Perfusion, Alteration in
 Urinary Elimination, Alteration in
 Violence, Potential for

   *Diagnoses accepted for Clinical Testing by the Fifth National Conference, April, 1982.

NURSING INTERVENTION

The lack of agreement about definitions and labels for steps of the nursing process was pointed out by Bloch (1974). Some of the terms used to label the treatment portion of the nursing process are listed here:

Term	Source
Intervention	Gordon (1982)
	Campbell (1978)
	Carlson, Craft, and McGuire (1982)
Nursing Actions	ANA Standards (1973)
	ANA Social Policy Statement (1980)
Implementation	Yura and Walsh (1983)
	Marriner (1983)
Nursing Order	Mayers (1983)

We prefer the term intervention; it seems to describe most adequately that portion of the nursing process which comes after nursing diagnosis.

A nursing intervention is an autonomous action based on scientific rationale that is executed to benefit the client in a predicted way related to the nursing diagnosis and the stated goals. Nursing interventions are treatments for nursing diagnoses. They are what nurses do with and for clients to solve a problem or prevent a possible problem. After a nursing diagnosis has been established, the nurse wants to alter the client's state of affairs with the aim of assisting the client to move toward desired goals. Establishment of the desired goals or outcomes is a crucial first step in the treatment plan. Projected outcomes serve as guideposts to the selection of nursing interventions and criteria in the evaluation of nursing interventions. Goals are derived from the data base underlying nursing diagnosis. They specify how a client can move toward promotion, maintenance, or restoration of health.

The nursing interventions described in this book can be implemented independently by the professional nurse. In our definition we have chosen to use the word autonomous to describe these independent actions to emphasize that the nurse has power and control over his or her own practice. "Such power and control allows for interdependence in the delivery of health care services while preserving the autonomy of one's own practice base" (Sills, 1983, p. 572). This book will not include activities that are carried out by the nurse in response to a physician's order. Campbell (1978) lists the activities identified by registered nurses and nursing students during a survey conducted in Texas that depend on directions from the physician, for example, changing intravenous fluids and passing medications. We recognize that nurses are responsible for this aspect of client care and that knowledge and decision-making skills are needed to make good judgments about dependent practices. However, it is our intent in this book to focus on the independent aspects of nursing practice.

We propose that nursing interventions are symbolic concepts that require a series of actions for implementation. Nursing has been using such concepts for about 20 years to assist with identifying the phenomena important to the discipline. As nursing has abandoned the medical model and adopted a nursing process model, concepts have served very well as organizers for the knowledge base for the field (Norris, 1982). "A concept expresses an abstraction formed by generalization from particulars" (Kerlinger, 1973, p. 28). It is "a generalized class name which represents certain generalized abstracted properties of a class"(Marx, 1965, p. 41). Acceptance of the conceptual approach in nursing was a prerequisite to the nursing diagnosis movement. A diagnosis requires that the nurse assess the client and identify the etiology and characteristics of a problem (the particulars). Naming the problem (generalization) completes the process of conceptualization. The intervention concepts for nursing have not been precisely clarified. This book is an attempt to move the conceptual approach into the intervention portion of the nursing process.

Four types of concepts were identified by Kaplan (1964) when he described the empirical-theoretical continuum.

Level 1	Level 2	Level 3	Level 4
directly observable	indirectly observable	constructs	theoretical terms

At one end of the continuum, which we have labeled Level 1, are concepts that are directly observable. These are the things which can be easily seen, felt, heard, or otherwise perceived through the senses. At Level 2, concepts are observed indirectly; they are inferred from certain evidence. At Level 3 the concepts, now called constructs, are not observable, either directly or indirectly. These higher level concepts are observable in principle: they are inferred from empirical referrents but symbolize a much more abstract idea. At Level 4 is the theoretical term, which has no meaning apart from the particular theory. In summary, Levels 1 and 2 are observational, whereas Levels 3 and 4 are symbolic. Jacox (1974) gives examples of concepts at each of the four levels and emphasizes the importance of concept development for building practice theory.

The diagnoses that appear in Table 1–4 are, in our view, concepts at the symbolic Levels 3 and 4. They are being empirically verified through validating the defining characteristics. The nursing interventions presented in this book are also concepts at the symbolic level. We are attempting to verify them empirically through operational definitions. In contrast, the interventions described by Campbell (1978) are concepts at the observational level. In fact, Campbell defined nursing intervention as "a single-action treatment designed to resolve, diminish, or prevent the needs that are inferred from the patient's problem" (p. 47). To illustrate this point, compare the intervention of Relaxation Training in this book with the intervention of "Massage" described in Campbell's book. It is, in fact, difficult to compare the interventions in this book, which are mostly psychosocial and more abstract, with Campbell's interventions, which are mostly physiological and less abstract. We view Campbell's interventions as the nursing orders, several of which would be needed to carry out each of the interventions described in this book (see *Implementation of Nursing Interventions* later in this chapter).

SELECTION OF NURSING INTERVENTIONS
The selection of a nursing intervention is based upon the following features:
1. The characteristics of the nursing diagnosis.
2. The research base associated with the intervention.

3. The feasibility of successfully implementing the intervention.
4. The acceptability of the intervention to the client.
5. The capability of the nurse.

Each of these will be discussed more fully in turn.

Characteristics of the Nursing Diagnosis

The primary consideration in selecting a nursing intervention to treat a nursing diagnosis is to identify one that will facilitate the client to move toward one or more desired outcomes. The intent is to direct the intervention toward altering the etiological factors associated with the diagnosis. If the cause is correctly identified during the nursing assessment and if the intervention is successful in altering the etiology, the client's status can be expected to improve. This improvement can be measured by a change in the signs and symptoms associated with the diagnosis. The predicted changes, specified in the goal statement, should serve as the outcome criteria used to evaluate the effectiveness of the intervention.

The following case study is presented to illustrate a nursing diagnosis in which the intervention would be directed toward altering the etiological factors:

Case Study 1

T.K. is a 22 year old man who has been diabetic for four years. He sought admission to his local hospital because of right upper quadrant abdominal pain. The following signs and symptoms were found on admission: Temperature, 98.5°F; pulse, 120; respirations, 24; blood pressure, 128/80; glucose, 450 mg/dl; urine, 4+/1 g; pH, 7.13. The medical diagnoses were diabetic ketoacidosis and possible cholelithiasis. Surgery was recommended. T. K. requested a second opinion and was transferred to a university medical center.

Nursing assessment revealed that T. K. is a high school dropout who works as a baker from 3 A.M. until noon. He eats breakfast at a local cafe around 9 A.M. and takes his insulin at that time. The present employer is aware of his diabetes, but T. K. states that he has been let go from previous jobs when the employer found out about his diabetes. He earns $4.50 per hour, lives alone, and has difficulty affording living expenses, proper food, insulin, and medical bills. He does not have health insurance and is reluctant to ask his parents for assistance. T. K. stated that he requested transfer to the university hospital in hope that the state would pay his medical expenses and also because he thought his diabetes should be brought into control before surgery.

T. K. was able to accurately discuss diabetes and his treatment regime. He scored very high on a paper and pencil test concerning diet. However, T. K. stated that for the past year he has not followed his diet or tested his urine. He related that he found it very repulsive to save and test his urine. He does take his insulin daily, increasing it when he plans to party with his friends. He checks his feet daily. Because of his work schedule he has erratic sleeping, eating, and exercise patterns. He states that he is depressed much of the time and when he is depressed he binges on sweets. He also states that he will probably not follow his regimen after discharge.

Nursing Diagnosis: Noncompliance.
Etiology:
1. Complex therapeutic regimen.
2. Inadequate financial resources.
3. Inadequate coping.
4. Stigma due to illness.
Signs and Symptoms:
1. Laboratory values that indicated ketoacidosis upon admission.
2. Knowledgable about therapeutic regime but only complies with some aspects of treatment plan.
3. States that he will probably not comply after discharge.

In this case study, the nursing treatment would be directed at the etiological factors. Anything that can be done to simplify the therapeutic regimen will help this client. For example, he could monitor his blood glucose level with an Autolet and Chemstrips and eliminate the need for urine testing. He is desperately in need of skills that will qualify him for a job with better pay, daytime hours, and insurance benefits. A referral to job training resources should be considered. This client needs to make many changes in his lifestyle to more adequately cope with his illness. Changes in diet, sleep, and exercise patterns are indicated. He needs assistance in ways that will be socially acceptable to him and his friends.

The following nursing interventions could be considered for implementation in this case: *Counseling* (Chapter 7); *Patient Contracting* (Chapter 6); *Cognitive Reappraisal* (Chapter 3); *Patient Teaching* (Chapter 12); *Self-Modification* (Chapter 5). The ultimate choice would depend upon the desires of the client and the capability of the nurse.

Although the prognosis for successfully treating a nursing diagnosis is better if the etiological factors can be changed, this is not always possible. In some instances the etiology cannot be altered and it is necessary to treat the signs and symptoms. In such instances it may be possible to achieve the desired outcome for a finite period of time. Case Study 2 is presented to illustrate a nursing diagnosis in which the nursing intervention must be directed toward the signs and symptoms.

Case Study 2

M.J. is a 63 year old woman admitted to the surgical oncology clinic for chemotherapy following a left-sided, modified mastectomy. Her surgical incision is well healed and she denies any pain. Her chemotherapy regime is a combination of two oral and one intravenous drugs, which will be administered on a rotating basis for two years. She consented to participate in a national drug study being conducted at the university medical center where she is receiving care and where she is employed as a unit clerk. She plans to keep her job while receiving chemotherapy and to retire at age 65. M.J. is divorced and has two grown sons whom she sees on a regular basis. Both M.J.'s mother and sister died from breast cancer. A close friend died within the past year from malignant melanoma. This friend experienced nausea and vomiting throughout her chemotherapy, resulting in anorexia and cachexia.

When asked about coping strategies M.J. reports, "My stomach is sensitive in stressful situations and I sometimes feel nauseated. I'm afraid I will be as sick as my friend was on chemotherapy." She reports that exercise is an effective way to relieve her anxiety and walks to and from work.

By the end of the first week, M.J. reports severe nausea and episodes of vomiting. She is able to tolerate some of her meals but has no appetite for candy or bananas, which are her favorite foods. She states, "Today it makes me sick just to walk in this place. I think it is the smell."

Nursing Diagnosis: Nausea and Vomiting.
Etiology:
1. Chemotherapy.
2. Negative past experience with chemotherapy through friend's experience.
3. History of nausea and vomiting in stressful situations.
Signs and Symptoms:
1. Persistent nausea and 10 episodes of vomiting over past 24 hours.
2. Gastric hypomotility on ausculation.
3. Sensitivity to olfactory stimuli in treatment area.
4. No appetite for favorite foods.

In this case it is not possible to eliminate the etiology. The client desires to continue the chemotherapy as recommended. Nursing intervention must focus upon helping her cope with the nausea and vomiting. The client has already identified that exercise helps her. The nurse could reinforce the client's use of this intervention, do an exercise assessment, and develop an *Exercise Program* (Chapter 15). *Relaxation Training* (Chapter 2) is another possible intervention for helping this client control her stress-related symptoms. *Nutritional Counseling* (Chapter 8) may be needed to assist this client maintain an adequate intake. Sound decisions about dependent nursing practice are also important in reducing the incidence of nausea and vomiting. What is the best time of day to administer the chemotherapy? When should prn antiemetics be given? Can the clinic environment be altered to minimize odor and waiting?

Nurses also treat clients with potential health problems. These clients display known risk factors that are predictive of future development of a health problem. The North American Nursing Diagnosis Association has identified several such diagnoses and has included the phrase "potential for" in the diagnostic label (Table 1–4). At this time the risk factors are considered to be the defining signs and symptoms, and an etiology is not specified or required (Gordon, 1983). In our opinion, it would be more accurate to call the risk factors the etiology of the nursing diagnosis to which the client is vulnerable and list the signs and symptoms that are predicted to appear. It is obvious that the preventive intervention is aimed at altering or eliminating the risk factors. Primary prevention encourages optimum health and personality development to strengthen the client's capacity to withstand physical and emotional stressors (Shamansky and Clausen, 1980). Examples of such health promotion interventions include *Exercise Program* (Chapter 15); *Patient Teaching* (Chapter 12); and *Self-Modification* (Chapter 5).

Research Base

A second consideration when selecting an intervention is the research base associated with it. Since the early 1960s, the profession has been attempting to produce clinical research that will give direction to nursing practice. Dumas and Leonard's classic study on preoperative preparation (1963) demonstrated that it is possible to test nursing interventions in the natural setting. Subsequently, many clinical studies have been produced by faculty, graduate students, and clinical specialists. The results of these studies have been slow to appear in practice for many reasons, which have been well described by other authors (Jacox, 1974; Aydelotte, 1976; Martinson, 1976; Smoyak, 1976).

In the mid-1970s, the Michigan Nurses' Association undertook a statewide, federally funded project to bridge the gap between research and practice. The Conduct and Utilization of Research in Nursing Project (CURN Project) developed and tested a model to facilitate the use of scientific nursing knowledge in clinical practice settings. Three categories of criteria were established for selecting research that was sufficiently developed to merit utilization in practice (Haller, Reynolds, and Horsley, 1979). The first category pertained to evaluation of the research base of the studies and included criteria on replication, scientific merit, and risk. The second category dealt with relevance to practice. Criteria included clinical significance, nursing control, feasibility, and cost. The third category dealt with potential for clinical evaluation by clinicians. Through application of these criteria, the CURN Project developed and field tested 10 research-based practice protocols:

1. Structured preoperative teaching.
2. Lactose-free diet.

   3. Sensory information: distress reduction.
   4. Sensory information: recovery rate.
   5. Nonsterile intermittent urinary catheterization.
   6. Prevention of catheter-associated urinary tract infections.
   7. Intravenous cannula change regimen.
   8. Prevention of decubiti by means of small shifts of body weight.
   9. Mutual goal setting.
  10. Deliberative nursing: pain reduction.

The research base associated with specific nursing interventions varies widely. *Preparatory Sensory Information* (Chapter 18) and *Preoperative Teaching* (Chapter 20) have been the subjects of extensive amounts of research, which is providing direction to the practitioner. Other interventions, such as *Presence* (Chapter 22) and *Patient Advocacy* (Chapter 24) are still at the stage of concept development and have had little empirical testing. Still other interventions, such as *Relaxation Training* (Chapter 2) and *Assertiveness Training* (Chapter 17) have been widely utilized but need more testing with specific nursing diagnoses. More work, such as the CURN project, is needed to help transfer research findings into practice. Publications by Stetler and Marram (1976) and Jacox and Prescott (1978) assist the practitioner in evaluating the quality and relevance of research for clinical practice.

Feasibility

Many factors contribute to concerns about feasibility when selecting a nursing intervention. Most clients will have several nursing diagnoses, and the order or priority in which to treat them must be decided. There may also be several medical diagnoses. It is probable that other health professionals in addition to the nurse are working with the client. Therefore, a total plan of care for the client is needed. Consideration must be given to interaction of the nursing interventions with treatments being provided by other health professionals. The nurse should recognize that such interactions may be either beneficial or detrimental to the client. A concerted effort by everyone involved is needed to achieve a successful outcome; at times the health team must establish a priority ranking of treatments to avoid overwhelming the client.

Cost and time are other feasibility concerns. Will there be third-party reimbursement for the treatment? Will the intervention be conducted in the hospital, clinic, or home? Can both the client and the nurse devote the amount of time required for the intervention? Today's consumer expects quality health care but is also concerned about the cost.

Acceptability to Client

Each client comes for health care with a perception of his or her problem and a notion of what should be done about it. Whatever the nurse assesses, diagnoses, and treats is going to be interpreted by the client within his frame of reference. The treatment plan must be congruent with the client's reality, or it is doomed to failure. If the nurse has established rapport during the assessment, the client should be ready to participate in goal setting. Whenever possible, it is important for the client to participate in both goal formulation and deciding goal priority. The nurse is frequently able to recommend a choice of nursing interventions to assist in reaching the goal. For each intervention the client should be given information about the conduct of the interaction and how he or she is expected to participate to help him or her make an informed choice. The client's values, beliefs, and culture must also be considered when selecting a nursing intervention.

Capability of the Nurse

There are three areas in which the nurse must be competent to successfully implement an intervention: (1) knowledge of the scientific rationale for the intervention; (2) the necessary psychomotor and interpersonal skills; and (3) ability to function within the setting to effectively utilize health care resources.

As our profession matures, we are becoming comfortable with the notion that not all nurses are alike. Each has unique knowledge with skills developed through education and experience. It is important for each nurse to differentiate the clients and nursing diagnoses he or she can treat from those that should be referred to other nurses or other health professionals. The American Nurses' Association's *Nursing: A Social Policy Statement* (1980) notes that specialization in nursing practice is developing. It presents criteria for specialists and addresses the role and function of specialists in nursing practice.

IMPLEMENTATION OF NURSING INTERVENTIONS

Once an intervention has been determined, the nurse and patient must implement it. Traditional methods for implementing interventions have included Kardex care plans, patient care conferences, treatment cards, and referrals. Generally, however, the nursing and medical professions have not faced up to the practical problems of implementation. In 1960, Weed designed the Problem-Oriented Medical Record to systematize what he considered the poor record keeping of physicians. The system, now called the POR system (the word "medical" was dropped to reflect today's use by all health professionals), is widespread and is easy to use with nursing diagnoses and interventions. Like all other care planning and record-keeping systems, this system does not ensure nursing action, however, unless the nurse writes orders. If nurses can derive independent treatments based on nursing diagnoses, then they should be able to "order" other nurses or assistants to provide them. McCloskey (1978, 1980) has advocated that nurses write orders on the same order sheet as physicians and that these be processed in the same way. Examples of nursing orders are:

○ Apply head lamp to decubitus on buttock 20 minutes tid.
○ I & O
○ Increase HOB when feeding
○ Teach patient and spouse how to give insulin

The orders can be viewed as lower level concepts, which Kaplan calls the observational level (see earlier discussion). For each of the interventions discussed in this book, several nursing orders would result. These are similar to medical orders but are derived from a nursing data base. They are made by the nurse, who should, of course, collaborate with the physician in all aspects of care but who does *not* need permission from the doctor to write such an order. Use of nursing orders have been reported in the literature (Carlson, 1972; Niland and Bentz, 1974), and they are seen as an acceptable and necessary aspect of primary nursing. Nevertheless, the use of nursing orders is still not widespread.

With the aid of computers, a problem-oriented record system that records, manipulates and retrieves all the health data on individuals over time is a reality. Computers can facilitate clinical decision making. In some institutions standardized care plans for patients with specific nursing diagnoses are being computerized. The challenge, however, is that nursing not use the computer as an expensive file for poor systems. As the saying goes, "Garbage in: garbage out." Nursing needs to first identify nursing interventions that work for specific diagnoses and then write standardized care plans which list specific actions (nursing orders) that outline the steps of the intervention and that, for each individual, will be modified as the situation dictates. The chapters in this book are a beginning attempt to standardize nursing interventions.

EVALUATION OF INTERVENTIONS

The expected outcomes, which were specified during the planning portion of the nursing intervention, serve as the criteria against which to judge the success of a nursing intervention. Mayers (1983) identifies four major categories of expected outcomes:

1. Patient verbalization regarding what he or she knows, understands, or feels about the situation.
2. Patient behavior pattern relating to a specific situation.
3. Patient signs or symptoms related to the disease process.
4. Patient management of the environment.

The patient may achieve the outcomes totally, partially, or not at all. If the criteria are achieved totally, the nurse must decide whether the nursing diagnosis has been alleviated or controlled. If it has been alleviated, no further nursing action is needed. If it has been controlled, the nurse should continue to monitor the patient's progress. If the criteria are met partially or not met at all, the nurse must reassess the situation and try to decide what went wrong. Was the diagnosis correct? Have new diagnoses occurred? Was the best intervention selected? Was the intervention consistently implemented? Is more time needed for the intervention to be effective? Was the expected outcome realistic? On the basis of this evaluation the nurse must decide whether to continue, modify, or stop the intervention. At this point a peer or more experienced person may offer valuable input. Involvement with an ongoing quality assurance program also provides the practitioner with experience in evaluating nursing care.

CURRENT PERSPECTIVES

Some disadvantages have been identified with regard to the nursing process and nursing diagnosis movement, which may also hold true for nursing interventions. Henderson (1982) cautions nurses that the nursing process, as it is presently conceived, (1) concentrates on the independent role of the nurse almost to the exclusion of the dependent and interdependent roles, (2) emphasizes the nurse's process rather than the nurse-client process, and (3) stresses problem-solving aspects of a nurse's work while ignoring subjective or intuitive aspects of nursing and the role of experience, logic, and expert opinion. Williams (1980) believes we should construct a taxonomy of nursing diagnoses, but "we should not claim that nursing diagnoses are the only diagnoses nurses can or should legitimately make" (p. 363).

Raising concerns such as these gives us directions for future work. Indeed, some of these concerns are being worked on now. For example, because they were concerned that diagnoses in critical care nursing would be excluded from the list because they were not deemed to be independent, a group of critical care nurses formed at the Fourth National Conference. Their purpose is to clarify the use of nursing diagnoses in critical care nursing (Popkess, 1980). At least three theses (Hubalik, 1981; Wessel, 1981; Dougherty, 1983) have resulted from these concerns.

Benner and Wrubel (1982a, 1982b) are concerned that the nursing process ignores subjective or intuitive aspects of nursing. They distinguish the beginner, who must rely on a deliberate analytical method to build a clinical picture from isolated pieces of information from the expert, who can grasp the situation rapidly and see the whole with a perceptual awareness that singles out relevant from irrelevant information. The perceptual awareness of the clinical expert is only developed from experience, Benner and Wrubel maintain.

In addition to aiding the beginner, the identification of nursing diagnoses and nursing treatments has many advantages. The client will benefit by having more problems identified and treated. Nursing care will be more standardized, which means that tomorrow's clients will benefit from the knowledge of what helped today's clients. The concern of nurses for prevention of disease and health maintenance should result in decreased health care costs. Gordon (1982) predicts what would happen if nurses were valued for their nursing diagnoses and treatments: Nurses would treat the inability to cope with a body image change after a leg amputation before it progressed to a severe depression; nurses would treat the poor coping pattern before it progressed to child abuse; nurses would treat the potential contracture before it occurred and required costly surgery. These are just a few examples of how nursing treatments can decrease the cost of health care. Another advantage to identifying and using nursing diagnoses and treatment is that nurse satisfaction increases. Studies have shown that nurses want more autonomy and participation in the decision making concerning patients' welfare (Stamps, 1978; Weisman, 1981). The identification of the body of knowledge that is uniquely and collaboratively nursing makes nurses for the first time in a century of organized nursing true colleagues of the physician. The concept of the health care team is closer to realization.

Special recognition is extended to Chris Ayers and Bonnie McDonald, Adult Health nursing students enrolled in the Master's Program at The University of Iowa College of Nursing, for the case study material in this chapter.

References

American Nurses' Association. *Standards of nursing practice.* Kansas City: American Nurses' Association, 1973.

American Nurses' Association. *Nursing: A social policy statement.* Kansas City: American Nurses' Association, 1980a.

American Nurses' Association. *The nursing practice act: suggested state legislation.* Kansas City: American Nurses' Association, 1980b.

Aydelotte, M. K. Nursing research in clinical settings: Problems and issues. *Reflections,* 1976, *2,* 3–6.

Benner, P., and Wrubel, J. Skilled clinical knowledge: The value of perceptual awareness, Part 1. *Journal of Nursing Administration,* 1982a, *12*(5), 11–14.

Benner, P., and Wrubel, J. Skilled clinical knowledge: The value of perceptual awareness, Part 2. *Journal of Nursing Administration,* 1982b, *12*(6), 28–32.

Bloch, D. Some crucial terms in nursing: What do they really mean? *Nursing Outlook,* 1974, *22*(11), 689–694.

Bruce, J. Implementation of nursing diagnoses: A nursing administrator's perspective. *Nursing Clinics of North America,* 1979, 14(3), 509–515.

Campbell, C. *Nursing diagnosis and intervention in nursing practice.* New York: John Wiley and Sons, 1978.

Carlson, J. H., Craft, C. A., and McGuire, A. D. *Nursing diagnosis.* Philadelphia: W. B. Saunders Company, 1982.

Carlson, S. A practical approach to the nursing process. *American Journal of Nursing*, 1972, *72*, 1589–1591.

Carrieri, V. K., and Sitzman, J. Components of the nursing process. *Nursing Clinics of North America*, 1971, *6*, 115–124.

CURN Project: *Distress reduction through sensory preparation*. New York: Grune & Stratton, 1981.

Dickoff, J., James, D., and Wiedenbach, E. Theory in practice discipline, I: Practice oriented theory. *Nursing Research*, 1968a, *17*, 415–435.

Dickoff, J., James, D., and Wiedenbach, E. Theory in practice discipline, II: Practice oriented theory. *Nursing Research*, 1968b, *17*, 545–554.

Dougherty, C. M. Defining the characteristics and interventions for the nursing diagnosis of decreased cardiac output (unpublished master's thesis). Iowa City: The University of Iowa, 1983.

Dumas, R. G., and Leonard, R. C. The effect of nursing on the incidence of post operative vomiting. *Nursing Research*, 1963, *12*, 12–15.

Gebbie, K. M. (Ed.). *Summary of the second national conference on classification of nursing diagnoses*. St. Louis: Clearinghouse for Nursing Diagnoses, 1976.

Gebbie, K. M., and Lavin, M. A. (Eds.). *Proceedings of the first national conference: Classification of nursing diagnoses*. St. Louis: C. V. Mosby Company, 1975.

Gordon, M. Nursing diagnosis and the diagnostic process. *American Journal of Nursing*, 1976, *76*, 1298–1300.

Gordon, M. *Nursing diagnosis: Process and application*. New York: McGraw-Hill Book Company, 1982.

Gordon, M. Conceptual issues in nursing diagnosis. In N. L. Chaska (Ed.), *The nursing profession: A time to speak*. New York: McGraw-Hill Book Company, 1983, 551–562.

Hall, L. E. Quality of nursing care. Address at Meeting of Department of Baccalaureate and Higher Degree Programs of the New Jersey League for Nursing, February 7, 1955. Seton Hall University, Newark, New Jersey. Published in Public Health Nursing, New Jersey State Department of Health, June 1955.

Haller, K. B., Reynolds, M. A., and Horsley, J. A. Developing research based innovation protocols: Process, criteria, and issues. Research in Nursing and Health, 1979, 2, 45–51.

Henderson, V. The nursing process—Is the title right? *Journal of Advanced Nursing*, 1982, *7*, 103–109.

Horsley, J., Crane, J., Crabtree, M. K., and Wood, D. J. *Using research to improve nursing practice: A guide*. New York: Grune & Stratton, 1982.

Hubalik, K. T. Nursing diagnosis associated with heart failure in critical care nursing (unpublished master's thesis). Chicago: University of Illinois, 1981.

Jacox, A. Theory construction in nursing: An overview. *Nursing Research*, 1974, *23*(1), 4–13.

Jacox, A., and Prescott, P. Determining a study's relevance for clinical practice. *American Journal of Nursing*, 1978, *78*, 1882–1889.

Kaplan, A. *The conduct of inquiry*. New York: Harper & Row, 1964.

Kelly, L. Y. Nursing practice acts. *American Journal of Nursing*, 1974, 74(7), 1310–1319.

Kerlinger, F. N. *Foundations of behavioral research*. New York: Holt, Rinehart & Winston, 1973.

Kim, M. J., McFarland, G. K., and McLane, A. M., *Classification of nursing diagnosis. Proceedings of the fifth national conference*, St. Louis: C. V. Mosby Company, 1984a.

Kim, M. J., McFarland, G. K., and McLane, A. M. *Pocket guide to nursing diagnoses*. St. Louis: C. V. Mosby Company, 1984b.

Kim, M. J., and Moritz, D. A. *Classification of nursing diagnoses: Proceedings of the third and fourth national conferences*. New York: McGraw-Hill Book Company, 1982.

Knowles, L. N. *Decision making in nursing—A necessity for doing*. ANA Clinical Sessions, 1966. New York: Appleton-Century-Crofts, 1967.

Lunney, M. Nursing diagnosis: Refining the system. *American Journal of Nursing*, 1982, *82*, 456–459.

Marriner, A. *The nursing process* (3rd ed.). St. Louis: C. V. Mosby Company, 1983.

Martinson, I. M. Nursing research: Obstacles and challenges. *Image*, 1976, *8*(1), 3–5.

Marx, M. General nature of theory construction. In M. Marx (Ed.), *Theories in contemporary psychology*. New York: Macmillan, 1965.

Mayers, M. G. *A systematic approach to the nursing care plan* (3rd ed.). New York: Appleton-Century-Crofts, 1983.

McCloskey, J. Teaching the nursing process. Paper presented at The Second Annual Nurse Educator Conference, New York City, December 4–6, 1978.

McCloskey, J. C. Nurses' orders: The next professional breakthrough? *RN*, 1980, February, 99–113.

Mintzberg, H. *The structuring of organizations*. Englewood Cliffs, N.J.: Prentice-Hall, 1979.

Mundinger, M. O., and Jauron, G. D. Developing a nursing diagnosis. *Nursing Outlook*, 1975, *23*, 94–98.

Niland, M. B., and Bentz, P. A problem-oriented approach to planning nursing care. *Nursing Clinics of North America*, 1974, *9*, 235–245.

Norris, C. M. *Concept clarification in nursing*. Rockville, Maryland: Aspen Systems Corporation, 1982.

Orlando, I. J. *The dynamic nurse-patient relationship*. New York: Putnam's, 1961.

Phipps, W. J., Long, B. C., and Woods, N. F. *Medical-surgical nursing*. St. Louis: C. V. Mosby Company, 1979.

Popkess, S. Nursing diagnosis—The key to professional autonomy. *FOCUS AACN*, 1980, *7*, 28–29.

Shamansky, S. L., and Clausen, C. L. Levels of prevention: Examination of the concept. *Nursing Outlook*, 1980, *28*(2), 104–108.

Sills, G. M. The role and function of the clinical nurse specialist. In Chaska, N. L. (Ed.) *The nursing profession: A time to speak*. New York: McGraw-Hill Book Company, 1983.

Smoyak, S. A. Is practice responding to research? *American Journal of Nursing*, 1976, *76*, 1146–1150.

Stamps, P. L., Piedmont, E. B., Slavitt, D. B., and Haase, H. M. Measurement of work satisfaction among health professionals. *Medical Care*, 1978, *16*(4), 337–352.

Stetler, C. B., and Marram, G. Evaluating research findings for applicability in practice. *Nursing Outlook*, 1976, *24*(9), 559–563.

United States Department of Health and Human Services: *Nurse planning information systems: A classification for client problems in community health nursing*. Washington, D.C.: U.S. Department of Health and Human Services, HRA 80–16, June 1980.

Weed, L. L. *Medical records, medical education and patient care*. Cleveland: Press of Case Western Reserve University, 1960.

Weisman, C. S., Alexander, C. S., and Chase, G. A. Patterns among newly hired hospital staff nurses: Comparison of nursing graduates and experienced nurses. *Nursing Research*, 1981, *30*(3), 188–191.

Wessel, S. L. Nursing functions related to the nursing diagnosis "decreased cardiac output" (unpublished master's thesis). Chicago: University of Illinois, 1981.

Williams, A. B. Rethinking nursing diagnoses. *Nursing Forum*, 1980, *19*(4), 357–363.

Yura, H., and Walsh, M. B. *The Nursing Process. Assessing, planning, implementing, evaluating*: New York: Appleton-Century-Crofts, 1978.

Yura, H., and Walsh, M. B. *The nursing process* (4th ed.). New York: Appleton-Century-Crofts, 1983.

Zimmerman, D. S., and Gohrke, C. The goal-directed nursing approach: It does work. *American Journal of Nursing*, 1970, *70*, 306–310.

STRESS MANAGEMENT

Overview: Preventing Stress Overload

GLORIA M. BULECHEK
JOANNE C. McCLOSKEY

The stress response is universal and prepares humans for "fight or flight." The considerable research on stress indicates that the stress response involves the endocrine, immunological, and nervous systems. Thus, all body organs are influenced. Specific characteristics of the stress response include the following:

○ Increased heart rate
○ Increased respiratory rate
○ Increased blood pressure
○ Dilation of pupils
○ Peripheral vasoconstriction
○ Increased muscle tension
○ Release of epinephrine
○ Increased blood glucose
○ Increased gastric motility
○ Increased metabolism

Nature intended the stress response to be protective and prepare humans to deal with imminent danger. The response, however, is the same whether triggered by a life-threatening situation or some aspect of modern living that the mind perceives as a threat. It is now believed that repeated and prolonged elicitation of the stress response, either by catastrophic life events or minor stressors, leads to disease. Symptoms or diseases often associated with stress

19

include headaches, heart disease, hypertension, back pain, allergies, peptic ulcers, overeating, fatigue, sexual dysfunction, and cancer. Thus, the stress response becomes maladaptive when there is prolonged and recurrent stress.

Stress management is a health goal for many clients. The nurse can assist the client learn this self-care activity. It is hoped that stress management can be initiated as a preventive measure and become a life habit. Unfortunately, many clients need to learn to control stress overload in order to cope with symptoms or diseases that have already occurred. Acutely ill clients often experience stress overload because of the technology needed to sustain them. Stress management can sometimes assist clients control long-term pain.

Three interventions for stress management are presented in this section. The first intervention, Relaxation Training, is defined in Chapter 2. The many relaxation techniques described in the literature are divided into two categories, external and internal. This classification is very useful to the reader because much of the literature on relaxation has been unclear about which relaxation technique is being utilized. The authors review both the general and nursing research related to Relaxation Training. An assessment guide for screening clients is presented as well as criteria for selection of appropriate clients. Associated nursing diagnoses are specified.

The chapter then presents a five-step nursing model for utilizing Relaxation Training drawing from the techniques discussed. This is an eclectic model utilizing both external and internal relaxation techniques. The model was developed by Scandrett and has been implemented by a group of psychiatric clinical nurse specialists at The University of Iowa. The intervention has been clearly defined and has been utilized with several hundred clients with a multitude of stress problems. The group is now in the process of testing the intervention, as is described in the chapter.

In Chapter 3, Scandrett presents an intervention, Cognitive Reappraisal, which nurses are beginning to use in assisting clients with stress management. The aim of this intervention is to assist the client reorganize the way in which he or she perceives stressors. If the stressors can be perceived as less threatening, the amount of stress experienced should be decreased. A five-step model for implementing Cognitive Reappraisal is presented. Scandrett points out that a behavioral intervention, such as Relaxation Training, can be used in combination with the cognitive approach to achieve an immediate and long-range reduction in stress. This is illustrated very effectively in her case study.

The third intervention presented in this section is Music Therapy. One of the primary uses of Music Therapy is stress management. However, it can also be used to stimulate clients, depending upon the mood and beat of the music and the musical preferences of the client. The authors present an historical review of the place of music in culture, describe the physical and psychological effects of music, and specify the goals of music therapy. Three nursing diagnoses are discussed in detail as the authors have tested Music Therapy as a treatment for these diagnoses. An assessment tool to identify the client's musical preferences is presented, as well as a tool to evaluate the client's response to the music therapy. The chapter concludes with two case studies.

The three interventions presented in this section are recommended for assistance in stress management. Other interventions in this book which might be appropriate include Exercise, Self-Modification, Patient Teaching, Sexual

Counseling, Role Supplementation, or Assertiveness Training, depending upon the cause of the stress-related diagnosis and the preferences of the client. Many popular publications and television programs have informed the public of the consequences of stress overload. Clients are seeking assistance with stress management both to promote wellness and to control undesired symptoms. Nurses have several treatments to offer in preventing stress overload.

2

RELAXATION TRAINING

SHARON SCANDRETT
SUSAN UECKER

DESCRIPTION OF INTERVENTION

Relaxation Training is composed of a group of varied and powerful techniques, but often in descriptions of Relaxation Training the literature does not specify which technique is being used. In this chapter the various relaxation training techniques are reviewed and organized into a framework. A five-step program drawing from these techniques is presented as an effective nursing model for intervention.

First, the techniques are classified into two basic categories: externally oriented Relaxation Training procedures and internally oriented ones. Externally oriented relaxation techniques rely on a more outward focus. Procedures included in this category are progressive muscle relaxation (PMR), biofeedback, and hypnosis. Internally oriented procedures have a more inner focus and include autogenic relaxation training, meditation, and self-hypnosis. The five-step program moves systematically from externally oriented relaxation techniques to internally oriented ones.

RELAXATION AS A RESPONSE TO STRESS

What is meant by relaxation? Is it lying around, resting? Benson, Associate Professor at Harvard Medical School and Director of the Hypertension Section of Boston's Beth Israel Hospital, described the relaxation response. He claims in this way:

> Each of us possesses a natural innate protective mechanism against "overstress," which allows us to turn off harmful bodily effects, to counter the effects of the fight or flight response. This response against "overstress" brings on bodily changes that decrease heart rate, lower metabolism, decrease the rate of breathing, and bring the body back into what is probably a healthier balance, (Benson and Klipper, 1976, p. 26.)

This response has the opposite effect from Selye's (1965) stress response. Early in the twentieth century, Cannon (1914) first described the fight or flight response or "emergency reaction." This response prepares the individual for fighting or running. Physiological changes include increases in heart rate, blood pressure, breathing rate, metabolism, and levels of epinephrine, other hormones, and blood glucose; peripheral vascular constriction, dilation of the pupils, and decreased testosterone levels (Cannon, 1914; Benson and Klipper, 1976; Budzynski, 1982; Mason, 1980; Selye, 1956). Benson and Klipper (1976) contend that when the fight or flight response is not used appropriately—for example, when minor stressors rather than catastrophic life events trigger this response—its repeated elicitation may lead to dire diseases such as heart attack or stroke. For example, although you may become stressed and worried over events such as paying the rent, it is unlikely that you will die from not paying the rent (unless your landlord or mortgage lender kills you when you file bankruptcy). Your body, however, cannot distinguish the hypothetical threat that you create in your mind from an imminent real catastrophic event, such as someone breaking into your home. In other words, the full stress response can be triggered by expectations, ideas, fears, memories, or emotions as well as by life-threatening events.

Mason (1980) reports that some people get addicted to the "rush of adrenaline" (epinephrine) and need to do stressful things to keep the epinephrine flowing. He even claims that some people so addicted will eat a lot of sugar quickly, which raises the blood glucose level, thus inducing a fight or flight physiological effect. This elevation causes the body to respond as if under threat; for example, "Eating a hot fudge sundae may elicit the same response as a roller coaster ride" (p. 3).

Many individuals tend to perpetuate or thrive on being tense or feeling this sense of rush. However, over time the body responds by creating physical symptoms in an attempt to notify the individual that something is going wrong, that there is need to change the living conditions. For example, the heart may develop symptoms of tachycardia since it was not designed to be in stress 90 per cent of the time. Symptoms or diseases often associated with stress include headaches, hypertension, tight or sore muscles, back pain, jaw tension, cold hands and feet, skin problems, allergies, asthma, arthritis, peptic ulcers, colitis, constipation, diarrhea, insomnia, fatigue, overeating, sexual dysfunction, fearfulness, forgetfulness, cancer, and others. The immune system weakens if stress is chronic, increasing susceptibility to disease (Budzynski, 1982; Zegans, 1982). When stress symptoms appear, the individual may seek medical help. Treatment may relieve a particular symptom, but the maladaptive response to stress is often left unattended.

In juxtaposition to the stress responses, relaxation elicits opposite physiological effects (Table 2–1). Other reported relaxation responses include an

Table 2–1. COMPARISON OF PHYSIOLOGICAL STRESS AND RELAXATION RESPONSES

Physiological Effect	Stress	Relaxation
Heart rate	Increased	Decreased
Breathing rate	Increased	Decreased
Metabolism	Increased	Decreased
Muscle tension	Increased	Decreased
Epinephrine	Increased	Decreased
Peripheral blood flow	Decreased	Increased
Blood pressure	Increased	Decreased

increase in alpha and theta brain waves, skin resistance, deep abdominal breathing, and decreased blood lactate levels. Pelletier (1978) suggests that healthy dealing with acute stressors includes four main states: baseline level, stress reaction (which corresponds to sympathetic nervous system stimulation), compensatory relaxation (which corresponds to parasympathetic stimulation), and return to baseline (Table 2–2). In chronically stressed individuals—for example, the chronic worrier—the stress response stays elevated, with frequent intermittent stress excitation and absence of compensatory relaxation. This pattern of high excitation, Pelletier proposes, leads to disease or exhaustion, which is one way to break the pattern. In an extreme way, after chronic stress, illness produces a relaxation response since the diseased person is forced to break the stress pattern and rest, allowing parasympathetic actuation to restore the body. Individuals who utilize relaxation or meditation procedures can induce the relaxation phase, "to let go of those excess levels of self-stressing neurophysogical activity and simply quiet themselves down" (Pelletfier, 1978, p. 5). By eliciting the relaxation response the chain of deleterious physiological effects can be broken, preventing the development of symptoms. Relaxation, by altering the physiological stress response, allows the body to heal and rebalance itself. In general, a calming of thoughts and emotions also occurs.

Benson and Klipper (1976) contend that there are four essential elements in eliciting the relaxation response:

(1) a quiet environment;
(2) a mental device such as a word or a phrase which should be repeated in a specific fashion over and over again;
(3) the adoption of a passive attitude. . .;
(4) a comfortable position (p. 27).

If various relaxation techniques are examined, usually all four elements are found to be present.

Table 2–2. HEALTHY RESPONSE TO STRESS

From Conversation with Ken Pelletier. *Medical Self-Care,* 1978, 5, 3–9. Reprinted with permission.

Externally Oriented Relaxation Techniques

The three types of externally oriented procedures—progressive muscular relaxation, biofeedback, and hypnosis—have an external component, For example, in progressive muscular relaxation there is externally visible active movement of gross muscle groups; with biofeedback, a biofeedback machine is used, and the external elements include the gauge, lights, or sound that indicates to the client the level of relaxation; and in hypnosis, there is the external dependence on another person to induce the state of relaxation.

Progressive Muscular Relaxation

Progressive muscular relaxation (PMR) is a systematic technique of tensing and releasing of gross muscle groups while attending to the differences in sensation of tension and relaxation (Bernstein and Borkovec, 1973). The goal is to increase the client's ability to identify even mild tension and to effectively reduce it. This awareness is an important aspect of relaxation that needs to be developed in the client. Muscle tension may not be recognized consciously. In fact, people would even be unaware of the tension needed to maintain their posture to read this page. PMR is a process by which clients become more aware of and, therefore, become more in control of, their tension levels. It can become a sensitivity program to increase the ability of the client to sense muscle tension and then more willfully let it go. Too often clients are not in touch with their bodies enough to sense tension until it is severe enough to create pain.

Progressive muscle relaxation began with the work of Jacobson in 1938 at Harvard University. He was looking for a technique that did not promote dependency on the part of the client. He also believed that "suggestive measures as a rule have failed to induce more than transitory emotional improvement" (Jacobson, 1970). Jacobson discovered that by systematically tensing and releasing the various muscle groups and by learning to discriminate between the resulting sensations of tension and relaxation, a person can almost completely eliminate muscle contraction and experience a feeling of deep relaxation. In this procedure, a cognition or awareness of the difference between tension and relaxation is developed and the cerebral effect is to attend to relaxation, which signals the muscle to relax.

PMR is based on the underlying assumption that anxiety and relaxation are mutually exclusive. Therefore, anxiety cannot exist if the muscles are truly relaxed. Jacobson defined anxiety from his later work in having people imagine triggering a telegraphic key with their finger, and then getting measurable electrical activity without actual motor activity. He viewed anxiety as the result of the person seeing or imagining the anxious situation consciously or subconsciously, which then sets the muscles of the person's body into a particular pattern of tension (Jacobson, 1970).

Jacobson's original program (1934) required too much time for practical application. Each of 15 muscle groups were worked on for one to nine hours daily for a total of 56 sessions. Wolpe modified Jacobson's program so that the basic training program could be completed in six 20 minute sessions with two 15 minute periods of daily home practice (Bernstein and Borkovec, 1973). Wolpe's technique generally dealt with phobias or fear response, but he helped to originate the modifications that make the technique so widely applicable today. Bernstein and Borkovec were major contributors in further refining and shortening the technique (1973). Since then, numerous authors have adapted Jacobson's progressive muscle relaxation technique.

Progressive muscle relaxation is a relatively simple technique that can be taught by a trained nurse in a short amount of time. It then becomes the client's responsibility to carry out the procedure rather than becoming dependent on the nurse.

Biofeedback

Biofeedback is a recent development evolving from animal experimentation (Miller, 1969) in which researchers discovered that "involuntary" responses mediated by the autonomic nervous system could be conditioned. Following World War II, technological advances devised instrumentation that could detect, record, and amplify the body's internally generated electrical impulses and provide a corresponding signal that could be interpreted by the subject. Discovered by individuals in separate laboratories (Budzynski and Stoyva, 1969; Green, Walters, Green, and Murphy, 1969), biofeedback in relaxation was recognized as helpful in learning deep muscle relaxation (Tarler-Benlolo, 1978). The biofeedback research and clinical applications have muschroomed and the Biofeedback Research Society was formed in 1969 (Gaardner and Montgomery, 1977). At present certification in biofeedback practice is offered through the Biofeedback Certification Institute of America.

In biofeedback an artificial closing of the external feedback loop occurs, for example, looking in a mirror provides information for the viewer. Information about biological functions of which an individual ordinarily is unaware is presented to the person so that it can be used to alter the biological function, e.g., reduce muscle tension or lower blood pressure. Voluntary control over autonomically regulated body functions allows the person to learn about and to alter the body's response in a more healthful way. In addition to the principle of feedback, Ashby's information theory (1963), which says that a variable cannot be controlled unless information about that variable is available to the controller, applies here. The information is delivered to the person in a neutral way, thus differentiating biofeedback from operant conditioning, in which feedback information is either reinforcing or aversive (Gaarder and Montgomery, 1977). The person can utilize the information received in any of several ways.

This feedback process is as simple or as complex as the feedback designer desires. Most feedback systems include physiological monitors, amplification of the physiological stimuli, a processor that selects pertinent physiological information, a feedback generator that alters information into meaningful units, and a feedback display (Breeden and Kondo, 1975). The feedback information can be continuous (analog) or discontinuous (digital). Physiological parameters utilized most often include electromyography (EMG), temperature, sound, electroencephalography (EEG), psychogalvanometer, and cardiovascular monitoring. In Relaxation Training, the physiological parameters utilized most often include muscle tension, heart rate, blood pressure, and hand temperature. Feedback information reported to be utilized most frequently in clinical settings involves continuous or discontinuous tones reflecting muscle tension, heart rate, blood pressure, or skin temperature.

An example of use of EMG biofeedback for relaxation training involves having the client sit in a comfortable position with limbs supported. Silver–silver chloride electrodes are placed over the client's frontalis muscle, which has been cleaned, removing loose epidermis and oil from the skin. EMG levels are then monitored prior to turning on the feedback machine so that a microvolt scale can be selected that allows fluctuation of muscle tension levels. The client is asked to listen to a continuous tone feedback in which the pitch reflects the tension in the muscle. The goal is for the client to lower the pitch of the sound, utilizing any relaxation technique he or she chooses. The client is asked to focus on how the body feels when the pitch is low. Home practice is encouraged and may involve utilizing a portable biofeedback machine or simulating the body sensations felt during the lowest pitched sounds of the training sessions. One of the difficulties with this approach is that transfer of learning from the machine must be carefully planned and reinforced. Dependence upon the biofeedback machinery has been noted and a return to previous tension patterns observed within a six-month period.

Hypnosis

Hypnosis is an intervention that can be very useful in nursing. Techniques are not discussed in detail here because the use of hypnosis does require supervised practice by qualified professionals. Unfortunately, hypnosis is a term that conjures up all kinds of misinterpretations, distortions, and fears. We all have experienced naturally occurring hypnotic states, for example, "spacing out" in a boring class or during a Sunday sermon (Grinder and Bandler, 1981). Also, most of us have some erroneous notions of what hypnosis is, according to our experiences with a stage hypnotist, television show, movie, or book, which have made hypnosis seem like magic or mind control.

According to LeCron (1971), it is difficult to define hypnosis but easy to describe it. It is perhaps this difficulty that contributes to the distortions and confusion. In a hypnotic state, subjects are aware of their environment but the focus is internal. Clients are more suggestible than at other times but still behave within the limits of their own moral codes. Persons who are hypnotized are actually quite protective of themselves but may be surprised at their resourcefulness in coming up with creative solutions to their problems or in seeing different perceptions of situations (LeCron, 1971). It is useful to think of hypnosis as an advanced stage of relaxation, as relaxation techniques are a usual part of the induction process.

Common phenomena in hypnosis are (1) hypermnesia—an ability to remember past details forgotten in the conscious mind; (2) age regression—the ability to reexperience a previous event; (3) increased suggestibility; (4) hypnotic anesthesia—the ability to block pain; and (5) time distortion—the sensation that time is contracted or lengthened (LeCron, 1971).

Although there are indications that hypnosis has been used throughout history, credit for the discovery is given to Franz Anton Mesmer in 1734. Mesmer, a Viennese physician, is reported to have learned this technique from a Catholic priest. Mesmer's theories were attacked by his colleagues and he died in obscurity in Austria (Daley and Greenspum, 1979; LeCron,1971). Interest in hypnosis has waxed and waned over the years.

Following World War I, use of hypnosis increased, as it did again after World War II, especially in the treatment of battle neurosis. More currently the influence of Erickson's hypnotic technique is being felt in the field as his followers carry on his work (Zeig, 1982). In addition, the work done by Grinder and Bandler (1981), who studied and analyzed Erickson's unique style, is having a widespread impact on the practice of hypnosis.

Hypnosis could be a powerful procedure for qualified nurses to use in acute situations, e.g., when clients are in such painful or anxious states that they cannot attend to learning PMR or autogenic techniques.

Internally Oriented Relaxation Techniques

The three internally oriented relaxation techniques—autogenic training, meditation, and self-hypnosis—rely on an inward focus. With these methods, the path to the relaxed state is more passive than with the methods of the externally oriented techniques. Once the internally oriented methods have been learned, clients are able to use the techniques without the nurse's further intervention. This fact is appealing to nurses in their goal of maintaining control by the client or returning it to the client. This type of intervention is also consistent with the nursing theory of self-care.

Autogenic Training

Autogenic training, derived from the self-suggestive techniques, was developed by the German psychiatrist and neurologist Schultz in the 1930s. Schultz had been influenced by Vogt, a brain physiologist, who noted that some of his hypnotic subjects had learned to place themselves in a state similar to hypnosis. He observed that if they practiced this technique several times a day, these subjects could overcome effects of stress such as tension, fatigue, and headaches (Green and Green, 1977).

Schultz was first attracted to this technique as he was looking for a way to achieve a similar state to hypnosis without the need for the hypnotist. He was intrigued by the idea that the technique did not promote a lack of responsibility by the client and overdependence on the therapist or hypnotist. Schultz found that subjects who experienced the hypnotic state reported two major physical responses, heaviness and warmth. In further work, it was found that the heaviness sensation correlates with relaxation of the muscles and the warmth is a psychophysiological perception of the vasodilatation of the peripheral vessels (Schultz and Luthe, 1969).

Autogenic training, then, consists of suggestions to oneself about the relaxing feelings of heaviness and warmth. It is viewed as a self-regulatory mechanism, a way to balance mental and physical functions. Autogenic training is built on the concept of "self-induced passivity or passive concentration" (Schultz and Luthe, p. 14, 1969). This idea is similar to that of "passive volition," which is often referred to in the literature on relaxation. Passive volition is simply allowing the sensations to take over rather than an active striving for the relaxation state. It is this passive opening up of the body to experience these physical sensations that is desired; an active pursuit of the desired state is not likely to meet with success.

Schultz and Luthe developed two basic series of exercises. The first series included six components: (1) heaviness (neuromuscular system), (2) warmth (vascular system), (3) heart rhythm (steady, strong), (4) respiration (effortless), (5) warmth (in the abdominal area), and (6) coolness (of the forehead). The second series consists of certain meditative procedures that are not generally used except by advanced followers of Schultz's methods.

Schultz's and Luthe's joint work was built on and modified by Kleinsorge and Klumbies (1964) who looked at specific symptoms and developed specific phrases to use. For example, with headaches they suggested such phrases as "My head feels free and light and my forehead pleasantly cool," or "I feel fresh air circulating around my head." The idea of warmth in the face and head is not usually suggested, especially with headaches, because of the resulting vasodilation and the possibility of increased pain.

Investigators accidentally discovered the usefulness of autogenic training in controlling migraine headaches. A subject, during a laboratory session on autogenic warmth, relieved her own migraine when she was able to warm her hands. It is thought that the vascular system tends to rebalance in response to the hand-warming exercise, pulling blood into peripheral circulation; that is, as the hand warms, the head cools and pain is decreased (Green and Green, 1977).

Meditation

In Eastern countries meditation has a religious as well as cultural connotation. In Western countries use of meditation practices has not been common but is increasing. Meditation is being recommended as a relaxation technique especially in the wellness or holistic health literature. Mason (1980) notes that meditation focuses the individual's attention and alters the level of awareness. During meditation the person's attention is specifically directed to an image or thought and the person is entirely involved in the technique.

LeShan(1974) states that meditation may be structured or unstructured. In one type of unstructured meditation, the individual chooses an idea and simply thinks about it and tries to fully experience the idea. This type of meditation requires discipline, as the person is to remain focused on the idea rather than allow the mind to go off on distracting thoughts. This is called reflective meditation, in which deeper meanings of an idea are revealed (*Meditation group for the new age*, 1978). LeShan (1974) suggests that an individual use his or her own response to a technique to determine which meditation is best. That is, if the person feels better doing a particular meditation, continue with it, and if he or she does not feel better, then do not use the procedure.

One type of structured meditation is to focus on specific objects, such as a seashell or candle. This type of meditation is called concentration and trains the individual to focus the mind at will and to attend to the present moment (*Meditation group for the new age*, 1978). Another form of this meditation makes use of a mantra, which is a word or phrase that is chanted over and over. An example of mantra meditation is transcendental meditation, commonly known as TM. Benson and Klipper (1976) chose to study TM subjects after they reviewed the numerous and various forms of meditation, finding TM to be basically a yoga technique that is done in a simple, consistent way. In TM, a trained instructor gives the individual a specific mantra, which is to be kept secret. The meditator repeats this mantra, which helps to prevent distracting thoughts, while sitting in a comfortable position. TM practitioners are usually instructed to meditate 20 minutes twice daily, 20 before breakfast and 20 before dinner.

Another type of meditation is called receptive. This meditative practice opens the individual's receptivity to intuition, insight, aspects of personality, guidance, inspiration, and knowledge. The person silences himself utilizing a mantra, breath, or visualization and then sits in quiet expectancy. Information may be received through seeing, hearing, feeling, inner knowing, or an urge to act (*Meditation group for the new age*, 1978).

Benson and Klipper (1976) studied TM subjects, noting that they produced a hypometabolic or restful state, in contrast to the physiological changes of the fight or flight (hypermetabolic) state. As noted earlier, they identified four basic elements of the hypometabolic state: a quiet environment, use of a mental device, a passive attitude, and a comfortable position.

In their book, *The Relaxation Response* (1976), Benson and Klipper propose the following meditative technique.

1. Sit quietly in a comfortable position.
2. Close your eyes.
3. Deeply relax all of your muscles, beginning at your feet and progressing up to your face. Keep them relaxed.
3. Breathe through your nose. Become aware of your breathing. As you breathe out, say the word "one" silently to yourself. Breathe easily and naturally.
5. Continue for 10 to 20 minutes. You may open your eyes to check the time, but do not use an alarm. When you finish, sit quietly for several

minutes, at first with eyes closed and later with your eyes opened. Do not stand up for a few minutes.

6. Do not worry about whether you are successful in achieving a deep state of relaxation. Maintain a passive attitude and permit relaxation to occur at its own pace. When distracting thoughts occur, try to ignore them by not dwelling upon them and return to repeating "one." With practice the response should come with little effort. Practice the technique once or twice daily, but not within two hours after any meal, since the digestive processes seem to interfere with the elicitation of the relaxation response (Benson and Klipper, 1976, p. 163).

Self-hypnosis

Self-hypnosis is the internal half of external hypnosis. That is, self-hypnosis is the result of returning the control and responsibility back to the client after the acuteness of the situation has ceased and the person is ready to learn the technique.

In self-hypnosis the individuals simply induce themselves into a hypnotic state. One way this may be done is by reading an induction script into a tape recorder and playing it back when the person wishes to do self-hypnosis. Another method is for the person to think or say aloud the hypnotic induction. Generally this technique requires disciplined practice for a person to become comfortable using it. The individual maintains self-control and, to end the hypnotic state, simply says something like, "I am ready to return to my normal state and on the count of four, I will open my eyes and feel alert."

Self-hypnosis is similar to autogenic training, but self-hypnosis is usually learned after the person has learned hypnosis. In addition, self-hypnosis, like hypnosis, allows for time in the altered state for the person to solve a problem or get a new perspective on a situation, rather than just experience relaxation.

LITERATURE REVIEW

General Research

A tremendous number of studies have been done in the area of relaxation. Some are symptom specific such as tension headaches (Beaty and Hagnes, 1979; Schlutter et al., 1980), migraine (Silver et al., 1979), or essential hypertension (Wadden and DeLatorre, 1980). Other studies have looked at combinations of particular relaxation techniques, such as progressive muscle relaxation and autogenic training (Schoot and Gregg, 1980; Shapiro and Lehere, 1980), biofeedback and progressive muscle relaxation (Belar and Cohen, 1979; Leedeauf and Lodge, 1980), biofeedback and hypnosis (Melzack and Perry, 1975), progressive muscle relaxation and meditation (Warrenburg et al., 1980), or meditation and self-hypnosis (Benson et al., 1978). However, subjective reports of feeling relaxed may be poorly or negatively correlated with low physiological measures, or may leave some question about what is occurring and how to more accurately measure feeling relaxed (Tarler-Benlolo, 1978).

Most studies use a combination of techniques or are unclear as to what specific type of relaxation is being used. Relaxation Training, therefore, may refer to progressive muscle relaxation or autogenic training or even meditation. Generally a distinction is made only among biofeedback, hypnosis, and Relaxation Training. Therefore, a general discussion of Relaxation Training literature follows, with distinctions made to the extent that is possible.

According to Tarler-Benlolo (1978), who reviewed 85 studies done in the relaxation field, evidence indicates that both biofeedback and autogenic or progressive muscular relaxation, alone or in combination, are effective in treating people with both tension and migraine headaches. More recently, Turner and Chapman's review (1982) of a number of studies came to the same conclusion. In addition, Turner and Chapman note that there is no evidence that biofeedback is superior to autogenic or PMR in treating headaches. This last conclusion was also reached in Beaty and Haynes' 1979 review article.

Common findings of the review articles indicate that home practice is important in maintaining reduction of tension headaches. Migraine headaches have responded well to finger-warming biofeedback, a procedure in which the subjects warm fingers using autogenic training and a feedback system to let subjects known temperature change. Migraines have also responded well to frontalis EMG biofeedback and progressive muscle relaxation as well as autogenic training (Agras et al., 1980; Tarler-Benlolo, 1978).

Hypnosis has been reported to be effective in reducing or eliminating pain, but many of the articles are in case study form and therefore comparisons are difficult. Turner and Chapman, in their review article on hyponosis, note that although hypnosis has been used longer than any other psychological intervention in pain, the research is sparse. They state that "until controlled research demonstrates otherwise, we are forced to take a posture of skepticism toward the clinical lore that hypnosis is a powerful method of chronic pain alleviation (Turner and Chapman, 1982, p. 30). Other researchers have found hypnosis to be useful in psychosomatic disorders such as asthma, hyperventilation, and insomnia (Wilkson, 1981). Benson and colleagues (1978) studied the effectiveness of self-hypnosis and a mediatational relaxation technique on anxiety and found both procedures to be equally effective.

Nursing Research

Nurses have begun to study the area of Relaxation Training. Two studies comparing EMG levels and anxiety symptom reduction with diverse Relaxation Training Procedures were conducted by nurses (Scandrett et al., 1976). The first study compared Bernstein and Borkovec's progressive relaxation (1973) with EMG auditory feedback of muscle tension on the frontalis muscle. No significant differences for EMG levels or for anxiety symptom reduction were found between the two groups (n = 23 subjects); however, within-group changes were found for the EMG feedback group across sessions. Also, progressive muscle relaxation subjects reported more anxiety symptom relief. In the second study, 65 subjects were randomly placed in three groups, one receiving two PMR sessions combined with EMG feedback, one receiving EMG feedback, and one receiving no treatment. No overall differences were found among the three groups; however, a significant difference in EMG levels was found between the fifth and tenth sessions for all groups. Subjects were then divided into high and low anxiety groups, which revealed that low anxiety subjects exhibited significant EMG differences at the fifth and tenth sessions. Anxiety symptom changes were equivalent for all groups. Investigators speculated that spontaneous changes across sessions may be associated with habituation to the situation and that lower anxiety levels may facilitate learning more than higher anxiety levels. A question was raised as to whether lower EMG frontalis levels are accompanied by reduction in anxiety-related symptoms.

Tamez and colleagues (1978) explored the effect of progressive muscle relaxation training on the frequency of use of medications to reduce tension.

They also compared the effect of "live" versus taped relaxation instructions. Sixty subjects were placed in three groups. One was a control group, treated as usual; the second received live instructions; and the third listened to taped instructions of modified progressive muscle relaxation. No significant differences were found in the three groups, but there were indications that live instructions were more effective than taped instructions. Bernstein and Borkovec (1973) also noted the superiority of live instruction.

Significant differences in incisional pain, body distress, consumption of analgesics and respiratory rate were found in a study on 42 acute postoperative elective surgical patients by Flaherty and Fitzpatrick (1977). Periods of data collection consisted of the first attempt to get out of bed and the immediate 24 hour period following surgery. The relaxation technique utilized was one of resting the jaw and focusing on a three-rhythm pattern of breathing. Wells (1982) studied use of a structured relaxation on six adult post-surgical cholecystectomy patients. The relaxation program consisted of concentration on breathing, awareness of muscle tension by alternating contracting and relaxing abdominal muscles while receiving EMG feedback from the rectus abdominis muscle, and a 5 minute exercise adapted from Jacobson's method. Results showed that relaxation did not alter abdominal muscle tension, physical intensity of pain, or use of analgesics, which differ from Flaherty and Fitzpatrick's findings. A significant difference was found for postoperative distress rating for the experimental group. Wells speculated that increased perceived control, a decrease in anxiety, or an interaction between these may explain this finding.

Aiken and Henricks (1971) studied progressive muscle relaxation as a preoperative intervention to decrease psychotic episodes in patients undergoing open heart surgery. There was lesser incidence of psychotic episodes in the experimental group than in the control group. The effects of progressive muscle relaxation on psychiatric inpatients was studied by Sheer (1980). No significant changes were found in the subjects' anxiety scores, which Sheer believed was due in part to the limitations of the study: a small sample size (12), only one Relaxation Training session, and self-report, which was of questionable reliability.

In 1979 Garrison and Scott reported on their finding of teaching patients a combined PMR and meditative technique as a coping skill. They noted that their clinical experience indicated satisfactory results even in heterogeneous groups. Bowles and colleagues (1979) found PMR plus biofeedback with home practice superior to PMR plus home practice alone. Results did diminish after 1 month, indicating a possible need for continued home practice.

From a methodological viewpoint, some of these research studies, both nursing and others, suffer from a lack of standardization of procedures, insufficient sample size, and other basic problems. Although some can be considered weak experimentally, enough sound studies exist to encourage the use of these techniques and further study. Findings indicate that live as opposed to taped instructions are best, and home practice is important in maintaining positive results. In addition, multiple training sessions appear to be a key factor in effectiveness (Bernstein and Borkovec, 1973; Bowles et al., 1979; Tamez et al., 1978). It is not now known whether PMR or autogenic relaxation is more effective or if a combination is best. Research is also needed to determine what techniques are best for what symptoms.

It is as yet unclear what influence, if any, personality traits have on determining what technique may work best. It is our belief that people respond differently to various techniques and may find one technique useful for one symptom and another procedure useful for other symptoms. Therefore, it is wise for the nurses desiring to use these interventions to educate and train themselves in as many different techniques as possible.

Nurses are begining to explore uses of these techniques. Although they are not research studies, many articles indicate increasing nursing usage. Several nurses have reported on their clinical use of relaxation techniques, such as Donovan (1980) in her description of Relaxation Training combined with guided imagery (brief description) to ease nause related to chemotherapy for cancer patients. Daley and Greenspun (1979) report on the use of hypnosis for stress management. Another nursing article reported on the use of PMR and meditation in stress management (Garrison and Scott, 1979). Kolkmeier (1982) reported on use of biofeedback and relaxation therapy for hypertension. Herrington (1983) explored the concept of relaxation in general, and Kern and Stejskal (1983) reported on use of relaxation to reduce students' tension in learning and recall. Blattner (1981), Brallier (1982), Flynn (1980), and Krieger (1981) note Relaxation Techniques in their books on holistic nursing. This is a new and exciting area that nurses are developing.

ASSESSMENT TOOLS

Before employing these techniques, a careful assessment of the client is essential. Symptoms need to be carefully identified. It is helpful to use an anxiety scale or anxiety symptom checklist. Baseline data on blood pressure, pulse, and respirations are recommended, as well as post-training measures of the same vital signs to validate the physiological changes associated with relaxation. In addition, it is vital to use an organized assessment guide. Essential components of an interview guide include the following:

1. Client's identification of the most bothersome symptoms.
2. Onset and duration of symptoms.
3. Full description of symptoms.
4. Family history of similar complaints.
5. What the client has previously tried that helped, what did not help.
6. What causes the client to seek relief now.
7. Current and past medications—include over-the-counter drugs.
9. Any physical illnesses.
9. Physical limitations, such as low back pain, neck pain, etc.
10. Previous experience with any relaxation training.
11. Pattern of alcohol use or use of any other mind-altering drugs.
12. Dietary pattern, including use of caffeine, sugar, and alcohol.
13. Sleep pattern.
14. Exercise pattern.
15. Overview of daily routine, including environmental and psychological stressors.
16. Any psychiatric history, including means to screen for major depressive disorders.
17. Motivation to learn and willingness to practice at home.

Number 16 is particularly important because people who also are severely depressed may be referred for Relaxation Training to relieve their anxiety. If the depression is not treated Relaxation Training will not be successful in relieving anxiety.

If the focus of the training is stress management, an assessment such as the Travis Wellness Inventory (Travis, 1977) or the Holmes-Rahe Social

Readjustment Rating Scale (Holmes and Rahe, 1967) may be useful. These tests may be repeated at the end of the training sessions to assist in evaluation.

All six of the Relaxation Training interventions presented in this chapter are skill-based and must be learned by nurses in an experiential format. Live training with specific feedback on technique delivery, voice tone, timing, and word choice are essential to training. This training is being offered in nursing continuing education programs as well as in college of nursing curricula. Other potential trainers are professionals from fields such as psychology.

The nurse's own belief and personal use of these techniques is essential in conveying to the client the effectiveness of the technique. Relaxation is not magic; learning it requires hard work. The reward of these interventions can be the effective modification of symptoms and the regaining of body control.

ASSOCIATED NURSING DIAGNOSIS AND APPROPRIATE CLIENT GROUPS

In determining the appropriate client group, it is useful to keep in mind the three basic criteria of being able to use Relaxation Training. The client needs to be able (1) to attend to body sensations, (2) to follow instructions, and (3) to follow through with home practice. One technique might be more effective over another with a particular client. The advantage of the Scandrett five-step relaxation training program is that it allows the nurse and the client to examine several techniques and to progress from gross motor movement to thought-induced relaxation.

Utilizing the previously outlined assessment guides, the nurse would likely arrive at one or more of the now more generally accepted nursing diagnoses. The ones that seem most likely include

- Anxiety
- Sleep Disturbance
- Activity Intolerance
- Powerlessness
- Ineffective Breathing Pattern
- Comfort Alterations in Pain
- Ineffectual Coping
- Impaired Physical Mobility
- Fear

Relaxation Training interventions would be useful in all of these diagnoses.

Because of the feature of muscular passivity, autogenic training has been most useful in patients who have pain, burns, traction, and bleeding tendencies. Active tensing and releasing of gross muscle groups, as in PMR, may be painful or impossible for these clients. All of the techniques can be used to combat the feelings of loss of control, powerlessness, and fear that can overwhelm clients and patients at times. For example, in working with a 54 year old man with testicular cancer who was feeling overwhelmed by the impact of numerous changes in his life created by his disease, autogenic training was used to help him to regain control of his response to his disease progression. He modified his work environment to more easily accommodate his relaxation practice sessions at work by having his secretary hold calls and setting aside a specific time to practice daily. He was able to carry on his work and as a result felt better about himself.

This example also illustrates how autogenic training is helpful in intervening in a pain-fear-anxiety cycle. The client can use the autogenic training to extend the period of pain relief and thereby decrease the amount of analgesics required. Another client, who had suffered from frequent headaches, was helped by a combination of PMR and autogenic relaxation. Autogenic training was used to reduce the pain after the headache developed. Progressive muscle relaxation was used during the day to release tension that built up in the client's muscles as a result of particular positions she had to maintain in her work.

Meditation has been reported to be particularly useful in stress management and in optimizing good health. Many regular meditators report an increased sense of well-being, increased energy levels, decreased anxiety, and an overall positive attitude (Benson and Klipper, 1976; LeShan, 1974). Many people using meditation regularly, as part of their daily routine, report that it helps to lessen the effects of the fight or flight response on the various body organs. One client, who prior to her admission to the hospital had practiced TM for a number of years, was concerned that the hospital routine would not allow her to continue this practice. In this situation, the client was not taught any new Relaxation Technique, but instead her existing one was reinforced by determining with her the best schedule and educating the staff about the technique to ensure their cooperation.

Hypnosis, on the other hand, seems more appropriate in situations in which there are acute time limitations, such as pain. Pain can impair the client's ability to concentrate on Relaxation Training. For example, in a situation with a young man, hypnosis helped him to cope with his back and neck pain caused by injuries in an automobile accident. The hypnosis provided relief initially; then throughout his hospitalization, he was taught other techniques as his ability to concentrate improved.

Possible Client Responses

There are some possible drawbacks to use of Relaxation Training techniques. These include a fear of loss of control. The clients need to be reassured that they are still in control and can choose to stop the procedure at any time by opening their eyes. Actually clients are less in control if they are unable to elicit the relaxation response. Some clients fall asleep before the procedure is completed. They may need to be instructed to get more sleep. In addition, a finger cue system may have to be set up in the training session to indicate whether a person is still alert or not. To use the finger cue the nurse simply makes a statement something like the following one during the training session: "As you continue to hear my voice, raise the index finger on your left hand to indicate you can still hear me" (Bernstein and Borkovec, 1973).

Another possible effect is becoming labile. Emotions are discharged when the body is more relaxed. The client may need to be reassured that this is normal and allowed an opportunity to deal with these feelings, either with the nurse or with another appropriate person.

Orthostatic hypotension may also occur. The client needs to be instructed to get up slowly and to flex and tighten muscles slightly before standing. Sometimes there are other unfamiliar body sensations, which may be unsettling to the client. These sensations include feeling very light, warm, heavy, floating or other responses. It is important to let the client know that these feelings are normal and are signs that the person is relaxing. It is useful to remind clients that they are always in control.

Guilt may also be in effect. Too often if a psychological intervention is used, assumptions are made that the symptoms are all in the client's head. It is important to accept the clients as they are, without judging their symptoms. It is unfair to induce guilt feelings in clients by implying they are causing their symptoms; instead, gently show them ways in which they can choose not to contribute to these symptoms and how to use relaxation methods to relieve symptoms and enhance their health.

FIVE-STEP RELAXATION PROCEDURE

A sequential learning procedure evolved from the senior author's years of studying relaxation procedures, especially comparing EMG biofeedback and progressive muscular relaxation (Breeden et al., 1974; Scandrett et al., 1976). Application of autogenic and meditative procedures ensued in clinical practice, and it was noted that many clients did best when relaxation techniques began with muscle tensing procedures. The progressive muscle procedures were especially helpful in instructing the clients to tune into their own body sensations. As the senior author began increasing the complexity of tasks, two autogenic procedures were added, which involved mental suggestion and autogenic switch-over. The sequence of autogenic instruction was expanded and modified to follow the same body routine, so there was consistency in training procedures. These short procedures were taught to elicit quick relaxation response in any setting. The five-stage procedure is as follows:

1. Progressive muscle relaxation.
2. Shortened muscle relaxation.
3. Autogenic heaviness.
4. Autogenic warmth.
5. Calming techniques.

Step One: Progressive Muscle Relaxation

Step one consists of tensing and releasing 12 major muscle groups, modified from Bernstein and Borkovec (1973). Jacobson first introduced this progressive relaxation procedure in 1938 in a book entitled *Progressive Relaxation*. Jacobson believed that a decrease in muscle tension would lead to a decrease of autonomic (especially sympathetic) nervous system activity. The outline of muscle systems utilized in the training program is presented in Appendix 2–1.

The therapist's goal is to have the client focus on the sensations in the muscles. Therefore the training might begin with the direction to "focus all of your attention on the muscles of your right hand." The therapist stimulates the onset of the tension cycle by saying, "make a tight fist *now*, noting how the muscles feel when they are tensed." This assists the client to pay attention to his body sensations. This tension is maintained for 7 to 10 seconds (with only 5 seconds for the feet).

At a predetermined cue, such as saying quickly "relax now," the muscle group is released. The client is encouraged to continue focusing on the muscle group as it relaxes, for example, "notice how the muscles feel as they relax." The therapist provides a relaxation "patter," such as "allow the muscles to relax," for about 20 to 30 seconds.

At this point, the state of relaxation can be assessed by having the therapist ask if the muscles are relaxed, i.e., "If the muscles in your right hand feel completely relaxed, signal by lifting the little finger of your left hand." After the initial check, the therapist can compare the muscle groups to determine the state of relaxation, for example: "If the muscles in your face are as deeply relaxed as those in your arm, lift the left little finger." Checking periodically with the client is extremely important, for having any muscles tensed can be distracting for the client. If tension remains in a muscle group, the same muscle group is tensed again for 7 seconds and then relaxed.

The next sequence of tensing occurs after the muscle relaxation check, or after the 20 to 30 seconds of relaxation "patter," depending on where one is in the training. The training occurs through all 12 muscle groups. The muscles of the feet should not be tensed longer than 5 seconds owing to the danger of cramping. It is best not to mention to the client that cramping might occur, but rather to simply shorten the time and lessen the intensity of the tensing. After one session, the nurse can recommend that the clients increase their consumption of calcium by adding a glass of milk. In some cases additional potassium is also needed. After all muscle groups appear relaxed, have the client take four deep breaths, releasing any remaining internal tension the client may have. Smooth muscle relaxes in approximately 20 minutes. This tensing-relaxing procedure takes about 15 to 20 minutes, and the client then sits relaxed for 10 to 20 minutes.

Clients gain several consistent results from this procedure. They report more awareness of their body and they learn with experience that they can control the tension response. Many clients are quite impressed with the dramatic differences between the two feeling states of tension and relaxation. This procedure is quite useful for an individual who has a short attention span or one who is agitated. Also, individuals with a lot of neck and shoulder tension often report a dramatic response to this procedure.

The nurse should carefully screen clients who have neck or back orthopedic injuries in which hyperextension of the upper spine would add discomfort and further complicate this condition. Also, clients with increased intracranial pressure, capillary fragility, bleeding tendencies, severe acute cardiac difficulties with hypertension, or any other condition in which tensing muscles might produce greater physiological injury need to be screened and taught more passive procedures. Some clients report some muscle soreness after beginning the procedure. Many clients have carried tension for years, and it takes a period of time to work out the various tensions in some parts of the body.

Step Two: Shortened Muscle Relaxation

The aim of this step in the training is to show the client that the relaxation response can be elicited more quickly by combining groups of muscles. It is taught after the client has mastered the first 12 muscle group procedures. Sometimes clients will mass the muscles on their own. The focus remains on how the muscles feel when tensed or relaxed, and the tensing-relaxation procedure usually takes about 5 to 10 minutes, after which the client relaxes for another 10 to 20 minutes.

The muscles are grouped in the following manner, utilizing the same tensing descriptions as in Step One.

SHORTENED MUSCLE RELAXATION

Both hands, upper and lower arms (Check for relaxation)

Face

Neck and upper back (Check for relaxation)

Abdomen and buttocks

Both legs (Check for complete relaxation)

Deep breaths are taken at the end of the procedure to again release inner tension. Clients are encouraged to keep the legs on the floor, chair, or bed instead of lifting both simultaneously, especially if they have low back pain. If it suits the client better, one leg can be lifted at a time.

Again checks are made for tension and any spots that still seem troublesome are again tensed and released several times. Certain muscle groups may continue to remain tense over several weeks. Persistent tension in certain muscle groups may need additional exercises prior to these procedures. Some clients have tremendous tension in their necks. They are encouraged to do gentle yoga neck stretches prior to beginning the relaxation procedure if they have no structural defects in the neck or spine.

Clients sometimes report that the relaxation is not as complete when the shortened procedure is used. However, encourage the client to practice daily, suspending judgment about the procedures until a week has passed. Usually satisfaction is reported after daily home practice. Slight setbacks in depth of relaxation response may occur as each new procedure is learned; however, increased proficiency usually occurs with consistent home practice.

Step Three: Autogenic Heaviness

When the client produces deep relaxing of the various muscle groups, physical tensing is dropped from the training procedures. At this point in the training, mental suggestion is emphasized, allowing the client to learn how the mind can facilitate a relaxed body. The purpose is to obtain a psychophysiological shift to an autogenic state fostering recuperative processes in the body through stimulating self-normalizing brain mechanisms.

This step requires an individual to concentrate on relaxation with various body parts eliciting a feeling of heaviness. Heaviness cues the muscular system specifically. The procedure consists of reading a statement, then pausing for enough time for the statement to be internally repeated (Appendix 2–2). The client is instructed to repeat the statement to himself and to elicit the feeling within the body part being directed. Leading with the script should take 15 to 20 minutes; then the client is to remain relaxed for another 20 minutes.

Heaviness is the first sensation emphasized because it seems to be a predominant feeling that accompanies deep relaxation. Most clients report this subjective feeling, although a few say they feel "lightness" or "floating" sensations instead of heaviness. For an obese client, a feeling of lightness may be more pleasing to them and lightness can be substituted for "heaviness." Usually clients report a deepened state of relaxation with this first autogenic procedure. Sometimes other mental imagery may be used. For example, to feel heaviness, "Imagine that your arm is as a sand bag—allow it to fall limp and loose."

Home practice instructions include having clients review the script, then making the suggestive statements to themselves. With clients who are highly distractible or who have difficulty concentrating, it is sometimes helpful to audiotape this session and have them practice once daily for three days with the tape. During the remainder of the week the client can try the procedure without the tape.

Step Four: Autogenic Warmth

The next step in this training program is autogenic warmth, which cues relaxation in the vascular system. The feeling of warmth is elicited after the person releases tension from the muscles, and senses a feeling of heaviness. The script for this step is given in Appendix 2–3. Some persons tend to have difficulty in eliciting warmth. Additional imagery is often helpful, in such cases, such as "Feel the sun shining upon your skin, "Feel the skin warming," or "Recall how your hands feel in warm dishwater." If someone is continuing to have difficulty, have them feel the warmth of their palm as it rests upon the arm of the chair. Let that warmth spread over and throughout the arm. Utilizing common, simple images seems to be more helpful than building more elaborate ones. This procedure takes the same amount of time as the third step and replaces that step.

A shortened list is provided for the client to review the key points for home practice. The key points include tension release, relaxation, heaviness, and warmth. We have found most clients are able to learn the procedure easily.

Step Five: Calming Techniques

When clients have mastered the previous steps, they are ready to learn the short procedures of eliciting the relaxation response. Three major procedures are taught (Appendix 2–4), allowing clients to select one that is most attractive and helpful to them. The first procedure combines yoga breathing with mental suggestions; the second procedure counts and relaxes the body parts; and the third uses repetition of a word that symbolizes relaxation to the client.

We have seen staff nurses attempt to train clients to relax by using quick procedures, such as tensing the whole body, then releasing it. From our experience, learning to relax is a reconditioning process which is most effectively trained by continued practice. When a person is first trained in relaxation, deep relaxation response occurs quickly. However, starting with the quick calming techniques bypasses the reconditioning of training and often fails to elicit as deep a relaxation response. In an emergency situation, 7 to 15 abdominal breaths can provide temporary relief.

APPROPRIATE CANDIDATES

The five-step procedure has been utilized for over eight years with a wide variety of inpatients and outpatients of a large university hospital. Successful training with positive patient self-reports has occurred in patients with orthopedic, neurological, blood dyscrasia, bone marrow transplant, psychiatric, obstetric, surgical, cardiac, pediatric, oncologic, and medical problems. The key symptoms utilized to select candidates from these patient populations are difficulties with tension and anxiety. Complete elimination of tension headaches, pain, and general tension have been noted repeatedly in individual cases.

We found it best to exclude persons with chronic pain, acute psychoses, spastic torticollis (stiff neck), alcohol, or drug problems and those taking psychotropic medications. However, if the trainer feels there is sufficient motivation by the clients to learn or to gain from the training, these clients need not be refused. We have successfully utilized tapes rather then live training with paranoid personalities. At this time, we are conducting research on the effect of internal-external locus of control on these Relaxation Training procedures. From clinical observation, it appears that a more externally controlled person (one who believes that others control his or her fate) seems to respond better with the muscle tensing procedures, whereas the more internally controlled person (one who is in charge of his or her own destiny) does best with autogenic or meditative procedures.

CASE STUDIES

Two client studies are presented. The first is that of a young woman who was in a severe automobile accident and suffered two crushed ankles and a broken arm in addition to facial lacerations. She experienced much physical discomfort and anxiety as the healing process ensued, and I (S.S.) was called to teach her relaxation techniques. She readily learned the five steps and found that her pain and discomfort were reduced as she elicited the relaxation response. In addition, she felt calmer and more in control of her situation. She utilized the Relaxation Training even after leaving the hospital to assist herself in dealing with anxieties related to her healing process.

The second client was a psychiatric outpatient who experienced much free-floating anxiety. This anxiety interfered with his ability to concentrate on his studies in his doctoral program. In addition, he tended to find it difficult to care for his son while his wife worked and would become very anxious and feel overwhelmed or irritable. Relaxation Training was a bit more difficult for him, but he practiced diligently and was able, with encouragement, to relax fairly well. He would use the relaxation to calm himself whenever he became anxious and he found that with regular practice, he had less anxiety and in general felt more in control.

GUIDELINES FOR PRACTICE

Certain guidelines or recurring themes help ensure the success of the Relaxation Training. One of these is the need for home practice once or twice a day, as mentioned earlier. Compliance with home practice becomes a key factor in motivation to learn. Another is to allow the client to progress to the next step only after the previous one was mastered. When possible (e.g., outpatients) it is preferable to let clients practice at one level for a week. In inpatient settings, clients have been trained in all five steps in a 10 day period with two days of practice between each session.

Occasionally a client masters only one stage, for example, PMR, and has great difficulty with the next step. Acknowledging that a client has learned a procedure well appears to be most helpful and allows the client to progress or maintain skills at his or her own rate. Some clients are doubtful or become discouraged easily and need reassurance that because their symptoms took years to develop, altering the symptoms or the habits of being tense also requires time. Reinforcement of daily home practice often assists to reduce this doubt.

Providing relaxation consultation in a variety of hospital settings often means modifying the basic training procedures to fit the client's needs. The selection of relaxation techniques must take into account the client's biological state, for example, offering only the autogenic and calming procedures to clients with high blood pressure, acute burns, increased intracranial pressure, or bleeding difficulties. In intensive care a client with C2 vertebral fracture on an automatic respirator was taught to use autogenic calming and warmth, visualizing her breath flowing easily and effortlessly. This procedure helped her feel that she had some control in her life and she left the rehabilitation hospital without respiratory assistance.

Some clients express fears or discomfort in being asked to relax. Some are fearful of losing control when they become relaxed. For the latter, have the client open his or her eyes, demonstrating that the client can maintain control at any time. We also suggest to the clients that if they cannot relax, they lack control over their range of responses.

Other persons occasionally report dizziness or orthostatic hypotension upon arising after the session. Have these persons tense their muscles by stretching and rising slowly. In fact, it is a good practice to have all clients stretch their muscles prior to walking.

Although audiotapes are often used, we believe in the value of having a client experience personal, individualized training and being able to observe the relaxed state of the trainer. Audiotapes are given to the client to take home only when difficulty with a particular procedure is encountered, and then the "in vivo" session is recorded. Budzynski (1982) claims that use of audiotapes works best with the Western oriented individual. Good response has occurred with our approach, which discourages dependence upon audiotapes. Usually use of the tape is suggested for only half of the week, with self-instruction encouraged for the remainder of time.

Some clients have difficulty controlling extraneous thoughts. Utilizing mental images, such as placing worries in a box in the mind or letting the thoughts drift by, as in the autogenic warmth script, or paying no attention to them, can reduce these. If a client, after several weeks, continues to experience trouble with intrusive thoughts, training the clients to "stop" thoughts may be indicated. Thought stopping is a behavioral procedure in which the client practices interrupting thought processes and replacing them with the desired state or thought. Intrusions may occur from disrupting external noises or family members. Encouraging the client to negotiate with family for uninter-rupted times and unplugging the phone are very helpful.

Another response the client may have is recalling emotionally painful situations, old conflicts, or emotional discharges. It is best not to bring this possibility to the client's attention beforehand, but if it occurs reassure the client that it is a normal response. The psyche will take advantage of the relaxed muscles and emotions by bringing to awareness unresolved conflicts for the person to release.

Providing a nondistracting and nondisrupting environment is critical for success in training clients in relaxation. Sitting in a recliner or comfortable chair with a footstool is the best position, although lying down also promotes relaxation (sometimes too much, so that the overtired client sleeps). Dim, nondirect lighting, quiet, and comfortable temperatures are important factors.

Training a person to relax takes a certain amount of self-discipline by the leader. The trainer produces the best effect if the pitch of the voice is lowered (unless the voice is already low), the pace of words is slowed, and speaking is rhythmical. Avoid speaking so softly that the client must strain to hear. Even more helpful (yet sometimes difficult in dimly lit rooms), is to pace the words with the client's breathing. In addition, going through the procedure with the client is helpful—using your body response to guide you. The nurse can also tape the instructions and note his or her own relaxation response to the directions. However, be quite careful to observe the client closely, utilizing the body's responses to pace the training. Difficulty with drowsiness, inatten-tion, and "drifting off" can occur in the trainer when experiencing the procedure simultaneously with the client.

One of our biggest concerns with Relaxation Training is the misuse of the procedures. Specifically, the client is trained in one procedure in only a single session with instructions to use this at home. This single session approach violates good learning principles because periodic training increases chances for successful behavioral alteration. Often the trainers themselves discredit relaxation as an intervention when the client does not show symptom change. Yet it is the trainer who has not offered optimal behavioral training. When we train in relaxation procedures we are altering chronic habits, which takes a period of time. Also, some trainers present relaxation as the final answer to the problem instead of acknowledging it as a part of a more holistic approach.

The five-step Relaxation Training procedure needs to be studied for effectiveness with a variety of clients. It has been utilized with differing clients in a major university hospital. Currently four research projects are under way to test this procedure with three populations: individuals with cardiac, oncologic, and psychiatric problems. Relaxation certainly is not a panacea for living stress-free, but it can provide an alternative to being "anxious." It also allows the client the opportunity to prevent more permanent structural problems in the body.

CONCLUDING REMARKS AND RECOMMENDATIONS

Nursing can certainly make a major contribution if nurses begin to practice and to train others in the use of relaxation techniques. Think of what it would be like if most nurses learned to relax. What a tremendous effect upon the climate of our hospitals, clinics, and health service agencies this would be. It could not help but be noticed by other members of our health teams as well as by clients. Perhaps some "real" healing and "refuge" could take place in our healing centers. Bustle, stress, and burdens on the part of nurses certainly don't uplift our clients; neither do they promote healing.

Perhaps the high medical costs could be a bit more justified if nurses helped provide an optimal healing environment for clients. Neither should it be overlooked that relaxation is being kind to oneself.

It is imperative that nursing clinicians as well as nursing researchers write and publish results of their work. There is greater wealth of knowledge than is apparent in the literature. Nurses practicing in a variety of settings need to report their use of and results with Relaxation Training. Because of the wide application of the Relaxation Training techniques and our own positive results in some similar situations, we see many opportunities for nurses to use relaxation techniques. For example, oncology nurses could use relaxation training interventions to help clients cope with the stress and anxiety accompanying changes caused by pain, radiation, chemotherapy and the disease itself. Psychiatric nurses could use relaxation in intervening with sleep disturbance and anxiety in their clients. Obstetrical nurses may use relaxation techniques in childbirth classes. Surgical nurses can explore the influence of relaxation on their patient's postoperative recovery. Some of these suggestions may already be in practice.

In the future, nurse clinicians and nurse academicians need to work together more to study the effects of Relaxation Training. Many research questions remain. What techniques are appropriate for which person? How long do the effects last? Is the technique effective to cope with symptoms only if home practice is continued even when symptoms are not present? Would regular and early use of Relaxation Training prevent stress-related disease? Nurses are the appropriate people to ask and answer these questions.

EDITORS' COMMENTS AND QUESTIONS

This chapter discusses the history of relaxation; reviews the related literature, and presents a practical five-step program for implementing Relaxation Training, which was developed by the authors over the past eight years in their practice as clinical nurse specialists. The chapter includes an assessment guide and criteria for selection of clients, specifies related nursing diagnoses, and presents case studies as well as implications for practice.

The various techniques for producing the relaxation response are divided into two categories, external and internal. This classification is based upon whether the stimulus to produce the response is located externally to or internally in the client.

Questions for Discussion

1. Where and how can nurses learn to do Relaxation Training?

2. The techniques to produce the relaxation response appear to fall on a level of consciousness continuum from muscular relaxation to hypnosis. Discuss how each of the techniques specified in this chapter relates to this continuum.

3. How do you inform a client that you intend to teach Relaxation Training and use techniques such as biofeedback and hypnosis?

4. Could you incorporate the five-step training program into your practice?

5. If you cannot do Relaxation Training yourself, how do you select appropriate clients for referral to an experienced therapist?

6. How could this intervention be evaluated? What would be relevant outcome measures?

References

Agras, W. S., Taylor, B., Kraemer, H. C., Allen, R. A., and Schneider, J. A. Relaxation training. *Archives of General Psychiatry, 1980, 37,* 859–863.

Aiken, L. H., and Henricks, T. F. Systemic relaxation as a nursing intervention technique with open heart surgery patients. *Nursing Research,* 1971, 20(3), 212–217.

Ashby, W. R. *An introduction to cybernetics.* New York: John Wiley & Sons, 1963.

Beaty, E. R., and Haynes, S. N. Behavioral intervention with muscle-contraction headache: A review. *Psychosomatic Medicine,* 1979, 41(2), 165–180.

Belar, C. D., and Cohen, J. L. The use of EMG feedback and progressive relaxation in the treatment of a woman with chronic back pain. *Biofeedback and Self Regulation,* 1979, 4, 345–353.

Benson, H., and Klipper, M. Z. The relaxation response. New York: Avon Books, 1976.

Benson, H., et al. Treatment of anxiety: A comparison of the usefulness of self-hypnosis and a meditational relaxation technique. *Psychotherapeutic Psychosomatics,* 1978, 30, 229–242.

Bernstein, D. A., and Borkovec, T. D. *Progressive relaxation training: A manual for the helping professions.* Champaign, Ill.: Research Press, 1973.

Blattner, B. *Holistic nursing.* Englewood Cliffs, N. J.: Prentice-Hall, 1981.

Bowles, C., Smith, J., and Parker, K. EMG biofeedback and progressive relaxation training: A comparative study of two groups of normal subjects. *Western Journal of Nursing Research,* 1979, 1(3), 179–189.

Brallier, L. *Transition and transformation: Successfully managing stress.* Los Altos, Calif.: National Nursing Review, 1982.

Breeden, S. A., Bean, J. A., Scandrett, S., and Kondo, C. EMG levels as indicators of relaxation (unpublished manuscript). A paper presented at Biofeedback Research Society, Monterey, California, 1974.

Breeden, S. A., and Kondo, C. Y. Using biofeedback to reduce tension. *American Journal of Nursing*, 1975, *75*(11) 2010–2012.

Budzynski, T. H. Presentations at the Memphis Medical Association Meeting. Memphis, Tennessee, Spring, 1982.

Budzynski, T. H., and Stoyva, J. M. An instrument for producing deep muscle relaxation by means of analog information feedback. *Journal of Applied Behavior Analysis*, 1969, *2*, 231–237.

Cannon, W. B. The emergency function of the adrenal medulla in pain and the major emotions. *American Journal of Physiology*, 1914, *33*, 356–372.

Conversation with Ken Pelletier. *Medical Self-care*, 1978, *5*, 3–9.

Daley, T. J., and Greenspun, E. L. Stress management through hypnosis. *Topics in Clinical Nursing*, 1979, *1*, 1.

Donovan, M. Relaxation with guided imagery: A useful technique. *Cancer Nursing*, February, 1980.

Flaherty, G. G., and Fitzpatrick, J. J. Relaxation technique to increase comfort level of postoperative patients. *Nursing Research*, 1977, *27*(6), 352–355.

Flynn, P. A. *Holistic health*. Bowie, Md.: Robert J. Brady Company, 1980.

Gaardner, K. R., and Montgomery, P. S. *Clinical biofeedback: A procedural manual*. Baltimore, Williams & Wilkins, 1977.

Garrison, J., and Scott, P. A. A group self-care approach to stress management. *Journal of Psychiatric Nursing*, 1979, *6*, 9–14.

Green, E., and Green, A. *Beyond biofeedback*. New York: Dell Publishing, 1977.

Green, E. E., Walters, E. D., Green, A. M., and Murphy, G. Feedback technique for deep relaxation. *Psychophysiology*, 1969, *6*, 371–377.

Grinder, J., and Bandler, R. *Trance-formation*. Moab, Utah: Real People Press, 1981.

Herrington, S. Exploration of the concept of relaxation. *Journal of Holistic Nursing*, 1983, *1*(1), 21–26.

Holmes, T. H., and Rahe, R. H. The social readjustment rating scale. *Journal of Psychosomatic Research*, 1967, *11*, 213–218.

Jacobson, E. *You must relax*. New York: McGraw-Hill Book Company, 1934.

Jacobson, E. *Progressive relaxation*. Chicago: University of Chicago Press, 1938.

Jacobson, E. *Modern treatment of tense patients*. Springfield, Ill., Charles C Thomas, 1970.

Kern, D. A., and Stejskal, J. Relaxation in the classroom: Reduce your student's anxiety while improving their learning and recall. *Journal of Holistic Nursing*, 1983, *1*(1), 17–20.

Kleinsorge, H., and Klumbies, G. *Technique of relaxation*. Bristol, England: John Wright, 1964.

Kolkmeier, L. Biofeedback—relaxation therapy for hypertension. *Topics in Clinical Nursing*, 1982, *3*(4), 69–73.

Kreiger, D. *Foundations for holistic health nursing practices: The renaissance nurse*. Philadelphia: J. B. Lippincott, 1981.

LeCron, L. *The complete guide to hypnosis*. New York: Harper & Row, 1971.

LeShan, L. *How to meditate*. New York: Bantam Books, 1974.

Leedeauf, A., and Lodge, J. Comparison of frontalis EMG feedback training and progressive relaxation in the treatment of chronic anxiety. *British Journal of Psychiatry*, 1980, *137*, 279–284.

Mason, L. J. *Guide to stress reduction*. Culver City, Calif.: Peace Press, 1980.

Meditation group for the new age. Kent, England: Courier Company, Ltd., 1978.

Melzack, R., and Perry, C. Self-regulation of pain: The use of alpha-feedback and hypnotic training for the control of chronic pain. *Experimental Neurology*, 1975, *46*, 451–469.

Miller, N. E. Learning of visceral and glandular responses. *Science*, 1969, *163*, 434–445.

Scandrett, S. L., Bean, J. A., Breeden, S., and Powell, S. A comparative study of biofeedback and progressive relaxation (unpublished manuscript). Presented at Sigma Theta Tau Research Day, University of Iowa, 1980.

Schlutter, L. C., Golden, C. J., and Blume, H. G. A comparison of treatments for prefrontal muscle contraction headache. *British Journal of Medical Psychology*, 1980, *53*(1), 47–52.

Schoot, D. S., and Gregg, J. M. Myofascial pain of the temporomandibular joint: A review of the behavioral relaxation therapies. *Pain*, 1980, *9*(2), 231–241.

Schultz, J. H., and Luthe, W. *Autogenic therapy* (vol. I). Autogenic Methods. New York: Grune & Stratton, 1969.

Selye, H. *The stress of life*. New York: McGraw-Hill Book Company, 1956.

Shapiro, S., and Lehrer, P. M. Psychophysiological effects of autogenic training and progressive relaxation. *Biofeedback and Self Regulation*. 1980, *5*(2), 249–255.

Sheer, B. The effects of relaxation training on psychiatric in-patients. *Issues in Mental Health Nursing* 1980, *2*(4), 1–15.

Silver, B. V., Blanchard, E. B., Williamson, D. A., Theobald, D. E., and Brown, D. A. Temperature biofeedback and relaxation training in the treatment of migraine headaches. One year follow-up. *Biofeedback and self regulation*, 1979, *4*(4), 359–366.

Tamez, E. G., Moore, M. J., and Brown, P. L. Relaxation training as a nursing intervention versus pro re nata medication. *Nursing Research*, 1978, *27*(3), 160–165.

Tarler-Benlolo, L. The role of relaxation in biofeedback training: A critical review of the literature. *Psychological Bulletin*, 1978, *85*(4), 727–755.

Travis, J. *Wellness workbook for health professionals.* Mill Valley, Calif.: John Travis Wellness Resource Center, 1977.

Turner, J., and Chapman, C. R. Psychological interventions for chronic pain: A critical review. II. Operant conditioning, hypnosis and cognitive-behavioral therapy. *Pain*, 1982, *12*, 23–46.

Wadden, T. A., and DeLaTorre, C. S. Relaxation therapy as an adjunct treatment for essential hypertension. *Journal of Family Practice*, 1980, *11*(6), 901–908.

Warrenburg, S., Pagano, R. R., Woods, M., and Hlastala, M. A comparison of somatic relaxation and EEG activity in classical progressive relaxation and transcendental meditation. *Journal of Behavioral Medicine*, 1980, *3*(1), 73–93.

Wells, N. The effect of relaxation on post-operative muscle tension and pain. *Nursing Research*, 1982, *31*(4), 236–238.

Wilkson, J. B. Hypnotherapy in the psychosomatic approach to illness: A review. *Journal of Royal Society of Medicine*, 1981, 525–530.

Zeig, J. *Ericksonian approaches to hypnosis and psychotherapy.* New York: Brunner/Mazel, 1982.

Zegans, L. S. Stress and the development of somatic disorders. In L. Goldberger and S. Brezwitz (eds.), *Handbook of stress: Theoretical and clinical aspects.* New York; Free Press, 1982.

Appendix 2–1. INSTRUCTIONS TO CLIENT FOR PROGRESSIVE MUSCLE RELAXATION

HAND: Tighten the dominant hand into a fist.
   Tighten the nondominant hand into a fist. (Check for relaxed state.)
UPPER AND LOWER ARM: Bend elbow of the dominant arm and point it to the ceiling, tensing both upper and lower arm.
   (Repeat with the nondominant arm. Check for relaxation.)
FOREHEAD: Raise eyebrows toward top of head.
EYES AND NOSE: Squint your eyes and wrinkle your nose.
MOUTH: Purse your lips into a little round "O" and push out in an accentuated "kiss."
   (Check for relaxation.)
NECK: Hyperextend your head, grit your teeth, and make wide smile.
UPPER BACK: Try to touch your shoulder blades, arch your back.
ABDOMEN: Suck in your abdomen.
BUTTOCKS: Tighten your buttocks.
   (Check for relaxation.)
THIGH: Raise your dominant leg about 6 inches from the floor, tighten your upper leg.
   Repeat with the nondominant leg.
CALF: Pull your dominant foot toward your head.
   Pull your nondominant foot toward your head.
FOOT: Point your dominant foot away and curl your toes.
   Point your nondominant foot away and curl your toes.
   (Check for relaxation.)

If tense, raise little finger of right or left hand.

Appendix 2–2. INSTRUCTIONS TO CLIENT FOR AUTOGENIC HEAVINESS

Please place yourself in a comfortable position; close your eyes.
Repeat to yourself the following statements and allow your body to experience the suggested feelings.
I am completely at rest, at rest, and my whole body is relaxed.
My thoughts are directed only at this rest, everything else is immaterial—insignificant—nothing can disturb me.
Rest and relaxation.
Each muscle is relaxed and limp.
Nothing can disturb me.
I am completely at rest.
My right arm is limp and relaxed.
My right arm feels heavy.
My right arm feels relaxed and heavy.
A leaden heaviness spreads throughout my whole right arm, through the upper arm, through the lower arm, through the hands, and into the fingertips.
My right arm feels pleasantly relaxed and heavy.
My left arm is limp and relaxed.
My left arm feels heavy.
My left arm feels relaxed and heavy.

Appendix 2–2. INSTRUCTIONS TO CLIENT FOR AUTOGENIC HEAVINESS
(Continued)

A leaden heaviness spreads throughout my whole left arm, through the upper arm, through the lower arm, through the hands, and into the fingertips.

My left arm is pleasantly relaxed and heavy.

The muscles in my head and face are limp and relaxed.

The muscles in my head feel heavy.

My head seems to sink into the couch.

My head is relaxed and heavy.

The muscles in my face grow limp and relaxed.

The muscles soften and a youthful quality comes over my face.

The muscles of my head and face are pleasantly relaxed.

The muscles of my neck and shoulders grow limp and relaxed.

These muscles feel heavy.

The muscles feel relaxed and heavy.

A leaden heaviness spreads throughout the muscles of the neck and shoulders, from the base of the skull, down the neck, out into the shoulders and upper back.

These muscles are pleasantly relaxed and heavy.

The muscles of my chest and middle back grow limp and relaxed.

These muscles feel heavy.

The muscles of my chest and middle back feel relaxed and heavy and a very pleasant heaviness spreads throughout all the muscles on my chest and around back to all the muscles of my back.

The muscles of my chest and of my middle back are pleasantly relaxed and heavy.

The muscles of my stomach and of my lower back grow limp and relaxed.

These muscles feel heavy.

The muscles of my stomach and lower back feel relaxed and heavy.

The muscles of my stomach and lower back are pleasantly relaxed and heavy.

The muscles of my buttocks and of my genitals are limp and relaxed.

These muscles feel heavy.

The muscles of my buttocks and my genitals feel relaxed and heavy.

A leaden heaviness spreads throughout all these muscles, relieving the tension.

The muscles in my buttocks and in my genitals are relaxed and heavy.

My right leg is limp and relaxed.

My right leg feels heavy.

My right leg feels relaxed and heavy.

A leaden heaviness spreads throughout my whole right leg, through the upper leg, through the lower leg, through my foot, and into my toes.

My right leg is pleasantly relaxed and heavy.

My left leg is limp and relaxed.

My left leg feels heavy.

My left leg feels relaxed and heavy.

A leaden heaviness spreads throughout my whole left leg, through my upper leg, through my lower leg, through my foot, and into my toes.

My right leg is pleasantly relaxed and heavy.

My left leg is limp and relaxed.

My left leg feels heavy.

My left leg feels relaxed and heavy.

A leaden heaviness spreads throughout my whole left leg, through my upper leg, through my lower leg, and into my foot and toes.

I am completely at rest.

A feeling of rest and well-being is coming over me.

Rest envelopes me like an ample cloak.

Rest protects me.

I surrender completely to the rest and relaxation—I am completely at rest.

This inner rest is of great benefit and helps me relax.

This process deepens with each exercise.

This inner rest will accompany me everywhere.

I will gain confidence and strength from it.

I will feel refreshed as if after a deep and peaceful sleep.

I will feel alert and renewed—ready to handle my tasks.

Breathe deeply.

Be aware of where your body is now, stretch and open your eyes.

Modified from: Kleinsorge, H., and Klumbies, G. *Technique of relaxation.* Bristol, England, John Wright, 1964. Used with permission.

Appendix 2–3. INSTRUCTION TO CLIENT FOR AUTOGENIC WARMTH

As before, place any concerns or worries in a little box in your mind so that you may now center yourself to help yourself relax. Take four deep breaths, sensing the deepness of your breath as you release any tension.

As before, repeat the following phrases to yourself, beginning with your dominant arm and hand. I focus on the tightness in my arm and hand, and I release it. I see the tension moving out from the body and feel again that slowing sense of relaxation. With the sense of heaviness, I feel my arm and hand become more and more limp. I allow a very gentle, comforting warmth to begin to slow down, starting at my shoulder and gently moving across my upper arm, down into my lower arm, and into my hand and fingertips. I move now to the other arm and hand, and again I release the tightness. I feel relaxation and heaviness flowing in. I allow the very limpness to become more and more accentuated. I again feel that gentle sense of warmth, beginning at my shoulder and moving down my arm, into my hand and into my fingertips. Now both of my arms are limp, and relaxed, and somewhat warmer than the rest of my body.

Moving now to my head and face, I release any tension, release any lingering worries away from my head and face. I know that my mind is powerful, and can do anything I choose to do. I feel the deep sense of relaxation flowing to the muscles of my head and face. I know that the heaviness of my head is too heavy to move or shift, unless I really want to. I allow the muscles of my face to become very smooth and very soft, taking on a youthful, creaseless quality. I do not warm my head, since I did not pull blood to that area, but instead I allow myself to feel a very gentle coolness, as if a breeze, a summer breeze, was caressing my face, bringing refreshment.

Next, I move down to the area of my neck and shoulders, again releasing the tension. With extra tightness in my shoulders and neck, I imagine that they are like knotted ropes, and I begin now to untie the knots, so that the fibers may lie lazily side by side. I feel the heaviness coming into these areas, and beginning at the base of my skull, I note the warmth slowly coming around and down the neck, bathing this area with deeper relaxation and increased blood flow.

I move now to the area of the shoulders, my upper chest, and upper back. I let go of my tension, and allow the relaxation to begin flooding this area. I feel the heaviness becoming more apparent, and I feel that comforting warmth flowing down my neck to my upper chest and across my upper back and shoulders. It is very comforting and warming.

I note that as I relax these areas, I feel less burdened. I now let go the tightness from my middle chest and abdomen, and my middle back and lower back, and I feel the relaxation flooding on down, bringing with it comforting heaviness. I allow the warmth to continue on down, bathing these areas with increased relaxation and rest. I now allow myself to release tightness in my buttocks and genitals, and again allow the relaxation to flow into these areas, bringing with it the sense of heaviness and comforting warmth. I'm aware now that the upper portion of my body feels relaxed, heavy, and very deliciously warm, except for my head and face, which feel refreshed.

I now release tightness and discomfort from my legs, and from all the joints in my legs, and my feet, and toes. I feel relaxation moving on down with a very comforting heaviness and limpness. I feel the warmth following, flowing on down into my legs and feet. I again take several deep breaths, feeling the fresh air flowing into my lungs, and releasing any remaining inner tension. I notice an increasing calmness coming over the center of my abdomen. This feeling grows, as if my stomach were the center of calmness within me. I feel its warmth. I feel how soothing it is. (At this point, the client is instructed to rest for 10 to 20 minutes).

Appendix 2–4. INSTRUCTIONS TO THE CLIENT: THREE ALTERNATIVES
FOR CALMING TECHNIQUES

Breath Control

Heaviness
1. Allow yourself to be comfortably supported by the chair (or couch or floor) with your arm on the armrests.
2. Close your eyes and begin to relax.
3. Take a deep breath, then another, overfilling your lungs.
4. As you slowly exhale, experience a band of heaviness move down through the body, from your head to your feet. It may take two to three breaths to complete this.

Warmth
1. Keep your eyes closed, again take a deep breath, then another, overfilling your lungs. Hold the breath.
2. As you slowly exhale, experience a band of warmth move down through your body from your head to your feet, taking a couple of breaths, if necessary, to complete

Appendix 2–4. INSTRUCTIONS TO THE CLIENT: THREE ALTERNATIVES FOR CALMING TECHNIQUES *(Continued)*

Count-back
Relax each body part as you count from 1 to 10.

Head	1
Face	2
Neck	3
Upper Back	4
Arms	5
Lower Back	6
Stomach	7
Buttocks	8
Legs	9
Release inner tension	10

Take two to three deep, cleansing breaths

Cue Word
Simply repeat one word such as "relax" or "calm" several times to yourself as you recall the feeling of being relaxed.

3

COGNITIVE REAPPRAISAL

SHARON SCANDRETT

DESCRIPTION OF INTERVENTION

Our minds are powerful. What we frame the world to look like through our perceptions strongly colors our actions. In essence, we create our world through our own thoughts. If we see it as threatening, then we relate to everything with caution and fear; if we see it as peaceful and loving, our actions correspond. Not only do our perceptions color our world, but people around us respond to our behavior, further amplifying the "vibrations" we initiate.

We create forces in our environment which amplify those stresses, because part of us thrives upon the fear. Mass media news reports are good examples; in these reports disaster and doom predominate. Advertising goes to the opposite extreme, portraying the "beautiful image," of which we often fall short.

Certainly actual threats do exist: divorce, crime, and unemployment are all realities which threaten us. We must learn to take care of ourselves just as the primitive people learned to protect themselves from the threats from their environment. Yet, we often react to small events as if they were immense. Being late for an appointment or a meeting may be met with the same intensity of emotion as lack of money to buy food; criticism from a colleague may be dealt with in the same depth as a major disaster, such as a fire or an accident.

In nursing, we tend to deal only with the physical effects of these indiscriminating cognitions. However, the physical effects are only the symptoms of the problem. Nurses can and should do more to deal with client's thoughts, feelings, and beliefs. Nurses need to go beyond treating symptoms and offer clients an opportunity to alter cognitions that contribute to the stress response in the body. As nurses see clients who experience stress, they can ask if the client desires to do anything about the situation causing the stress. If so, the nurse can offer the client assistance in several ways: by exploring and

49

evaluating the causes of the stress; by teaching how to relax in response to the stress; and by changing the perception of the situation.

The intervention whereby a nurse helps the client deal with stress by changing the perception of the situation is termed *Cognitive* Reappraisal. Reappraisal is an evaluative process in which stressful stimuli are examined for their impact and meaning and are placed in perspective of the whole. Thought patterns are consciously altered by reinforcing responses that are more holistically adaptive. Pragmatic strategies for facilitating alternative ways of coping are explored and rehearsed. Other names for this approach are cognitive restructuring and cognitive therapy.

LITERATURE REVIEW

Cognitive theory has ancient origins dating to Greek philosophers such as Epictetus, who wrote, "Men are distressed not by things, but by the views which they take of them" (Epictetus, 1948, p. 19). The scientific community has refocused its attention on cognitive theory in the last two decades. Rotter (1954), Kelly (1955), and Beck (1963) are early cognitive learning cultivators who developed theories, conducted research, and taught these notions. They are considered the founding fathers of the current cognitive revolution in psychotherapy. Ellis (1962) brought the client's belief systems to the forefront and gained lay popularity with his rational-emotive therapy. Some other "thought management" writers who emphasized positive thinking were Bain (1928), Carnegie (1948), Coué (1922), Dubois (1909), Maltz (1960), and Peale (1960). Bandura (1969) ushered in the shift in behavior therapy to a cognitive and information processing model of behavior change. Other behaviorists supported the cognitive approach, e.g., Lazarus (1971), Goldfried (1971), and Meichenbaum (1972).

Most writers on cognitive theory believe that maladaptive feelings are caused by maladaptive thoughts. Some basic assumptions of cognitive theory include the following:

1. adaptive and maladaptive behavior and affective patterns are developed through cognitive patterns;

2. moods and feelings are influenced by current thoughts;

3. cognitions include inner dialogue, perceptions, and fantasies, which represent meanings the client attaches to his experiences;

4. pessimistic thoughts that cause anxiety are frequently unrealistic, illogical, and distorted; and

5. many clients have underlying assumptions or cognitive schema that predispose them to anxiety or depression (Childress and Burns, 1981).

The cognitive approach to emotion emphasizes the appraisal of the situation as a kind of mediator between the environmental stimulus and the emotional response (Murray, 1964). The appraisal of a situation depends on information available to the person, contextual as well as immediately relevant, and how a person processes and deals with that information. The emotional response, whether it be positive or negative, is viewed as part of adaptation to a situation.

If, for example, a person who is turned down for a desired job claims, "This shows how undesirable I am, I'll never amount to anything," the resulting emotions most likely will be feelings of being worthless, hopeless, and guilt-ridden. Others might perceive the rejection differently—as an opportunity to learn why they were not selected for the job—and will utilize the feedback to seek a position that is better suited for them. This person may feel disappointed, but will not feel overwhelmed or have a compromised self-esteem because of the episode.

Burns (1980) identified some cognitions that were self-defeating for a person. Cognitive distortions, include all-or-nothing thinking (black or white), overgeneralization (seeing one negative event as evidence for defeat in other areas), dwelling on a single negative detail excluding other things, disqualifying positive experiences, jumping to conclusions (such as predicting negative outcomes), catastrophizing or minimizing, assuming one's negative emotions are a valid reflection of the world, using "should" statements, labeling oneself negatively, and personalizing (claiming things are caused by oneself).

Cognitive appraisals may be influenced by information from multiple sources, with resulting bodily reactions and emotions. Bodily reactions can be seen as preparatory for upcoming behavioral demands. The person must appraise the bodily arousal itself for consistency with other information being processed. In addition, the person evaluates his or her own ability to cope with the threat. The anxious client, in general, distorts the world view in terms of imminent danger from future events, predicting dire consequences and treating them as fact. The client is often blind to these negative predictions, which can become self-fulfilling prophecies. For example, a person who sees himself as unlovable may not interact with other people even on brief occasions. Avoidance of others further creates a sense of loneliness, undesirability, and lack of love. Physical sensations of emptiness, agitation, and general discomfort may result. Reinforcement of the irrational belief that one is unlovable is supported.

Cognitive Reappraisal or Therapy is a "structured short-term treatment for depression and anxiety, based on helping the client to identify and change distorted thought patterns that trigger and perpetuate one's distress" (Childress and Burns, 1981, p. 1024). Clients are taught to recognize cognitive distortions and to observe their bodily reactions. Awareness is the first step in gaining control over one's behaviors. Alteration of a person's reaction to a seemingly threatening stimulus can occur by providing a benign interpretation of the event. If people view a stressor as manageable with their coping abilities, their defensive behavior is no longer necessary. Mastering one problem area increases a person's confidence in being able to cope with other problems, including those that are more threatening (Murray and Jacobson, 1978).

Behavioral techniques are then used to assist clients to reinforce changes in their beliefs about the feared stimuli and to reduce anxiety response habits. It is important to develop coping skills. Those encouraged are relaxation training, meditation, self-distraction, assertion, and behavior rehearsal. In essence, what is being encouraged by this approach is behavioral self-control—an act which the individual regulates.

Little research was done on self-control therapies prior to the 1960s. One phenomenon that may be operating in positive self-control is *self-reward*, which researchers have found effective. This self-reward can simply be self-praise (Mahoney and Arnkoff, 1978). A sizable amount of research shows that "self-talk," messages one tells oneself—can dramatically influence an individual's performance of widely varying tasks (Meichenbaum, 1974, 1977).

In his cognitive approach, Ellis focused on "core irrational ideas" (Ellis and Harper, 1975), whereas Meichenbaum was most interested in idiosyncratic thoughts. Beck (1970, 1977) successfully utilized cognitive therapy with depressed patients. He emphasized self-discovery by the patient more than direct confrontations by the therapist, which were emphasized by Ellis. Other studies support the use of a cognitive approach with depressed patients. The National Institute of Mental Health (NIMH) is studying the efficacy of cognitive therapy in relation to other treatment modalities (Blackburn et al., 1981; Kovacs, 1980; Kolata, 1981). The use of cognitive therapy has been studied with other pathological conditions, such as psychosomatic illnesses, pain, and anxiety states (Blinchik and Grezesiak, 1979; Kolata, 1981; Biran and Wilson, 1981). While psychiatric nurses have long used both cognitive (e.g., Assertiveness Training) and behavioral (e.g., Relaxation Training) interventions, no studies report the effectiveness of cognitive approach.

REAPPRAISAL TOOLS

Five steps are presented which the nurse can use to assist clients in reappraising their thoughts and perceptions.

1. Stress Identification

The first part of this intervention consists of an evaluation process—an assessment of the stresses, fears, hurts, and problems of the client. Stress identification tools, such as Holmes and Rahe's Life Change Scale (1967) or Wolpe and Lang's Fear Survey (1969), can assist the client to identify problematic areas. "While all stressors represent change of some sort, many of them involve the loss of something valued" (Brallier, 1982, p. 6). Listing of the specific stressors allows clients to more fully examine their world and the forces impinging upon them. Sometimes individuals cannot define what is upsetting them, perhaps because they are unable or unwilling to examine the disturbing force. Often the vagueness of a stressor is distressing in itself. Frequently examination of all the things the client is attempting to deal with brings charity and focus to the client's thoughts. This clarity by itself may reduce tension. In addition, the clients may relax their self expectations when the amount of stressors is seen in perspective. Of course, some clients may find themselves even more overwhelmed and feel unable to move beyond the emotion.

2. Stress Evaluation

Examination of specific stressors is indicated at this point. The nurse can assist the client in this exploration by listening and by clarifying areas that seem vague. Information can be obtained about the following areas: incidence of stressors, frequency of occurrence, meaning of the stressor to the client, pervasiveness of threat or amount of actual risk to client's well-being, and the placement of stimuli in relation to other things in life. Brallier (1982) claimed that generally individuals "give in" to the cumulative effects of stress, whereas some may utilize defense mechanisms or healthy adaptations to a long-term stressor. Often some stressors will be defused in the process of evaluation as the client sees the amount of focus or energy already expended on a stressor. Clients tend to put the stressors into perspective and may decrease the amount of energy wasted on unimportant stressors.

3. Stress Hierarchy

Stressors are then assigned priorities by the client, from the most upsetting to the least upsetting. At times the client may actually be able to "let go" of minimally disturbing stressors at this time. This allows the client to focus more fully upon the most important stresses.

4. Assessment of Coping

Clients can then focus upon the ways they handle particular important stressors. The facilitative skills that allow healthy adaptation in relation to a specific stressor can be seen and their own resources and strengths are recognized more consciously. Brallier (1982) suggests that the client's perceptions of his or her ability to control a stressor is an important factor. Individuals who have a strong sense of internal control are able to prevent distressing experiences, and those with only a moderate sense of control manage a stressor more adaptively. In addition, clients can examine the weakness in their coping styles. These coping styles may include avoidance of stressors, accommodation to stressors, or adjusting mentally and emotionally to stressors (Brallier, 1982). The nurse can assist the client to learn more facilitative coping strategies or can refer the client to another resource, which can offer such information and training. This step assists the client to move from being a passive "victim" to an active participant in handling life. Another component of this step is allowing the client to see what aspects of the stressor can be altered through individual action and which things are beyond change. Once the person has acknowledged what can and what cannot be changed, the process of acceptance of unchangeable events can begin. Sometimes clients learn that they like to scare themselves and thrive on fear. The "rush of adrenalin" can be addicting. Others may seem themselves as crisis-prone, living as victims most of the time, and may create crises when life becomes too quiet.

5. Behavior Management Techniques

Alteration of socially and symbolically threatening situations sometimes involves specific techniques that assist the client in letting go of these stressors. Some of these releasing techniques include extinction procedures, persuasion, vicarious experiences, imagery, and problem solving (Table 3–1). Referral to counselors or other psychotherapists may be necessary with some of these techniques. With the decrease in stressors, alteration of one's life adaption style is required. Long-term personality factors, such as a tendency to appraise every setback as a catastrophe, may have to be dealt with to produce significant emotional changes. In particular, individuals with psychosomatic disorders tend to deny that emotional factors are connected with their physical symptoms. The nurse in some cases may only "plant seeds" about contributory

Table 3–1. DESCRIPTION OF BEHAVIOR ALTERATION APPROACHES

Extinction: Learning through consequences of a response in which no aversion or strong reinforcers occur

Persuasion or Direct Guidance: Encouraging the client to utilize more adaptive behavior methods

Vicarious Learning: Observing successful handling of a stressful situation by others

Imagery or Covert Modeling: Utilizing mental images to experience or rehearse behaviors prior to real-life attempts

Desensitization: Using relaxation to cope with real life and imaginary anxiety-arousing situations

Problem Solving: Resolving situational difficulties in life utilizing a specified process

factors to a particular psychosomatic condition, and actual change may occur much later in the client's life through another helper or psychotherapist.

SELF-CONTROL TECHNIQUES

The nurse can assist the client to modify either the stressor or the response. The stressor can be defused by clarification and examination from a broader perspective. The stressor can also be modified by assisting the client to focus on more adaptive thoughts or desired behaviors, such as the use of affirmations or positive thoughts. Another technique involves reconditioning the stressor through systematic desensitization (Wolpe and Lazarus, 1967). In this reconditioning process, the stressor is paired with the relaxation response, thus counteracting the anxiety response. Through relaxation, the client gains control over the physical response to a stressor. Another tool that can assist in gaining control of responses is to keep a journal in which self-negating statements are written and expounded on and their opposites explored (Burns, 1980). Use of imagery—that is; visualizing oneself as successfully handling stressors—can also be of assistance, as can the use of role playing. The nurse can teach the client these techniques.

NURSING DIAGNOSES AND CASE STUDY

Nursing diagnoses pertinent to this intervention include

- Fear
- Powerlessness
- Ineffective Individual Coping
- Alteration in Thought Processes
- Health Maintenance Alteration

Any client who suffers from stress and anxiety may benefit from consideration of this intervention. In particular, clients who have incorporated stress into their lives so much that they have developed psychosomatic illness or experience chronic anxiety are prime candidates. Often the symptoms these clients experience are treated without any attempt being made to eliminate the cause or contributory factors. Reappraisal can lessen fear by shifting perspective and allowing the individual to regain maximum control of his or her response to the fearful stimuli. A sense of powerlessness can be reduced if the person clarifies a stressor and his or her response to it. Identification of areas in which to seek assistance, to grow, or to make decisions certainly assists people to see where they have control over a stressor. Health maintenance alteration is also addressed by this intervention. Any individual attempting to facilitate health by changing a life style is susceptible to stressors that may be perceived as blocks to living harmoniously with oneself. The life changes necessary for health maintenance are often seen as stressful in themselves. Interventions that may alter these perceptions can ensure greater success in producing the desired life style change. Methods of reappraisal allow the individuals to change their cognitive frame or "glasses," permitting them to see the world differently.

Case Study

A 34 year old, moderately overweight male dentist was referred to me for relaxation training and stress management. He was interested in reducing his hypertension, which began one year ago when he found his work situation becoming highly stressful. Even

Table 3–2. SUBJECT'S REPORTED BLOOD PRESSURE LEVELS DURING RELAXATION TRAINING AND REAPPRAISAL

mm Hg	2/1 (Baseline)	2/9 1	2/17 2	2/23 3	3/10 4	3/17 5	3/31 Post
160							
150							
140	S		S				
130		S			S	S	
120				S			S
110							
100			D				
90	D	D		D	D	D	
80							D

though he was in supportive counseling with a psychiatrist and planned major life changes to alleviate the situation, he continued to be anxious. Although his blood pressure had been reduced by medications (Inderal, Diazoxide, and Minipress) and a weight reduction diet, it still fluctuated to high levels whenever some upsetting incident occurred at work. To help the client gain control of both the stressors and his response, two interventions were used: Relaxation Training and Cognitive Reappraisal.

A five-step Relaxation Training program was instituted (see Chapter 2). His blood pressure levels during the training period are presented in Table 3–2.

Initially the dentist was impatient for his blood pressure to become lower. In general, his blood pressure fluctuated less with stress as he continued to practice the relaxation at least five times a week, e.g., on February 10 his blood pressure was 190/120 following a very stressful event at work, whereas by mid-March, his blood pressure was 130/90 after a very stressful clinic morning. By the end of March he reported feeling much more relaxed a greater percentage of the time and he could quiet himself within 3 to 5 minutes when previously it had taken him 20 to 30 minutes. In April his hypertensive medications were reduced and in May he could maintain his blood pressure at 130/90 in upsetting events.

Concurrently with Relaxation Therapy, Cognitive Reappraisal was used. The client identified listed all stressors that were plaguing him at the time (Table 3–3). The list was prioritized for work and for home from the most stressful to least stressful. After reviewing each of these items, in-depth work was done on two main areas: interactions with his father and interactions with his department chairman. Imagery was enlisted to assist him to have meaningful conversations with these individuals and he was able to use the relaxation response to counter upsetting stimuli. In addition, keeping his focus on the here and now was encouraged, since fear is often anticipatory. A third area was also addressed: his impatience with the slowness of the sale of his house. His typical response to this problem was reviewed in depth. His pattern was first to worry and do nothing. Second, to rationalize that it takes time to sell houses now, and third, to feel helplessness and anger about failing to effectively influence his realtor. Using Cognitive Reappraisal he cited all of the good points about his house and argued with himself that it should sell easily. After this process of reviewing his feelings and examining all he had done about the house, he was able to relax and let go of the worry. By the end of March he reported that while many upsetting stimuli still existed, his response

Table 3–3. SUBJECT'S LIST OF STRESSORS

Work: (Most Stressful)
1. Interactions with department chairman and dean.
2. An individual at work.
3. Some dealing with a passive-aggressive hygienist.

Home: (Most Stressful)
1. All interactions with parents, especially father.
2. Arguments with wife (infrequent).
3. Selling of house and moving.
4. Children vying for attention, especially at meal times.
5. Misplacing things.

to them had changed. His list of stressors became shorter. It still included stressful interactions with his parents, which he decided he did not want to change, his children still seeking attention at meals, and avoidance of his department chairman. Signs of his anxiety were reflected mainly in the shallowness of his breathing which we worked on with Relaxation Training, encouraging him to breathe deeply of life in each moment. In general, he reported feeling better and calmer. The relaxation assisted him to gain control over his physical response and to see that he could control anxiety, at least at the physical level. However, if we dealt only with that level, he would most likely still feel hurt by the emotionally painful stressors. Cognitive Reappraisal has reduced the emotional pain.

RECOMMENDATIONS FOR RESEARCH

Research is needed on the utilization of cognitive approaches in nursing practice. Some questions that should be studied are the following: What types of clients respond best to Cognitive Reappraisal? What cognitive techniques are most helpful with illogical versus valid thoughts? Are symptoms reduced by changed thinking? What coping styles are most helpful in reducing signs of stress? For what types of clients do combined approaches of cognitive and behavioral approaches work best? Does a person gain more internal control using these procedures? Methods of diffusing stress or releasing fear and stress also need to be validated. Efficacy for nursing practice in various clinical settings also needs to be studied.

EDITORS' COMMENTS AND QUESTIONS

Stress management has traditionally emphasized behavioral therapy: those techniques that treat a stress response. The intervention in this chapter, Cognitive Reappraisal, treats the stimulus that produces the stress response. Cognitive Reappraisal is a way of helping the client reorganize the way stressors are perceived. This is a new intervention that has appeared in the literature during the past ten years. More health workers, including nurses, are learning the intervention.

Questions for Discussion

1. *How do behavioral and cognitive therapies complement each other?*

2. *Can you use the five-step model for implementing Cognitive Reappraisal in your practice?*

3. *How would you learn more about this intervention?*

4. *What are the stressors in your life? How do you perceive them?*

5. *Is Cognitive Reappraisal a nursing intervention?*

References

Bain, J. A. *Thought control in everyday life.* New York: Funk and Wagnalls, 1928.

Bandura, A. *Principles of behavior modification.* New York: Holt, Rinehart and Winston, 1969.

Bandura, A. Self efficacy: Toward a unifying theory of behavioral change. *Psychological Review,* 1977, *84,* 191–215.

Beck, A. T. Thinking and depression. I. Idiosyncratic content and cognitive distortions. *Archives of General Psychiatry,* 1963, *9,* 324–333.

Beck, A. T. *Cognitive therapy and the emotional disorders.* New York: International Universities Press, 1976.

Beck, A. T., Cognitive therapy: Nature and relation to behavior therapy. *Behavior Therapy,* 1970a, *1.* 184–200.

Beck, A. T. Role of fantasies in psychotherapy and psychopathology. *Journal of Nervous and Mental Disease,* 1970b, *150,* 3–17.

Biran, M., and Wilson, G. T. Treatment of phobic disorders using cognitive and exposure methods: A self-efficacy analysis. Journal of *Consulting Clinical Psychology,* 1981, *49*(6), 886–899.

Blackburn, I. M., Bishop, S., Glen, A. I.M., Whalley, L. J., and Christie, J. E. The efficacy of cognitive therapy in depression: A treatment trial using cognitive therapy and pharmacology, each alone and in combination. *British Journal of Psychiatry,* 1981, *139,* 181–189.

Blinchik, E. R. and Grzesiak, R. C. Reinterpretative Cognitive Strategies in Chronic Pain Management. Archives of Physical Medical Rehabilitation, 60 (Dec. 1979). 609–612.

Brallier, L. *Transition and transformation: Successfully managing stress.* Los Altos, Calif.: National Nursing Review, 1982.

Burns, D. D. *Feeling good: The new mood therapy.* New York: William Morrow and Company, 1980.

Carnegie, D. *How to stop worrying and start living.* New York: Simon and Schuster, 1948.

Cautela, J. R. Covert Conditioning. In A. Jacobs and L. B. Socks (Eds.), *The psychology of private events: Perspectives on covert responses systems.* New York: Academic Press, 1971.

Childress, A. R., and Burns, D. D. The basics of cognitive therapy. *Psychosomatics,* 1981, *22*(12), 1017–1020, 1023–1024, 1027.

Coué, E. *The practice of autosuggestion.* New York: Doubleday, 1922.

Dubois, P. C. *The psychic treatment of nervous disorders.* New York: Funk and Wagnalls, 1909.

Ellis, A. *Reason and emotion in psychotherapy.* New York: Stuart, 1962.

Ellis, A., and Harper, R. A. *A new guide to rational living.* Englewood Cliffs, N. J.: Prentice Hall, 1975.

Epictetus. *The enchiridon.* New York: Bobbs-Merrill, 1948, p. 19.

Gelb, L. A., and Ullman, M. Instant psychotherapy offered at an outpatient psychiatric clinic. *Frontiers of Hospital Psychiatry,* 1967, *4,* 14.

Goldfried, M. R. Systematic densensitization as training self-control. *Journal of Consulting and Clinical Psychology,* 1967, *11,* 213–218.

Holmes, T. H. and Kahe, R. H. The social readjustment rating scale. *Journal of Psychosomatic Research.* 1967, *11,* 213–218.

Kelly, G. A. *The psychology of personal constructs.* New York: Norton, 1955.

Kolata, G. B. Clinical trial of psychotherapies is under way. *Science,* 1981, *212* (4493), 432–433.

Kovacs, M. The efficacy of cognitive and behavior therapies for depression. *American Journal of Psychiatry,* 1980, *137* (12), 1495–1501.

Lazarus, A. A. *Behavior therapy and beyond.* New York: McGraw-Hill, 1971.

Mahoney, M. J., and Arnkoff, D. B. Cognitive and self-control therapies." In S. L. Garfield and A. E. Bergins (Eds.), *Handbook of psychotherapy and behavior change.* New York: John Wiley and Sons, 1978, pp. 689–722.

Maltz, M. *Psycho-cybernetics.* Englewood Cliffs, N. J.: Prentice-Hall, 1960.

Meichenbaum, D. Cognitive modification of test anxious college students. *Journal of Consulting and Clinical Psychology,* 1972, *1,* 39, 370–380.

Meichenbaum, D. *Cognitive behavior modification.* Morristown, N. J.: General Learning Press, 1974.

Meichenbaum, D. *Cognitive behavior modification.* New York: Plenum, 1977.

Murray, E. J. Sociotropic-learning approach to psychotherapy. In P. Worchel and D. Byrne (Eds.), *Personality change.* New York: John Wiley and Sons, 1964.

Murray, E. J., and L. I. Jacobson. Cognition and learning in traditional and behavioral therapy. In S. L. Garfield and A. E. Bergins (Eds.), *Handbook of psychotherapy and behavior change.* New York: John Wiley and Sons, 1978, pp. 661–687.

Peale, N. V. *The power of positive thinking.* Englewood Cliffs, N. J.: Prentice-Hall, 1960.

Platt, J., and Spicack, G. Problem-solving thinking of psychiatric patients. *Journal of Consulting and Clinical Psychology,* 1972a, *39,* 148–151.

Rotter, J. B. *Social learning and clinical psychology.* Englewood Cliffs, N. J.: Prentice-Hall, 1954.

Strupp, H. H. A multidimensional analysis of techniques in brief psychotherapy. *Psychiatry,* 1957, *20,* 387–397.

Waring, E. M. Marital intimacy, psychosomatic symptoms and cognitive therapy. *Psychosomatics,* 1980, *21*(7), 595–601.

Wolpe, J. *Psychotherapy by reciprocal inhibition.* Stanford, Calif.: Stanford University Press, 1958.

Wolpe, J., and Lang, P. J. *Fear survey schedule.* San Diego, Calif.: Educational and Industrial Testing Services, 1969.

Wolpe, J., and Lazarus, A. A. *Behavior therapy techniques.* New York: Pergamon Press, 1967.

4

MUSIC THERAPY

KATHLEEN BUCKWALTER
JANE HARTSOCK
JILL GAFFNEY

There is a charm: a Power that sways the breast;
Bids every Passion revel or be still;
Inspires with Rage, or all your Cares dissolves;
Can sooth Distraction, and almost Despair.
That Power is Music.

JOHN ARMSTRONG (1744) (Schullian and Schoen, 1948, p. v)

Throughout history, music has been used to ease the suffering of people; its influence on history, morals, and culture has long been noted. The Greeks and Romans believed music had magical charm and power to aid the body and soul in healing (Schullian and Schoen, 1948). However, it was not until the twentieth century that music as a form of treatment was investigated, and only after World War II did colleges begin educating music therapists. Music as a form of therapy has been used mainly in psychiatric and rehabilitative settings (Herth, 1978), but can be utilized to help many types of individuals, including the aged, hearing impaired, cerebral palsied, blind, mentally retarded, culturally deprived, speech handicapped, physically handicapped, gifted, or learning disabled (Dolan, 1973).

DESCRIPTION OF INTERVENTION

Music, a combination of rhythmic, harmonic, and melodic sounds, is simply the tool used to attain certain therapeutic goals. Music therapists are interested in the effects of music upon the individual and not in the individual's ability to become an accomplished musician (Dolan, 1973). Therapeutic activities may include playing instruments, singing, listening, and creative moving or dance.

Music Therapy has been defined as "the controlled use of music, its elements, and their influences on the human being to aid the physiologic,

58

psychologic, and emotional integration of the individual during the treatment of an illness or disability" (Munro and Mount, 1978, p. 1029).

The National Association for Music Therapy (1977) suggests that music therapy is "the use of music in the accomplishment of therapeutic aims, the restoration, maintenance, and improvement of mental and physical health" (p. 2).

Hadsell (1974) emphasized a more sociological approach, whereby music is used to assist persons in coping with social problems. She defines music therapy as "the use of the unique properties and potential of music in a therapeutic situation for the purpose of changing human behavior so that the individual affected will be more able to function as a worthwhile member of today's as well as tomorrow's society" (p. 114). Dolan (1973) also includes the notion of behavioral change in her concept of music therapy as "the scientific functional application of music by a therapist who is seeking specific changes in an individual's behavior" (p. 11). Similarly, Gaston (1968) views music therapy as a "gently insistent but dynamic persuasion of man to change his behavior, to share with and to expect fearlessly from his fellowman, and in so doing to achieve a happy confidence and satisfaction in himself" (p. 7).

Sears (1968) developed a theoretical framework encompassing three processes of music therapy: (1) experience within structure; (2) experience in self-organization; and (3) experience in relating to others. The content of Sears' framework can be individualized for a patient's own needs and abilities and is summarized later in this chapter. "Experience within structure refers to those behaviors of an individual that are required by and are inherent in musical experience" (Sears, 1968, p. 34). Music is an aural stimulant that takes place in time and evokes physical and psychological responses. Music provides for self-expression and allows individuals to communicate attitudes, feelings, and moods nonverbally, all of which can lead to an enhanced self-image. Musical activities often occur in groups and necessitate cooperation that fosters social interaction in addition to providing entertainment and recreation.

Nurses do not have to be polished musicians to use Music Therapy effectively as an intervention. With better knowledge of this relatively new treatment modality, they can participate in and encourage musical activities with selected patients or make appropriate referrals to trained music therapists. The nurse's role can be both diversionary and therapeutic (Forrest, 1972).

Historical Perspectives

Music has been utilized throughout history as a therapeutic influence. Early archaeological findings revealed crude musical instruments, although among primitive people music was primarily associated with dance and words. Altshuler (1948) stated that "the study of folk legends, fairy tales and myths . . . indicates that man has always attributed great power to music" (p. 269). Similarly, Herth (1978) found that "accounts of the use of music in medicine date from the earliest times when music had a social function in every phase of life, civil and religious." When a primitive person became ill or injured, it was believed that a taboo had been broken or that a deity was angry. Music was then used to appease the "gods" (Radin, 1948).

Egyptians of 1500 B.C. referred to music as "physic for the soul" and their priest-doctors used musical incantations to increase fertility (Diserens and Fine, 1939; Paul and Staudt, 1958).

The ancient Persians and Hebrews also employed music to cure various physical and mental illnesses. The Persians believed music was an expression of Ahura-Mazda (spirit of good) and utilized the lute for curing illness. The most famous recorded Hebrew incident concerning the healing power of music involved King Saul, who listened to music to preserve his reason:

> When the evil spirit from God was upon Saul, then David took up a harp and played with his hands so that Saul was refreshed and well, and the evil spirit departed from him (I Samuel, 16:23).

The Greeks were particularly known for their attention to music. Apollo was the god of music, and his son Aesculapius, the patron of medicine, provided an early medicine-music linkage (Diserens and Fine, 1939). It was reported that music was employed in stopping the nearly fatal hemorrhage of the Greek hero Odysseus (Podolsky, 1939), and that Hippocrates took mental patients to the temple to hear music (Paul and Staudt, 1958). Podolsky (1939) suggests that the first regular use of music as a therapeutic factor was by three Greeks, Zenocrates, Sarpander, and Arion. They utilized music in decreasing the outbursts of the "violently insane" (Podolsky, 1939, p. 3). Pythagoras also used music in treating mental disorders, as did Plato (Diserens and Fine, 1939).

Tarantism, a disease rampant in the Middle Ages, and characterized by screaming and convulsions, was treated with music. Podolsky (1939) reports that "musicians were hired . . . to carry the St. Vitus dancers more quickly through the attacks" (p. 150).

The Renaissance inaugurated the modern age and applied the characteristics of individualism and naturalism to the sciences as well as the arts. Scientists and physicians were often poets and musicians.

Just as the dominant theory in medicine supported the existence of four elements or humors of the body, so also were there four elements dominant in music theory. These four elements (bass, tenor, alto, and soprano) were the parts forming complete harmony. During the Renaissance illness was thought to be due to a disruption in the harmonious balance between the four body elements (blood, phlegm, yellow bile, black bile). Music was used to restore this harmony. Musical beat and rhythm were related to the beat of the heart. The Renaissance philosopher Zarlino stated that just as medicine has systole (contraction) and diastole (dilation), music also has systole or thesis (accented notes) and diastole or arsis (the unaccented part of a measure or upbeat) (Carapetyan, 1948).

During the eighteenth and nineteenth centuries, the effects of music continued to be valued. Napoleon allegedly attributed his defeat in Russia to the combination of the Russian winter and Russian military music. The "barbaric" tunes incited the Muscovites to furious attacks (Podolsky, 1954).

Philip V of Spain, George II of England, and Ludwig of Bavaria were all reported to have suffered from melancholia and depression, and music proved to be a curative factor. An eighteenth century Englishman, Pargiter, studied the effects of music on mania, and asylums in France were the first to utilize music in the course of treatment of the mentally ill. During the Crimean War, Florence Nightingale utilized the healing power of music to aid the injured and ill, and in 1891 the Guild of St. Cecilia was formed to provide music for the ill (Diserens and Fine, 1939).

Munro and Mount (1978) noted that

> while the traditional close association between music and medical practice was largely forgotten in the technologic explosion of the 20th Century the

last two decades have seen a resurgence in interest and research to evaluate the physiologic and psychologic effects of music. (p. 1029)

LITERATURE REVIEW

The poets did well to conjoin music and medicine in Apollo, because the office of medicine is but to tune this curious harp of man's body, and to reduce it to harmony.

FRANCIS BACON

The latter half of the nineteenth and early twentieth centuries saw the beginnings of systematic study of music and its possible therapeutic benefits. In the following sections, research conducted during the present century will be identified as it relates to the physiological and psychological therapeutic effects of music in various health care settings.

Physical Effects

Research has shown that music affects the cardiovascular, respiratory, musculoskeletal, neurological, and metabolic systems of the body. Respiratory rate, heart rate, and blood pressure are affected by music, with variations dependent on the pitch, intensity, and timbre of sound (Diserens and Fine, 1939; Podolsky 1954).

Some of the earliest research in this area was conducted by Shepard, who studied the effects of music on blood flow to the brain, and found that lively music increased circulation to the brain (Walters, 1954). Similarly, Ellis and Brighouse (1954) determined that music affected respiratory rate, which increased with all types of music.

Research conducted on musculoskeletal and neurological responses indicates that music affects muscular contraction and relaxation, muscle strength, and reflex action. Diserens and Fine (1939) found that muscular strength increased with the intensity and pitch of sound stimuli. Further studies concluded that the rhythm of the body responds to the rhythm of the music, which Van de Wall (1946) described as the "kinesthetic response." This response is due to the interrelation and influence of sound vibration present in the body (McMahon, 1978). Other neurological effects appear to be due to the stimulation of the autonomic nervous system (Grunewald, 1953; Paul and Staudt, 1958).

Music is believed to exert a powerful influence upon the higher cerebral centers, as evidenced by its effects on attention, motivation, memory, and dreams (McMahon, 1978; Pickerell, Metzger, Wilde, Broadkent, and Edwards, 1954). Persons listening to music can have a decreased or an increased response to external sensory stimuli (Diserens and Fine, 1939; Gillman and Paperte, 1949). These sensory responses, in addition to the other musculoskeletal and neurological effects noted, can be very useful in the treatment of different types of mental illness. Table 4–1 summarizes the physical and psychological effects of music.

Psychological Effects

The psychosocial benefits of music have been studied extensively in psychiatric hospitals and clinics. Forrest (1972) states that music therapy helps the

Table 4–1. PHYSICAL AND PSYCHOLOGICAL EFFECTS OF MUSIC THERAPY*

Physical	Psychological
Causes muscle contraction	Subjective responses
Increases muscle strength	Stimulates memory (past & present)
Physical motion	Increases motivation
Increases or decreases response to external sensory stimuli	Increases attention span
Decreases HCl produced by stomach	Mood changes
Depression of H^+ ion concentration in stomach	Strong positive emotions
Local ischemia to gastric mucosa	Removes depression
Increases gastric secretion response	Stimulates abstract thought
Increases or decreases muscular tonicity and motor activity	Decreases hallucinations
Increases or decreases work output	Decreases delusions
Intensifies and accelerates muscular coordination	Decreases compulsions
Increases or decreases respiratory rate and regularity	Decreases obsessions
Delays fatigue	Increases concentration and discrimination
Increases physical endurance and perserverence	Increases imagination and self-discipline
Increases secretion of epinephrine	Decreases state anxiety
Increases extent and energy of reflexes	Increases creativity
Increases oxygen to tissues	Decreases illusions
Increases oxygen consumption	Allows nonverbal expression of feelings
Decreases muscular tension	Decreases feelings of isolation
Improves testing scores	Decreases stress
Increases internal secretion of hormones	
Increases or decreases basal metabolic rate	

*Table courtesy of Dougherty, Walker, and Schug, unpublished.

ill individual to

> develop concentration and discrimination, self-discipline and imagination, as well as stimulating abstract thought. At the same time the moods of the individual can be radically altered, preventing hallucinations, delusions, obsessions and compulsions taking over from conscious activity. (p. 40)

Experiments have confirmed that music directs the attention of patients from themselves, thus increasing their interaction with the world around them (Pickerell et al., 1954). The motivation and attention span of patients can also be greatly influenced by music (McMahon, 1978). Studies conducted by Diserens and Fine (1939) showed that music was capable of lowering the threshold of sensory perception of sights and sounds. The effects exhibited correlated with the type of music used and the preference of the listener. The greater the person's interest in music, the more influence is exerted on his or her behavior (Herth, 1978). Research has also shown that music can influence and may change moods (Altshuler, 1948; Capurso, 1952; Schullian and Schoen, 1948; Simon, Holzberg, Alessi, and Garrity, 1954).

To initiate psychotherapy, it is essential to remove states of inattention, anxiety, tension, and morbid moods (Altshuler, 1948). Research has shown that music can help to accomplish this (Altshuler, 1948; Browne, 1954; Dickens and Sharpe, 1970; Diserens and Fine, 1939). Herman (1954) identified the following therapeutic effects of music:

> 1. It has the property of attracting attention and prolonging its span. This is important in treating depression because it distracts the patient from depressive thought.
> 2. Music has the property of replacing one mood with another.

3. It has the ability to relieve inner tensions and conflicts.

4. The rhythmic stimuli produce physical motion which draws attention of patients to things around them. (p. 115)

Music therapy has also been used in an effort to decrease anxiety, a major psychological problem. Gaston (1951) discussed music in terms of stimulative versus sedative music. He stated that "percussive music . . . stimulates and demands physical activity . . . it is uninhibited" (p. 42). In contrast,

> melodic passages of a sustained nature in which the percussive element is lacking produce a very different response. . .the responses are not physical, not tension of the striped musculature, but more intellectual, more contemplative. . . . When a quiet, simple rhythm is repeated over and over again in the same style, and a sustained melody is superimposed, it will produce a sedative, often hypnotic effect. (Gaston, 1951; pp. 42–43)

Brickman (1950) investigated the effects of different types of music on moods and activities of a group of mentally ill patients. He reported that slow, even rhythms had a sedative effect on patients, to the extent that less medication was required to calm them. Rapid rhythms resulted in increased activity, as evidenced by an increased attendance at shop and gymnasium activities. Preuter and Mezanno (1973) also found that soothing music promoted more interaction in counseling interviews than did stimulating music.

Stimulative music has been shown to produce higher levels of state anxiety, physiological arousal, and aggression compared with sedative music (Biller, Olson, and Breen, 1974; Fisher and Greenberg, 1972; Smith and Morris, 1976). A second study by Smith and Morris (1977) confirmed that "the incremental effects of stimulative music on anxiety is as great or greater than the decremental effects of sedative music . . . and effects of music on the cognitive component are as great or greater than on the affective component of anxiety" (p. 1053).

Additional studies have reported the effects of music on decreasing test anxiety (Peretti, 1975, Stanton, 1975). Stoudenmire (1975) showed that relaxing music was as effective as muscle relaxation for reducing state anxiety.

In examining the psychological benefits of music therapy, Gutheil (1954) stated "music—like language—can be a vehicle of therapeutic communication" (p. 106). He further identified the therapeutic value of music as depending on "psychophysiological effects, particularly those involving tension and relaxation, and . . . psychologic effects, particularly those involving the mood" (p. 106).

Kerr (1942) pioneered a study to determine the psychological effects of music. Results demonstrated an overwhelming confidence in its psychological powers: 96 per cent of his male subjects reported a favorable belief in the psychological effects of music; 77 per cent thought it improved feelings toward associates; 90 per cent felt it helped them when they were tired; 88 per cent believed it soothed their nerves; 56 per cent thought it helped their digestion; 90 per cent thought it helped them in performing monotonous tasks; and 85 per cent believed it helped them forget worries.

Studies in brain hemisphere function provide some insight as to why music may be considered a therapeutic intervention in alleviating anxiety. Bennett (1970) and Dimond (1972) noted that the left hemisphere has generally been considered rational, propositional, and analytical, whereas the right hemisphere has been considered more intuitive, appositional, and gestalt-oriented. Similarly, Brydon and Nugent (1979) stated that the dominant hemisphere (which generally is the left hemisphere for right-handed individuals) understood the language of logic and rational analysis, whereas the nondominant hemisphere understood a language of symbols and imagery. Milner (1971) and King and Kimura (1972) reported that the right hemisphere (the nondominant hemisphere for most individuals) was concerned with melodic patterns. In the words of Altshuler (1948),

> music, even more than the spoken word, lends itself as a therapy because it meets with little or no intellectual resistance, and does not need to appeal to logic to initiate action. . .is more subtle and more primitive, and therefore its appeal is wider and greater. (p. 267)

Additional psychological effects of music include facilitating the ability to aid recall of past and present events; reinforcing identity, self-concept, and reality; and remitting the expression of fantasy (Diephouse, 1968; Munro and Mount, 1978; Van de Wall, 1946).

Music is thought to accomplish these effects in various ways. Musculoskeletal and neurological influences of music explain some of these responses (affecting attention span, memory, physical motion, and possibly inner tension). Another explanation is offered by Van de Wall (1946), who states that music initiates associational responses which connect or associate ideas and emotions that are not directed cognitively or necessarily consciously. This type of mental response is highly subjective and emotional rather than intellectual. The processes of association may explain music's ability to change moods and initiate recall of past and present events (Van de Wall, 1946).

A third possible explanation for music's behavioral effects may be related to Altshuler's theory of "thalamic response." Altshuler (1948) states that the thalamus is the seat of emotions, feelings, and sensations, and it is influenced by the pitch and rhythm of music, which in turn affect emotion and feelings.

These theories explain to some extent the effects of music on mental health, but the exact mechanism remains unknown. However, the responses to musical stimuli are rich in variation and subject to sociocultural influences. Choice of music and type of pitch preferred are often determined by the patient's sociocultural background. Music has a very personal and intimate meaning for each person, and this aspect is important when using music therapeutically. Favorite music usually elicits strongly positive emotional reactions (Maultsby, 1977).

Therapeutic Use of Music in Various Health Settings

A review of the use of therapeutic music revealed many diversified and positive outcomes. Scott (1970), in his study with minimally brain-damaged children and the effects of background music on level of productivity, found that productivity was enhanced. Gatewood (1921) reported that anesthesia was accepted more calmly when music was used as a diversion. Herth (1978) found a 30 per cent decrease in the use of pain medication when music therapy was utilized. She also noted a kinesthetic response of decreased lightheadedness with the application of music therapy. Munro and Mount (1978) showed that music therapy was useful in palliative care. Their findings included the ability of music to bring comfort when words were inadequate, and the facilitation of positive interactions and expression of feelings. Hinds (1980) noted that music increased the number of social interactions of children in a group situation at a small mental health unit. Dickens and Sharpe (1970) similarly reported that music therapy augmented the group psychotherapy of neurotic patients, in that it stimulated emotional release. Table 4–2 summa-

Table 4–2. GOALS OF MUSIC THERAPY

Podolsky (1954)
By Listening:
- improve attention
- maintain interest
- influence mood (to produce acceleration)
- produce sedation
- release energy

By Participation (in group singing, dancing):
- bring about communal cooperation
- release energy
- arouse interest

By Creation of Sound:
- increase self-respect by accomplishment and success
- increase personal happiness by ability to please others
- release energy

Munro and Mount (1978) and Michel (1976)
Physical:
- promote muscular relaxation
- break the vicious circle of chronic pain by relieving anxiety and depression and thus alter the perception of pain
- facilitate physical participation in activities to the greatest degree possible

Psychological:
- reinforce identity and self-concept, increase self-esteem
- alter the patient's mood, including easing anxiety and lessening depression and fear of others
- increase attention span and concentration
- help the patient recall past significant events
- provide a nonverbal means of expressing a broad range of recognized and intense feelings
- reinforce reality
- express fantasy
- direct appeal to the emotions
- increase tolerance of criticism

Social:
- a means of socially acceptable self-expression
- a bridge across cultural differences and isolation
- a bond and sense of community with family members and others past and present, through the mental associations aroused
- a link to the patient's life before the illness
- an opportunity to participate in a group, increasing social interaction
- entertainment and diversion, to develop constructive use of leisure time
- increase responsibility to self, to others

Spiritual:
- provide means of expressing spiritual feelings and feeling comforted and reassured
- provide an avenue for expression of anger, fear, punishment and questions on the meaning of life.

rizes the physical, psychological, social, and spiritual goals of music therapy, as identified in the literature, by type of musical activity.

MUSIC AS A NURSING INTERVENTION

Nursing has historically focused on the whole person and his or her interaction with the environment. From this holistic perspective, Altshuler (1948) reported that "music has always been an important factor in the instinctual, emotional, cultural, and spiritual life of people and as such . . . exercised a sort of therapeutic influence" (p. 267). Music, with its potential harmonizing and balancing effects, is an appropriate approach for nursing because of help in achieving the holistic health goal of harmonious integration of mind, body, and spirit.

Ryan and Travis (1981) stated that "just as sound can cause illness and

Table 4–3. MODIFIED HARTSOCK MUSIC PREFERENCE QUESTIONNAIRE (MPQ)*

The following questions are concerned with music likes. All information will be kept confidential.

1. The following is a list of different types of music. Please indicate your three (3) most favorite types with 1 being the most favorite, 2 the next, and 3 your third choice.

   _____1. Country and Western
   _____2. Classical
   _____3. Spiritual/Religious
   _____4. Rock
   _____5. Folk
   _____6. Blues
   _____7. Jazz
   _____8. Disco
   _____9. Other: _____

Please put a check (√) beside your choice in the following questions.

2. What form does your favorite music take?

   _____1. Vocal
   _____2. Nonvocal
   _____3. Both

3. What type of music makes you feel the *most* happy?

   _____ Country and Western
   _____ Classical
   _____ Spiritual/Religious
   _____ Rock
   _____ Folk
   _____ Blues
   _____ Jazz
   _____ Disco
   _____ Other: _____
   _____ None

4. Are there any specific songs/selections which make you feel happy?

injury and set you on edge, so it can be one of the easiest ways to relax you" (p. 79). The balancing and harmonizing effects of music on body, mind, and spirit have long been noted. Music therapy is easily initiated and self-regulated, allowing the individual to assume responsibility.

The literature acknowledges and supports a wide variety of therapeutic uses of music. Although research has been done on the use of music therapy, there is little documentation of music as a therapeutic intervention in nursing. Nightingale (1946) in her discussion of the nurse as a regulator of the environment, noted the importance of music and reported "the effect of music upon the sick has been scarcely at all noted . . . wind instruments, including the human voice and stringed instruments . . . have generally a beneficent effect." Furthermore, Herth (1978) suggests:

> We have been able to use music in many different ways as an adjunct in providing total care for our patients. It is an area which seems to have many possibilities and is open to further research. . . . We also need to recognize how we in nursing can play a valuable role in the judicious integration of music into total, individualized patient care. (p. 23)

Music Therapy can be used in a wide variety of health care settings (e.g., a pediatrics ward, a psychiatric hospital, a rehabilitation center, a medical-surgical department) to alleviate a variety of conditions (e.g., pain, anxiety, depression) and to enhance others (self-expression, self-esteem, relaxation, and so forth).

5. When listening to music that makes you feel happy, is there any particular artist/performer you enjoy listening to *most*?

6. What type of music makes you feel the *most* sad?

_____ Country and Western
_____ Spiritual/Religious
_____ Rock
_____ Folk
_____ Blues
_____ Jazz
_____ Disco
_____ Other:_____
_____ None

7. Before your hospitalization, how important a role did music play in your life?

_____1. Very important
_____2. Moderately important
_____3. Slightly important
_____4. Not important

8. Before your hospitalization, how often did you enjoy listening to music in a typical 24-hour period (day)?

_____1. Less than 1 hour
_____2. 1–3 hours
_____3. 4–6 hours
_____4. 7–9 hours
_____5. Over 10 hours

9. During your hospitalization, how often do you enjoy listening to music during a 24-hour period (day)?

_____1. less than one l hour
_____2. 1–3 hours
_____3. 4–6 hours
_____4. 7–9 hours
_____5. Over 10 hours

*From Hartsock, 1982.

A major objective of Music Therapy is "to help the patient to verbalize phantasy and express emotion" (Dickens and Sharpe, 1970, p. 83). Gatewood (1921) stated that to obtain the greatest benefits from use of music, it is important to keep the mood of the music the same as the mood desired by the therapist. Conversely, Altshuler (1948) advocated the use of the "iso" principle, which simply means that the mood or tempo must match the mood of the patient. Music chosen by the patient may be reflective of his or her moods, and a shift in musical taste may indicate changes in mood (Munro and Mount, 1978). Both approaches are considered valid by music therapists today.

Music preference appears to be influenced by emotional associations and learned response and is an important consideration in the selection of intervention tools for use in Music Therapy. Together, the nurse and patient can explore the option of using a musical intervention, taking into consideration the patient's background, musical interests, and abilities.

To assess a patient's musical preference, nurses can use the Hartsock (1982) Music Preference Questionnaire (MPQ) (Table 4–3). The questionnaire was used by Hartsock to determine patients' musical preferences in her study of the effects of music on depression levels in immobilized patients.

The MPQ requires approximately 15 minutes to complete. After assessment of musical preference, the nurse will need to choose particular music selections representative of the preferences expressed and prepare tapes if none are commercially available. Hartsock (1982) collected music from personal and library resources and recorded the records onto cassette tapes. A pilot study determined the degrees of quality of cassette tapes, and she selected Maxwell Ultra-Dynamic tapes. A Wollensak machine was used to create the tapes without the interference of extraneous sounds. Approximately 2 to 3 days were allowed for the collection and preparation of the intervention tapes, and copyright laws were adhered to.

In addition to the taped music, patients were given portable tape cassette players equipped with headphones. The cassette players and tapes can be left at the patients' bedsides for the duration of their hospital stay, or, if there is not enough equipment to meet patient demands, they can be checked from a central location, such as the nurses' station. Patients should be instructed to listen to the music whenever and for as long as they desire.

Nurses should consider developing a portable patient listening library that houses tapes covering a broad spectrum of musical tastes. Philanthropic groups can be approached to purchase cassettes for the patient music library, and hospital volunteers can successfully run the administrative and maintenance aspects of the library, thus freeing nurses for more professional activities, which include the identification of patients likely to benefit from music therapy and the implementation of such a nursing order (Table 4–4).

In addition to tapes or radio music, nurses may also elect to lead patients in singing, dancing, or playing musical instruments. Potential variables in the selection of music therapy as a nursing intervention include the patient's sex, previous experience and familiarity with music, and musical interests and abilities.

Nurses should also evaluate the effects of the music intervention on a continual basis to assess the impact of the music on the patient as well as changes in musical preference. This can best be done using an interview schedule, such as the one developed by Hartsock (1982) for research purposes (Table 4–5).

Nurses who introduce Music Therapy in an effort to change a particular aspect of patient care (e.g., pain, anxiety, depression) may wish to measure systematically the influence of the intervention on the variable of interest using standardized tools (e.g., Melzack-Wall's Pain Scales, Spielberger's State-Trait Anxiety Inventory, or the Beck Depression Inventory).

NURSING DIAGNOSES ASSOCIATED WITH THE USE OF MUSIC THERAPY

Music Therapy is a nursing intervention that may be applicable to several nursing diagnoses (see Table 4–4). This section will focus on three diagnoses accepted at the fourth national conference in 1980:

  o Coping, Ineffective Individual
  o Diversional Activity Deficit
  o Mobility, Impaired Physical

Research conducted by the authors is cited in relation to each of these diagnoses.

Hartsock (1982) and Gaffney (1982) investigated the effectiveness of Music Therapy as a nursing intervention for patients with impaired physical mobility (orthopedic patients confined to bed for more than seven days). Although Hartsock studied the effect of music in terms of mood changes (alleviation of

Table 4–4. NURSING DIAGNOSES FOR WHICH MUSIC THERAPY CAN BE USED AS A NURSING INTERVENTION

Alteration in comfort; pain	Ineffective coping
Anxiety	Reactive depression (situational)
Diversional activity deficit	Self-concept disturbance
Fear	Sexual dysfunction
Grieving	Sleep-pattern disturbance
Impaired physical mobility	Social isolation
Impaired thought processes	Spiritual distress
Impaired verbal communication	

depression) and Gaffney analyzed the effects of music on state anxiety, both approached the musical intervention as a technique to help patients cope with the depression and anxiety they experienced as a result of being immobilized. The Music Therapy intervention was also conceptualized as a diversionary activity for this patient population confined to bed and thus experiencing a deficit.

Although the adverse psychological effects of immobilization—specifically increased state anxiety—are well documented in the literature (Bexton, Heron, and Scott, 1954; Browse, 1965; Dietrich, Whedon, and Schorr, 1948; Kottke, 1966; Levy, 1966; Lilly, 1956; Zubek et al., 1963, 1968, 1969a and b), Gaffney (1982) failed to support her hypothesis that patients on prolonged bedrest would have decreased state anxiety when listening to relaxing, nonstimulative music. However, subjects in this study listened to these tapes when they were relaxed rather than anxious, in direct opposition

Table 4–5. INTERVIEW QUESTIONNAIRE TO EVALUATE EFFECTS OF MUSIC THERAPY*

May I tape this interview with you? All information will be kept strictly confidential.
How many minutes or hours did you listen to the music during a 24-hour period?
Did you listen more during the day or the night?
Was there any time when you felt like listening to music and were unable to?
Was there any time you would rather not have listened to your music?
Did you feel sad any time during the week?
Can you tell me about any event that occurred this week that has made you feel sad?
Did you feel like listening to music when you were sad?
What type?
Did you feel happy any time during the past week?
Was there any event that occurred which made you feel happy?
Did you listen to music when you felt happy?
What type?
Has there been any change in your music likes?
The type of music?
The songs?
Any other comments about the music?

*From Hartsock, 1982.

to the investigator's intended use of the tapes. Gaffney's (1982) sample also included a high percentage of elderly (over 65) patients on prolonged bedrest because of total hip replacements. She recommends further research to determine appropriate nursing interventions to decrease anxiety with the following modifications:

1. Build into the study controls for the length of time per shift that a subject can be out of bed.

2. Specify a minimum amount of time and frequency for listening to the taped music.

3. Pretest and posttest various types of "relaxing" music to verify the assumption that a particular type of music is indeed perceived as relaxing by subjects.

4. Include a different sample of patients (a wider variety of ages, settings, and types of immobilization) to develop greater generalizability to the populations of immobilized patients.

5. Build into the study a control by instructing subjects to listen to the taped relaxation music when feeling anxious, as opposed to when feeling relaxed. When given instructions to play the taped music "whenever and for as long as they want to," it was found that the subjects listened more frequently when feeling relaxed than when feeling anxious.

Nurses must continue to investigate creative alternative health practices that decrease state anxiety in immobilized patients.

Hartsock (1982) also failed to support her hypothesis that listening to favorite music would significantly decrease depression levels in immobilized patients. However, her experimental and control groups were not equivalent prior to the start of the intervention period, with subjects in the experimental group experiencing baseline depression levels three times higher than subjects in the control group. Hartsock (1982) noted an interesting trend in that experimental subjects who listened to their favorite taped music showed a steady drop in their average depression levels throughout the intervention period. Based on her interviews, Hartsock (1982) suggests that three extraneous factors affected the moods of her subjects and may have interacted with the musical intervention: (1) change in prognosis, (2) visiting of significant others, and (3) perceived role changes of subjects. Because of the small sample size of her study (n = 12) Hartsock also recommends further research with music therapy and its effect on patients with limited mobility.

Buckwalter (1976) evaluated the use of Music Therapy in a variety of settings and with varied clinical populations. While serving as a member of an "on-call" pain intervention team, she was frequently summoned by nurses to deal with "problem pain patients." Music Therapy was one of the nursing interventions found to be particularly effective when anxiety was a major component of the pain problem. For example, Music Therapy positively influenced the course of treatment for patients with Crohn's disease and was also effective with adolescent trauma victims recuperating in Stryker frames. Because of the unusual and frequently awkward positioning associated with this latter treatment, these young patients were unable to watch television, read, or enjoy other diversionary activities for long periods of time. However, taped music (for this age group usually rock) could provide distraction from the pain as well as diversionary activity regardless of the position of the bed frame, and when headphones were used, the music could be enjoyed literally around the clock. Other examples of effective nursing interventions using Music Therapy are presented in the form of case studies.

CASE STUDIES

Case Study 1

L.R., a 42 year old black male, had suffered a massive abdominal wound from being shot at close range. The front and back dressings on L.R.'s wound had to be changed and irrigated every 4 hours, and this event was a painful ordeal for both the patient and the nurse. L.R. was irritable and restless in anticipation of the dressing change which he dreaded. He was abusive to the staff throughout the experience and sullen and withdrawn at other times. His only other interaction with the nurses consisted of frequent and excessive demands for pain medications following the dressing changes. One of the authors (K.B.) was contacted by the nursing staff in an effort to help them deal with this "problem pain patient," and music therapy was tested as an intervention. An initial interview with L.R. determined that his favorite type of music was rhythm and blues, and cassette tapes of this genre were recorded for his use. Approximately 30 minutes prior to each dressing change L.R. began listening to the music on headphones attached to a bedside cassette player. He listened throughout the course of the dressing change (another 30 to 45 minutes) and for a short time afterward. Subjectively, L.R. reported being better able to cope with the experience of the dressing changes, feeling more relaxed and painfree because he could concentrate on the music rather than on the activity of the nurses. Objectively, a significant decrease was noted in amount of prn pain medications L.R. requested and significant increases were documented in terms of L.R.'s hours of sleep per day, amount of food consumed, and positive interactions with the nursing staff. It is of further interest that L.R. requested his family to provide him with additional tapes to enable him to successfully cope with the painful and anxiety-laden experience of the dressing changes.

Case Study 2

P.M. was a 19 year old man who had undergone resection of a poorly differentiated diffuse lymphocytic lymphoma. Palliative abdominal irradiation and chemotherapy were used with varying effects. At the time of last admission to the hospital he had severe colicky abdominal pain and back pain. His symptoms worsened, with intractable nausea, vomiting, and pain and extreme emotional distress for P.M., his family, and the nursing staff. P.M. expressed a wish to die rather than suffer more pain.

A program of music therapy had extremely good results in relieving his pain and enhancing his ability to relax. The intervention used consisted of playing taped music selections of Bach, Schubert, and Mozart. During previous admissions P.M. had insisted on listening only to an FM radio station playing rock music. P.M. was often frantic to get more medication and was afraid that he couldn't relax at all anymore. He became intolerant of his former choice of music. The classical music helped to calm him in approximately 10 minutes without extra medication and decreased musculoskeletal tension. During the last week of his life he continued to have intractable vomiting of large amounts of gastric secretion because of complete gastric outlet obstruction. Subsequently renal failure developed.

In the last days of his life P.M. repeatedly requested the taped music. Analgesics were discontinued and he was managed on music therapy only. He was quite comfortable, not anxious or tense, and able to talk with his family and many visitors.

SUMMARY

Music has a long tradition of easing human suffering. More recently, Music Therapy has been used effectively to promote both physiological and psychological integration in the treatment of many illnesses and disabilities. Nurses can use music as a diversionary or therapeutic intervention in a variety of health care settings and patient populations. In particular, Music Therapy has been associated with the nursing diagnoses of Ineffective Coping, Diversional Activity Deficits, and Impaired Physical Mobility. It is an area with great potential, and nurses need to conduct further research on the application of music therapy to individualized, holistic patient care.

The authors are grateful for the conceptual contributions of Cindy Dougherty, Vicki Hertig Walker, and Vicki Schug, graduate students at The University of Iowa College of Nursing, and to Steven Warner and Becky Latta for assistance with preparation of the chapter.

EDITORS' COMMENTS AND QUESTIONS
This chapter discusses the use of music to accomplish therapeutic aims for restoring, maintaining, and improving mental and physical health. The chapter includes a historical review of the place of music in culture. From this perspective, music has always been an important factor in the life of people. Nursing's holistic perspective can take advantage of this intervenion to accomplish a variety of goals, which the authors set forth in Table 4–2.

Questions for Discussion
1. *Is Music Therapy the primary intervention, or an adjunct intervention, for each of the suggested nursing diagnoses?*
2. *Have you used music with clients? Was it done as a purposeful intervention? What happened?*
3. *Select five clients and administer the Hartsock Music Preference Questionnaire. Is this a useful tool for structuring the intervention?*

References

Altshuler, I. A psychiatrist's experience with music as a therapeutic agent. In D. Schullian and M. Schoen (Eds.), *Music as medicine.* New York: Henry Schuman, 1948.

Bennett, J. The difference between right and left. *American Philosophical Quarterly,* 1970, *1,* 175–191.

Bexton, W. H., Heron, W., and Scott, T. H. Effects of decreased variation in the sensory environment. *Canadian Journal of Psychology,* 1954, *8,* 70–76.

Biller, J. D., Olson, P. J., and Breen, T. The effect of "happy" versus "sad" music and participation on anxiety. *Journal of Music Therapy,* 1974, *11,* 68–73.

Brickman, H. R. Psychiatric implications of functional music for education. *Music Educator's Journal,* 1950, *36,* 29–30.

Browne, H. The use of music as therapy. In E. Podolsky (Ed.), *Music therapy.* New York: Philosophical Library, 1954.

Browse, N. L. *The physiology and pathology of bedrest.* Springfield, Ill.: Charles C Thomas, 1965.

Brydon, K. A., and Nugent, W. R. Musical metaphor as a means of therapeutic communication. *Journal of Music Therapy,* 1979, *16*(3), 149–153.

Buckwalter, K. C. Use of music therapy in patients with pain (unpublished manuscript), 1976.

Capurso, A. The Capurso study. In E. Guthiel (Ed.), *Music and your emotions.* New York: Liveright Publishing Corporation, 1952.

Carapetyan, A. Music and medicine in the Renaissance and in the 17th and 18th centuries. In D. Schullian and M. Schoen (Eds.), *Music as medicine.* New York: Henry Schuman, 1948.

Dickens, G., and Sharpe, M. Music therapy in the setting of a psychotherapeutic center. *British Journal of Medical Psychology,* 1970, *43,* 83–94.

Diephouse, J. Music therapy: A valuable adjunct to psychotherapy with children. *Psychiatric Quarterly* (suppl.), 1968, *42,* 75–85.

Dietrich, J., Whedon, G., and Schorr, E. Effects of immobilization upon various metabolic and physiologic functions of normal men. *American Journal of Medicine,* 1948, *3,* 3–36.

Dimond, S. *The double brain.* Baltimore: Williams & Wilkins, 1972.

Diserens, C., and Fine, H. *A psychology of music.* Cincinnati: College of Music, 1939.

Dolan, M. S. Music therapy: An explanation. *Journal of Music Therapy,* 1973, *10,* 172–176.

Ellis, D., and Brighouse, G. Effects of music on respirations and heart rate. In E. Podolsky (Ed.), *Music therapy.* New York: Philosophical Library, 1954.

Fisher, S., and Greenberg, R. P. Selective effects upon women of exciting and calm music. *Perceptual and Motor Skills,* 1972, *34,* 987–990.

Forrest, C. Music and the psychiatric nurse. *Nursing Times,* 1972, *68,* 410–411.

Gaffney, J. M. The use of music therapy to decrease state anxiety in immobilized patients (unpublished master's thesis). Iowa City: University of Iowa, 1982.

Gaston, E. T. Dynamic music factors in mood change. *Music Educator's Journal,* 1951, *37,* 42–44.

Gaston, E. T. *Music in therapy.* New York: Macmillan Company, 1968.

Gatewood, E. L. The psychology of music in relation to anesthesia. *American Journal of Surgery*, 1921, *35*(4), 47–50.

Gillman, L., and Paperte, F. Music as a psychotherapeutic agent. *Journal of Clinical Psychopathology*, 1949, *10*, 286–303.

Gordon, M. *Nursing diagnosis: Process and application.* New York: McGraw-Hill Book Company, 1982.

Grunewald, M. A physiological aspect of experiencing music. *American Journal of Psychotherapy*, 1953, *7*, 59–67.

Gutheil, E. A. Music as adjunct to psychotherapy. *American Journal of Psychotherapy*, 1954, *8*, 94–109.

Hadsell, N. A sociological theory and approach to music therapy with adult psychiatric patients. *Journal of Music Therapy*, 1974, *11*, 113–124.

Hartsock, J. The effects of music on levels of depression in orthopedic patients on prolonged bedrest (unpublished master's thesis). Iowa City: University of Iowa, 1982.

Herman, E. P. Music therapy in depression. In E. Podolsky (Ed.), *Music therapy*. New York: Philosophical Library, 1954.

Herth, K. The therapeutic use of music. *Supervisor Nurse*, October 1978, pp. 22–23.

Hinds, P. S. Music: A milieu factor with implications for the nurse therapist. *Journal of Psychiatric Nursing*, 1980, *18*, 28–33.

Kerr, W. A. Psychological effects of music as reported by 162 defense trainers. *Psychological Record*, 1942, *5*, 205–210.

King, F., and Kimura, D. Left-ear superiority in dichotic perception in vocal nonverbal sounds. *Canadian Journal of Psychology/Review of Canadian Psychology*, 1972, *26*(2), 111–117.

Kottke, F. J. The effects of limitation of activity upon the human body. *Journal of the American Medical Association*, 1966, *196*, 117–120.

Levy, R. The immobilized patient and his psychologic well-being. *Postgraduate Medicine*, 1966, *40*, 73–77.

Lilly, J. C. Mental effects of reduction of ordinary levels of physical stimuli on intact, healthy persons. *Psychiatric Research Reports*, March 9, 1956, pp. 1–28.

Maultsby, M. Combining music therapy with rational behavior therapy. *Journal of Music Therapy*, 1977, *14*(2), 89–96.

McMahon, T. Music therapy for training and growth. *Australian Nurses Journal*, 1978, *7*(11), 5–6.

Michel, D. E. *Music Therapy*. Springfield, Ill. Charles C Thomas, 1976.

Milner, B. Interhemispheric differences in the localization of psychological processes in man. *British Medical Bulletin*, 1971, *27*(3), 272–277.

Munro, S., and Mount, B. Music therapy in palliative care. *CMA Journal*, 1978, *119*, 1029–1034.

National Association for Music Therapy, Inc. *Music therapy as a career.* Lawrence, Kansas: National Association for Music Therapy, 1977.

Nightingale, F. *Notes on nursing: What it is and what it is not.* Philadelphia: J. B. Lippincott, 1946. (Originally published 1860).

Paul, R., and Staudt, V. M. Music therapy for the mentally ill: I. A historical sketch and a brief review of the literature on the physiological effects and an analysis of the elements of music. *Journal of General Psychology*, 1958, *59*, 167–176.

Peretti, P. O. Changes in galvanic skin response as affected by musical selection, sex, and academic discipline. *The Journal of Psychology*, 1975, *89*, 183–187.

Pickerell, K., Metzger, J., Wilde, N. J., Broadkent, T. R., and Edwards, B. The use and therapeutic value of music in the hospital and operating room. In E. Podolsky (Ed.), *Music therapy*. New York: Philosophical Library, 1954.

Podolsky, E. *The doctor prescribes music.* New York: n.p., 1939.

Podolsky, E. (Ed.). *Music therapy.* New York: Philsophical Library, 1954.

Prueter, B. A., and Mezzano, J. Effects of background music upon initial counseling interaction. *Journal of Music Therapy*, 1973, *10*, 205–212.

Radin, P. Music and medicine among primitive peoples. In D. Schullian and M. Schoen (Eds.), *Music as medicine*. New York: Henry Schuman, 1948.

Ryan, R. S., and Travis, J. W. *The wellness workbook.* Berkeley: T. Speed Press, 1981.

Schullian, D., and Schoen, M. (Eds.). *Music as medicine.* New York: Henry Schuman, 1948.

Scott, T. J. The use of music to reduce hyperactivity in children. *American Journal of Orthopsychiatry*, 1970, *40*(4), 677–680.

Sears, W. W. Process in music therapy. In E. T. Gaston (Ed.), *Music in therapy*. New York: Macmillan Company, 1968, 30–44.

Simon, B., Holzberg, J., Alessi, S., and Garrity, D. The recognition and acceptance of mood in music by psychiatric patients. In E. Podolsky (Ed.), *Music therapy*. New York: Philosophical Library, 1954.

Smith, C. A., and Morris, L. W. Effects of stimulative and sedative music on cognitive and emotional components of anxiety. *Psychological Reports*, 1976, *38*, 1187–1193.

Smith, C. A., and Morris, L. W. Differential effects of stimulative and sedative music on anxiety, concentration, and performance. *Psychological Reports*, 1977, *41*, 1047–1053.

Stanton, H. E. Music and test anxiety: Further evidence for an interaction. *British Journal of Educational Psychology*, 1975, *45*, 80–82.

Stoudenmire, J. A comparison of muscle relaxation training and music in the reduction of state and trait anxiety. *Journal of Clinical Psychology*, 1975, *31*(3), 490–492.

Van de Wall, W. *Music in hospitals*. New York: Russell Sage Foundation, 1946.

Walters, L. How music produces its effects on the brain and mind. In E. Podolsky (Ed.), *Music therapy*. New York: Philosophical Library, 1954.

Zubek, J., and MacNeil, R. Effects of immobilization: Behavioral and EEG changes. In J. Zubek (Ed.), *Sensory deprivation: Fifteen years of research*. New York: Appleton-Century-Crofts, 1969a.

Zubek, J., and Wilgosh, L. Prolonged immobilization of the body: Changes in performance and in the electroencephalogram. *Science*, 1963, *140*, 306–308.

Zubek, J., Bayer, L., Milstein, S., and Shephard, J. M. Behavioral and physiological changes during prolonged immobilization plus perceptual deprivation. *Journal of Abnormal Psychology*, 1969b, *74*, 230–236.

LIFESTYLE ALTERATION

Overview: Assisting with Changes in Behavior

GLORIA M. BULECHEK
JOANNE C. McCLOSKEY

Nurses routinely work with clients who desire or need to alter their lifestyles. The aim may be a desire to promote wellness or it may be an attempt to control chronic illness. Most of us find security and comfort in our daily routines and altering health behavior means change in familiar habits. The need for change often comes coupled with the grief and stress associated with catastrophic illness or injury. Changing behavior, especially long-term patterns, is never easy for the client.

Psychologists continue the debate about what produces individual behavior change. Cognitive theorists believe that a change in behavior is preceded by an internal change in attitudes, values, or beliefs. Rosenstock's Health Belief Model is a cognitive model that focuses on decisions made by the client based upon his or her perceived susceptibility to disease or illness and the likelihood of goal attainment. On the other side of the debate, behaviorists argue that behavior is shaped externally through reinforcement. Operant conditioning research has demonstrated that it is positive reinforcement rather than negative reinforcement or punishment that is accompanied by behavioral change.

The professional practitioner is forced to conclude that the theory to explain lifestyle change is inadequate. The challenge for the nurse is to develop skills that will facilitate self-directed change in the client. Lifestyle alteration can be viewed as a three-step process: (1) goal setting; (2) goal achievement; and (3) goal maintenance. This section of the book presents thirteen interventions to assist with this process. The authors of the respective chapters draw from both cognitive and behaviorist theories to formulate treatments to assist the client with changes in behavior.

Chapter 5 presents the intervention of Self-Modification. This intervention consists of assisting the client to learn the internal and external conditions for changing personal behavior. Pender discusses how three principles of learning—operant conditioning, stimulus control, and associative learning—can assist the client to modify behavior. Pender emphasizes that in Self-Modification the individual is making voluntary changes in selected personal behaviors. This is a distinct difference from behavior modification in which the principles of operant conditioning are applied to change behavior toward goals valued by the therapist. Self-Modification can be used as a nursing intervention with illness behavior, sick role behavior, or health behavior. Pender focuses on health behavior in discussing the strategies for achieving Self-Modification. Two case studies, one on helping a man to reestablish an exercise program and another on assisting a woman to stop smoking, illustrate the application of the Self-Modification intervention.

Patient Contracting, presented in Chapter 6, is an intervention to assist the client increase desirable behavior. The contract terms are mutually agreed upon by the client and the nurse. Jensen emphasizes that the greater the client input into the contract, the more likely it is that the client will achieve the desirable behavior. It is recommended that the contract be written, dated, and signed by both the client and the nurse. A reinforcer is given the client when the contract is achieved. This intervention incorporates one of the principles of behaviorism, that behavior can be increased when it is followed by positive reinforcement. Jensen pilot tested the intervention of Patient Contracting with a small group of diabetic clients and reports the outcome in her chapter.

Counseling, presented in Chapter 7, involves a series of interactions over time in which the counselor helps the client to focus on feelings and behaviors that have interfered with usual adaptive behavior. Banks lists the numerous approaches to Counseling as falling in either of two major camps: (1) cognitive, which emphasizes factual knowledge and increased awareness of the client; and (2) affective, which focuses on exploration of the client's attitudes, emotions, and feelings. Banks herself favors an eclectic approach and her definition of counseling reflects this. A case study of a brain-injured young woman with the nursing diagnoses of Self-Care Deficit, Dependent Coping, and Ineffective Family Coping illustrates the three stages of Counseling. In the initial stage, goals are set; in the working stage, specific counseling activities (e.g., listening, questioning, clarifying, confronting) are used to achieve the goals. In the closure stage, progress is reviewed.

Banks differentiates Counseling from the related intervention of Patient Teaching by pointing out that with Counseling the responsibility for the outcome rests with the client. An attentive reader will note that in this chapter Banks includes active listening as a counseling strategy, whereas in Section IV of this book Active Listening is included as a nursing intervention. Likewise, the reader may feel some confusion as to whether Counseling is an intervention or a theory of nursing. Unfortunately, we cannot provide clarification; only research and more thoughtful analysis by nurses will resolve these issues.

The next two chapters are about two specific kinds of Counseling: Nutritional (Chapter 8) and Sexual (Chapter 9). Whereas nurses have long done Nutritional Counseling and only recently have begun Sexual Counseling, the nurse's role in both areas is controversial. In the first instance, the nurse's role has to be distinguished from the dietitian's; in the second, the nurse's role has to be distinguished from the sex therapist's.

These two chapters also have other things in common: both can be viewed as interventions that combine counseling and teaching; both emphasize the importance of assessment. (Note that the assessment of details of the problem differs from the assessment done to make the nursing diagnosis. In these chapters, the assessment is an important aspect of the *intervention*). Both chapters emphasize the treatment effect of the nurse-patient relationship; both outline how important it is for the nurse to have knowledge of the problem and available resources; and both frequently require team planning. In response to the question concerning which of the health team members should do Sexual Counseling, Kerfoot and Buckwalter give an answer that is appropriate for both Sexual and Nutritional Counseling: the person who is best prepared and has the best relationship with the patient.

Nutritional Counseling requires the nurse to be knowledgeable of nutrition and human behavior. Every nursing curriculum includes content on nutrition, and the resources available to the nurse are many. In her chapter, Busse emphasizes the complexity of the nutrition assessment, the importance of goal setting, and the provision for client control of outcomes. She, like Banks, favors an eclectic counseling approach and her chapter on nutrition demonstrates many of the counseling strategies listed by Banks. The richness of Busse's chapter lies in the multiple illustrations of what the nurse can do through Nutritional Counseling.

Sexual Counseling requires the nurse to be knowledgeable of sexuality and human behavior. Content on sexuality was not included in schools of nursing until the 1970s, so it is not surprising that little research has been done on this intervention. Kerfoot and Buckwalter differentiate Sexual Counseling, which focuses on normal sexual functioning and response, from Sexual Therapy, which focuses on specific sexual disorders. Sexual Therapy requires specialized training. The techniques of Sexual Counseling include some noted by Banks and some others. Kerfoot and Buckwalter carefully discuss listening, including significant others, noting response to body image change, use of humor, permission, query, use of groups, and early intervention.

Reminiscence Therapy, described in Chapter 10, has developed to take advantage of the aged individual's normal developmental tendency to think about and relate personally significant past experiences. The aim is to enhance wellness in the aged client who is lonely, depressed, and withdrawn. Hamilton indicates that Reminiscence Therapy can be used with the individual client or in small groups. The social sciences have studied reminiscence as a phenomenon, but have merely tried to describe it. Nursing is interested in Reminiscence Therapy as an intervention, and nursing research has focused on the outcome of the intervention. Favorable outcomes demonstrated through research include decreases in depression and in the amount of required medication and increases in socialization and self-care activities. Hamilton gives many suggestions for implementing the intervention. Topics, objects, and activities to stimulate reminiscence are presented. Related nursing diagnoses and possible outcomes of Reminiscence Therapy are discussed. The chapter concludes with a case study of an elderly couple. Hamilton suggests that Reminiscence Therapy might be appropriate for age groups other than the elderly, as relating past events tends to occur after the age of 10 years.

Nurses frequently work with clients who are involved in a transition of roles either because of developmental circumstances or because of changes in their health status. The behavioral changes required because of this role transition are very difficult for many individuals. Moorhead describes the intervention of Role Supplementation (Chapter 11) as a possible way the nurse can assist. This intervention first appeared in the nursing literature in 1975 and has had minimal testing. Moorhead describes the process and strategies for utilizing the intervention and suggests nursing diagnoses for which it would be appropriate. She emphasizes the potential wide applicability of this intervention and urges further testing.

Redman and Thomas define Patient Teaching (Chapter 12) as an intervention that uses a stimulus to help the patient develop a new thought, skill, or attitude that is permanent enough to be useful in behavior change. They state that Patient Teaching is used in situations in which a combination of cognitive, affective, and psychomotor skills are to be developed, and that the nurse's role in Patient Teaching requires counseling skills, but they distinguish between the counseling and teaching interventions. They believe the primary focus of the counseling intervention is the affective domain. Redman and Thomas dealt with a body of literature related to the intervention that was larger than for any of the other interventions in the book. This is the only intervention in which meta analysis of some of the research findings has occurred. Redman and Thomas do a superb job of synthesizing the various reports on Patient Teaching from the health care field. They present a current state-of-the-art report on Patient Teaching and give direction for future practice and research development. There are more intervention tools available for Patient Teaching than for any of the other interventions described in the book. Redman and Thomas present a method for classifying these several kinds of tools. An in-depth look at education for diabetic individuals illustrates some of their concerns about tools. Application of the Patient Teaching intervention is illustrated through the presentation of three case studies.

Values Clarification (Chapter 13) is an intervention that can assist a client in making important decisions about his or her personal lifestyle. Many clients are ambivalent about changing their behavior to deal effectively with health promotion or chronic illness. Self-understanding of the personal value system may be a first step in helping to establish realistic goals. Wilberding defines values, describes the process of valuing, and outlines the use of Values Clarification in nursing. Nurses have tested use of the intervention with clients with heart disease and adolescents in a public school. The literature relating to the field of education contains a number of intervention tools. Wilberding recommends two of these that are applicable in nursing. The chapter concludes with a case study in which Wilberding implemented Values Clarification in helping a young man with leukemia face a decision about whether to have a bone marrow transplant.

Newspapers and other publications are filled with announcements for meetings of various self-help groups. These groups form around some common theme, such as a handicapping condition or a stressful life experience. In their chapter Kinney, Mannetter, and Carpenter present a framework that can be used by the professional nurse to determine the type of Support Group (Chapter 14) most appropriate for a given client. The framework is based on social support needs, and these authors give guidance in assessing the needs of the individual client. The framework also describes the characteristics of groups that are effective in providing social support. These authors present a unique model that demonstrates how nursing diagnoses result from a social support need and how group benefits can assist in treating the diagnoses. The model should help the reader see how much of the nursing literature that is organized around needs can be utilized in deriving and treating nursing diagnoses. The recommendations for practice can assist both the nurse who is assessing a client for possible referral to an appropriate Support Group and the nurse who will be serving as a leader for a group. Matching of client and group and timing of the intervention appear to be crucial to a successful outcome. The authors present recommendations for research and conclude with a case study example of a Support Group for individuals with multiple sclerosis.

Exercise is a frequently recommended health promotion intervention. Nurses are becoming increasingly involved in helping clients initiate and monitor an Exercise Program such as that described in Chapter 15. Allan, an adult health nurse practitioner, gives concrete guidance for assessing clients' suitability to undertake an Exercise Program. She describes the eight components of an exercise prescription and provides a format for writing the exercise prescription. She stresses the importance of helping the client develop a positive attitude toward this lifestyle change before initiating any activity. She acknowledges that long-term adherence to an Exercise Program is difficult to achieve, and the time spent with motivation activities and in assisting the client with goal setting is crucial. Tables are presented that give guidance for the progression of activity in a program of walking, jogging, or swimming. Strategies for maintaining the Exercise Program are presented, including an example of how a patient contract could help with maintenance. The chapter concludes with a case study of a 40 year old man who desires to initiate a jogging program.

The purpose of Group Psychotherapy (Chapter 16) is to help the client develop abilities and strengths that can be used in interpersonal relationships both within and outside of the group. Weiland and Cummings outline a five-step intervention for which the nurse provides group members with an experience that allows them to develop new skills and abilities in understanding themselves in relating to others. This intervention is based upon the stages of group development. The authors describe two interaction tools which the nurse can utilize to help the group progress through the developmental stages. Clinical examples of each of the five stages of the intervention are given, along with illustrations of application of the two tools.

Sadler defines assertive behavior as setting goals, acting on these goals in a clear and consistent manner, and taking responsibility for the consequences of those actions. She traces the history of Assertiveness Training (Chapter 17) from the 1950s and discusses the influence of various theoretical camps. Criteria are given for selection of clients. The intervention is presented in four steps. A case study is interwoven throughout the chapter to illustrate the various techniques. Sadler maintains that the nurse can utilize Assertiveness Training to assist clients and to improve relationships with co-workers.

In conclusion, Section II presents thirteen interventions that can be used by nurses to facilitate self-directed change in their clients. The need for lifestyle alteration is great among the escalating numbers of chronically ill and those who wish to emphasize health promotion activities in order to prevent chronic illness. Nurses are key professionals in assisting with the changes in behavior that will foster healthy lifestyles in clients.

5

SELF-MODIFICATION

NOLA J. PENDER

DESCRIPTION OF INTERVENTION

Considering current understanding of the significant impact of lifestyle on health, professional nurses should be proficient in assisting clients to acquire the requisite knowledge and skills for self-modification of health behavior. Self-Modification can be defined as self-directed change that individuals undertake voluntarily to achieve personally important goals or desired outcomes (Pender, 1982, p. 207). In Self-Modification, principles of learning are applied by individuals to create the right set of internal and external conditions for changing personal behavior.

It is important to differentiate between behavior modification as a general concept and the more specific term *Self-Modification*. Historically, behavior modification, based on principles of operant conditioning from psychology, was formulated as an approach to change the behavior of others through manipulation of extrinsic rewards and punishments. Writings by LeBow (1973) and Berni and Fordyce (1977) describe behavior modification as an appropriate nursing intervention in acute and ambulatory care settings. Rottkamp (1976) found that positioning behavior of spinal cord–injured patients could be shaped by a nurse-managed behavior modification protocol. Swain and Steckel (1981) used behavior modification to influence adherence to therapeutic regimens among hypertensive clients attending an ambulatory care clinic. Traditional approaches to behavior modification place the responsibility for decisions about behavior change and the power to control behavior with a person other than the client, usually a health professional.

In contrast, Self-Modification is the application of principles of behavior modification by individuals themselves to make voluntary changes in selected aspects of their own behavior. Self-Modification enhances the self-reliance and personal freedom of clients by providing them with the tools that they need to make desired changes in lifestyle. Individuals who undertake Self-Modification are responsible to themselves, and it is they, not health professionals, who decide what behaviors they will change and what approaches they will use (Martin and Poland, 1980, p. 9).

While Self-Modification as a nursing intervention can be applied to illness behaviors, sick-role behaviors, and health behaviors, the focus of the present chapter is health behavior, both health-protecting and health-promoting actions. Given the chronic nature of prevalent illnesses and the lack of effective curative therapies, increasing attention has been given by lay persons and health professionals alike to prevention of illness and the promotion of health. Health-protecting behaviors (prevention) are activities directed toward decreasing the probability of occurrence of specific health threats, while health-promoting behaviors focus on developing the resources of clients that enhance well-being, self-actualization, and realization of human potential. "Approach" rather than "avoidance" is the underlying motivation for health-promoting behavior. Some overt actions may be both health protective and health promotive. Other health behaviors, such as immunization of a child for measles, can be more easily classified into one category or the other.

Factors that need to be considered in working with clients to facilitate Self-Modification of health behaviors include the following: client's reasons for wanting to change, present knowledge and skills of client to be used in initiating and sustaining change, perceived ratio of payoffs for present behavior in relation to anticipated payoffs for new behaviors, and the extent of support for new behaviors in the client's social and physical environment (Kanfer and Karoly, 1972). By carefully assessing clients and their level of motivation for change as well as their support network for facilitating change, the nurse can assist clients in identifying the most effective strategies for self-modification.

STRATEGIES FOR SELF-MODIFICATION

The strategies to achieve Self-Modification that will be described in this chapter include operant conditioning, stimulus control, and associative learning. The consequences of behavior are the primary focus for *operant conditioning*, which is based on the premise that a behavior followed by positive consequences is likely to be repeated, whereas a behavior followed by negative or neutral consequences will be unlikely to recur. In *stimulus control*, antecedents of behavior are the targets for intervention. By focusing on the events that precede behavior, it is possible to decrease the frequency of undesirable behavior and increase the incidence of desirable behavior. On the other hand, *associative learning* is the development of habits as a result of repeated linking of specific stimuli with a given response sequence. Associative learning results in stable patterns of behavior that are partially independent of reinforcement contingencies (Hunt, Matarazzo, Weiss, and Gentry, 1979). Each of these strategies for Self-Modification will be described and case study examples presented to illustrate their applicability to clinical practice.

Operant Conditioning

Operant conditioning is one of the most effective strategies for Self-Modification. This intervention focuses on the consequences or outcomes of behavior. It is through manipulation of these consequences that the client is able to modify personal health behavior. Operant conditioning consists of five phases: self-monitoring; developing a reward or reinforcement list; shaping behavior; fading; and evaluating outcomes.

Self-Monitoring. The primary purpose of self-monitoring is to make the client aware of the frequency with which health-damaging or health-promoting behaviors occur. A preintervention record of the incidence of the behavior of concern is essential to evaluate the effectiveness of operant conditioning.

Behavior may be coded or graphed to determine its frequency. Examples of two intervention tools, a self-observation sheet and a cumulative graph to depict frequency of behavior, are provided by Pender (1982, pp. 219 and 220). The form on which behavior is recorded must be portable so that it is readily available when the behavior occurs. A coding sheet should clearly identify the behavior to be observed; time intervals for observation, e.g., morning, afternoon, and evening; and the coding system to be used for ease of recording. Most behaviors should be observed for at least three days, other behaviors for one to two weeks. Length of observation for baseline data depends on the frequency with which the behavior occurs and the stability of the behavior. The more infrequent and variable the occurrence of the behavior across coding periods, the longer the behavior must be observed to identify consistent patterns.

One of the problems that should be recognized in self-monitoring is the potential for inaccurate recording. Particularly when behaviors are habitual, they may occur without awareness on the part of the client. For example, lighting a cigarette may occur unconsciously. How is the nurse to assist the client in obtaining an accurate baseline assessment of such behavior? One approach, suggested by Martin and Poland (1980), is to have the client save the matches used in a small container and count them later to determine how many cigarettes have been smoked. They also suggest that if the setting for smoking is to be recorded, this can be written on the shaft of the match. Thus, while smoking may begin automatically, sometime during the course of smoking the cigarette awareness of the behavior is likely to occur, and it can be recorded. Self-Monitoring is an important skill to develop because the target behavior is then less automatic and more subject to conscious control.

Developing a Reward or Reinforcement List. An essential step in Self-Modification is assisting the client to develop a list of rewards that are optimally effective for that individual. An example of a reward or reinforcement list similar to the one shown in Table 5–1 should be developed for each client. In the list, valued extrinsic and intrinsic rewards are itemized. Extrinsic rewards refer to concrete objects (such as a bottle of shaving lotion) or social experiences (taking the family to a movie) that are rewarding for the client. Intrinsic rewards are produced by the client and are therefore more immedi-

Table 5–1. REWARD AND REINFORCEMENT LIST

Extrinsic Rewards	Intrinsic Rewards
Objects	
Bottle of shaving lotion	Praise myself for appropriate behavior
Golf balls	Tell myself I am a more responsible person
Paperback book	Compliment myself for being able to control
Golf club covers	my own behavior
Tie tack	
Cufflinks	
Social Experiences	
Requiring advance planning	
Take family to a movie	
Go to a play with friends	
Take children to an amusement park	
Not requiring advance planning	
Watch a favorite television program with my wife	
Play basketball outside with my children	
Spend time reading a book of my choice	
Call a friend with whom I have not talked lately	

ately available than extrinsic rewards; examples include self-praise and self-satisfaction. The approach to operant conditioning that appears to be most effective is to begin with extrinsic rewards that are clearly visible to the client and progress to intrinsic rewards, which are less tangible but under the client's immediate control.

Objects chosen for reinforcement should be available to the client. Experiences used for rewards should be divided into those that require advance planning and those that do not. The reward or reinforcement list can be used as a basis for determining how the nurse, family members or friends can assist the client in behavior change.

Shaping Behavior. Many behaviors are too complex to be acquired all at once. Acquiring desired health behaviors gradually is likely to be more successful in the long run than attempts to make major changes abruptly. The gradual acquisition of desired behavior is called shaping (Panyan, 1980). Clients often need to be reassured that beginning slowly and gradually is prudent and appropriate. A systematic plan for behavior change should be formulated, with successive steps identified. This allows the client to experience success at each stage of behavior change. A sample plan for shaping behavior appears in Table 5–2.

A critical aspect of shaping is to reinforce successive approximations of the desired behavior. The shaping program should be flexible so that it can be adjusted as necessary, depending on the tolerance of the client and the extent to which the client is moving along the successive steps of the program. The size of each step should not be so large that successful accomplishment cannot occur. Repeated experience of failure can result in the client's becoming disillusioned and giving up on his or her own ability to make the desired alterations in lifestyle. Realistic planning for shaping behavior can help the client estimate the time frame required for developing the desired behavior.

Fading. Weaning the client from dependency on others for reinforcement is one way to accomplish fading. While the nurse may actively participate in the client's reward system early in the course of behavior change if the client prefers, the nurse should decrease participation over time. The client should be encouraged to move from dependency on the nurse or family for rewards to primary reliance on self-reinforcement, such as self-praise or complimentary

Table 5–2. SAMPLE PLAN FOR SHAPING BEHAVIOR

Day	Behavior	Check if Completed	Reward
1	Brisk walk for 15 minutes	—	Buy golf balls
2	Brisk walk for 15 minutes	—	Call Dan and visit
3	Do 2 warm-up exercises and take brisk walk for 30 minutes	—	Buy a new book
4	Do 2 warm-up exercises and take brisk walk for 30 minutes	—	Watch TV with my wife
5	Do 3 warm-up exercises and take brisk walk for 45 minutes	—	Spend time reading a favorite book
6	Do 3 warm-up exercises and take brisk walk for 45 minutes	—	Buy shaving lotion
7	Do 3 warm-up exercises and take brisk walk for 50 minutes	—	Play basketball with the children
8	Do 3 warm-up exercises and take brisk walk for 50 minutes	—	Take family to a movie
9	Do 4 warm-up exercises and take brisk walk for 1 hour		Invite friends over to visit
10	Do 4 warm-up exercises and take brisk walk for 1 hour, 15 minutes	—	Relax outside in my favorite chair for 30 minutes

thoughts. Having the client be the source of reward has the following advantages: all occurrences of the behavior can be reinforced, behavior can be reinforced immediately, and the client develops a sense of personal control over lifestyle.

Fading is also accomplished by the client's moving from continuous reinforcement to intermittent reinforcement. The primary goal is to make the behavior less "reinforcement-dependent" and more habitual in occurrence. During the stage of shaping and acquisition of desired behavior, continuous reinforcement is important. Intermittent reinforcement is desirable at the point where the goal is to stabilize the new behavior and make it resistant to extinction (discontinuation). There is evidence from empirical studies that behaviors reinforced periodically are more resistant to extinction than are behaviors reinforced consistently once the behaviors have been learned.

Evaluating Outcomes. Periodical evaluation of client behavior is important to determine if operant conditioning is working. Data collected during self-monitoring should be used as a record of past performance, with which present behavior can be contrasted. Panyan (1980) has suggested the following indices for evaluating program effectiveness: (1) rate—the number of times a behavior occurs during a given time period; and (2) duration—total amount of time spent in a behavior during a designated time interval. For example, if a client is attempting to quit smoking, rate of smoking should be less at any point during shaping than during the initial period of self-monitoring. If duration is used as the evaluation measure, time spent smoking should progressively decrease over time.

Graphing the rate or duration of behavior either daily or at intervals provides the client with a visual depiction of success in changing behavior. The graph can indicate whether operant conditioning is working. Aspects of the shaping schedule that may need to be adjusted if change in behavior is not occurring include the following: size of shaping steps, type or amount of reward, or immediacy of reward. Tailoring the shaping schedule to each client's needs will maximize the probability of successful behavior change through operant conditioning.

Stimulus Control

Stimulus control is another strategy that clients can use for Self-Modification. In stimulus control, attention is focused on the antecedents of behavior as opposed to the consequences that are the focus in operant conditioning. The client must have a clear understanding of the circumstances or situations in which specific desirable or undesirable behaviors occur if the frequency of health-promoting behavior is to be increased or health-damaging behavior decreased. Antecedents of behavior are those cues in a given circumstance or situation that appear to trigger the behavior. These configurations of cues are important aspects of the environment that must be taken into consideration when planning for stimulus control.

When assisting a client in structuring an environment to promote behavior change through stimulus control, the following aspects of the environment must be considered: physical setting in which the desirable or undesirable behavior occurs, social setting that prompts the behavior, and the intrapersonal setting, that is, what the client is thinking, feeling, or doing at the time at which the behavior occurs. The goal of the client is to modify both the external and the internal environments (thoughts, feelings) so that cues promoting positive health practices are encountered on a regular basis.

Table 5–3. CUE ANALYSIS SHEET: OVEREATING

Cues (Stimuli) that Trigger the Behavior	Setting
Presence of candy and cookies	Home
Eating out	Restaurant
Passing vending machines	Canteen at work
Preparing my favorite dessert	Home
Cleaning up the dishes after a meal	Home
Buying bread at the bakery	Bakery
Fixing my children an ice cream cone	Home
Thinking about a hot fudge sundae	Anywhere

Cues may be action specific. That is, cues that trigger daily practice of deep relaxation may not be the same cues that trigger brisk walking for a given client. Table 5–3 provides an example of a Cue Analysis Sheet for determining cues that prompt either desirable or undesirable behaviors in a particular client. The environment, family members, and friends, as well as the client, are important sources of cues that may trigger either health-damaging or health-promoting behavior.

There are two basic techniques of stimulus control: cue expansion and cue restriction or elimination. Cue expansion is a technique in which the client is assisted to increase the number of cues that prompt a desired behavior. For instance, a client may prepare nutritious foods when eating at home but consume "junk food" when eating at the office where vending machines with foods high in carbohydrates are present. Expanding cues that elicit healthy eating behaviors to the office may be the client's goal. This can be accomplished by requesting more nutritious choices in vending machines or by bringing nutritious snack foods from home. Eating snacks and meals in an area away from vending machines may also expand the situations in which appropriate eating behaviors occur. By increasing the number of settings (range of cues) that elicit health-promoting behaviors, clients will find that they can engage in such behaviors with greater frequency and regularity.

Cue restriction or elimination decreases the frequency of cues that elicit undesirable behaviors. When such cues cannot be eliminated totally they often can be reduced considerably in frequency. For instance, cues for smoking may be reduced to one area of the house, with smoking not being permitted in any other location. A setting can also be selected that is incompatible with the behavior that the client wishes to eliminate. As an example, an individual who is attempting to quit smoking can ask for a seat assignment on an airplane in the "No Smoking" area or routinely sit in the "No Smoking" section of a restaurant. Making telephone calls at a location away from the desk where the client generally lights up a cigarette can also eliminate cues for smoking behavior. Through cue restriction, an action is elicited by fewer and fewer cues. By localizing the cues that prompt an undesirable behavior, the client can control the extent to which such cues are encountered. If total elimination of cues for the behavior is achieved, the behavior should be extinguished. However, in most cases cue restriction rather than total elimination is the more realistic goal.

Associative Learning

Developing positive health habits that are an integral part of lifestyle is the goal of any client who seriously undertakes Self-Modification in the area of health promotion. The client who practices health-promoting behaviors erratically does not achieve the long-term benefits that are possible through regular and sustained practice. Associative learning has been proposed as one approach in maintaining consistency in health-promoting behaviors and avoiding recidivism or backsliding into less desirable or even health-damaging behaviors.

Associative learning has occurred when behaviors become automatic and are maintained on an immediate stimulus-response level. Many activities of daily living that individuals engage in with little conscious thought are automatic or habitual behaviors, e.g., brushing teeth, showering, dressing. These habits are formed through associative learning, that is, the repeated pairing of a given stimulus with a given set of responses. Getting out of bed in the morning and walking into the bathroom may repeatedly prompt starting to shower and brushing teeth. Habituation of behavior through associative learning results in stable patterns of behavior that are partially independent of reinforcement contingencies. When a behavior is stabilized to the point that it no longer needs reinforcement or requires only intermittent reinforcement, a habit has been developed.

The nurse can assist clients in associative learning by helping them plan for certain health-promoting activities to occur repeatedly in the same situation or context. For example, if the client has a consistent work schedule, the best way to promote a regular exercise program may be to refer the client to a physical fitness activity where exercise sessions are held at the same time daily. This may be a fitness center where he or she works or a local "Y" program. Getting into the routine of exercising on a regular schedule during lunch hour or immediately after work can result in habituation of that behavior.

A basic assumption undergirding associative learning is that a client's behavior comes to be governed by a relatively broad strategy of health promotion that, once adopted, then dictates complex response sequences—in this example, regular exercise—as opposed to behavior being under the control of the anticipated consequences of specific actions. When associative learning has occcurred, behaviors become partially independent of their immediate reinforcements or rewards. A sequence of responses is initiated automatically in response to a given stimulus when the stimulus and response have been paired repeatedly.

For example, once a client arrives at the fitness center, the stimuli of exercise equipment, the running track, other people jogging, and locker rooms will prompt the client to get into appropriate attire, warm up, and start to exercise. After a period of time, if associative learning has occurred, exercising at noon or immediately after work becomes a habit just like brushing teeth or showering. Habitual health-promoting behaviors can improve the quality of life for the client and can even increase life span.

In summary, three approaches to Self-Modification have been discussed: operant conditioning, stimulus control, and associative learning. These strategies can be used singly or in combination by the client under the guidance of the nurse to achieve Self-Modification and a healthier lifestyle. The nurse can provide clients with an overview of each strategy but should allow clients to decide not only what behaviors they will change but what specific strategy or strategies appear most useful to them. The final decisions in structuring a Self-Modification program rest with the client.

NURSING DIAGNOSES AND SELF-MODIFICATION

Self-Modification of health behavior is an appropriate intervention to prescribe for any of the following diagnoses:

○ Health Maintenance Alteration
○ Alterations in Nutrition (Less than Body Requirements)
○ Alterations in Nutrition (More than Body Requirements)

A diagnosis of Health Maintenance Alteration can be defined as inability to manage or sustain health promotion activities as an integral part of lifestyle. This diagnosis identifies the client's need for assistance in adopting positive health practices or a need to reacquire health habits previously practiced but no longer a part of one's behavior repertoire. Areas of behavior that might be the focus for Self-Modification following diagnosis of a Health Maintenance Alteration include stress management; physical fitness; building social support systems; or eliminating addictive behaviors, such as smoking, drinking alcoholic beverages, or drug use.

Alterations in Nutrition can occur from consuming either fewer or more calories than required to maintain weight. In adults in the U.S.A., excess caloric intake relative to metabolic needs is a common problem. Brailey (1982) indicates that many weight reduction programs fail because of too much emphasis on amount of food consumed and number of pounds to be lost. Use of Self-Modification as a nursing intervention to promote weight loss focuses the client's attention instead on behavioral aspects of eating, such as rewards for eating, circumstances surrounding eating, and psychological and environmental cues that trigger eating. Clients assume responsibility for Self-Modification of eating behavior and work toward developing permanent improvements in eating habits.

Self-Modification as an intervention is applicable to a wide age range of client groups. However, children and adolescents need special consideration in structuring Self-Modification programs, as they generally are much more susceptible to counter forces that work against behavior change, such as peer pressure and desire for freedom from structure in patterns of everyday living, than are adults. This does not mean that problems of social pressure from significant others should not receive thoughtful attention for adults undertaking Self-Modification. However, adults are often more autonomous and self-reliant than children or adolescents, who have not securely established their own identity. Evidence from a number of studies indicates that peer pressure can be used productively to facilitate change by incorporating peer support as a dominant feature of the Self-Modification program.

CASE STUDIES

Case study examples illustrate the use of Self-Modification as a nursing intervention. Two clients with differing manifestations of the nursing diagnosis Health Maintenance Alteration will be described. One case focuses on reactivation of a physical fitness program for a client, the other on helping a client stop smoking.

Case Study 1

Mr. H., 28 years old, had been a jogger during his college years but owing to the pressures of work in an accounting firm in which he is a junior partner, he had become very sedentary for the past five years. Realizing the lack of activity that he experienced on the job and the absence of recreational sports in his daily schedule, he contacted the Nursing Center, a service provided to the community by nursing faculty and graduate students at a local university, to make an appointment for professional guidance in structuring an individualized physical fitness program that would meet his personal needs.

At his first appointment, the nurse clinician explored with Mr. H. his interest in health and his level of motivation to exercise regularly. She conducted a physical fitness evaluation and made arrangements for stress testing to determine his cardiovascular status. At the next appointment, the nurse discussed with Mr. H. the possibility of using a Self-Modification program to increase level of physical activity and make exercise an integral part of his lifestyle. The basic components of the program were explained to Mr. H., and he decided that such a tailored program might be most beneficial. He was encouraged to keep baseline data (self-monitoring) on his level of physical activity for the next two weeks and was given a coding card to carry with him at all times to permit immediate recording of any physical activity in which he engaged.

The coding card was divided into three time periods during the day (morning, afternoon, and evening). In addition, a coding format was developed for him based on his usual reported physical activities, including the following codes: S = climbing stairs, W = walking (one block or more), M = mowing the lawn, B = bicycling. The nurse told Mr. H. that he could add other activities to the coding list as the need arose during the week. She explained the importance of carefully assessing current level of physical activity before planning a program of Self-Modification.

On his next visit to the Nursing Center, the nurse reviewed with Mr. H. his pattern of physical activity from his self-observation sheet. In addition, she assisted him in developing a reward or reinforcement list. She also continued the collection of other assessment data that would give Mr. H. a more comprehensive view of his health status. Additional areas of assessment were physical examination, health history, major risk factors, current dietary patterns, lifestyle and health habits, stress status, and perceived control of health. The nurse also assessed and reinforced Mr. H.'s self-care strengths. Together they formulated a health protection and promotion plan that identified personal health goals and areas for improvement in self-care, including specific behavioral changes to be accomplished.

A plan for shaping jogging behavior was developed in progressive steps that the client considered attainable. The plan was based on consideration of the current level of physical fitness of Mr. H. determined during the assessment phase. Both the nurse and client were aware that experiencing success at each step of progressive behavior change was critical to Mr. H.'s continuing involvement in the program. Mr. H. began brisk walking for four laps (½ mile) on two days of the week in the field house of a nearby university that had a running and walking track. He was also taught specific warm-up exercises to do prior to walking. His activity program was gradually increased from brisk walking to walk-jog with the eventual goal of jogging two miles three to four times per week. An exercise physiologist who collaborated with nurses at the Nursing Center monitored Mr. H.'s activities at the field house, helping him keep a log of his progress.

As Mr. H. advanced in his fitness program, he used the reward or reinforcement list to plan for both extrinsic and intrinsic reinforcement. Although he did contract with the nurse for rewards during the first four weeks of the program, Mr. H. then assumed responsibility for his own reward plan, obtaining assistance from family members as needed to carry out his reinforcement system. Because the nurse knew that associative learning in addition to operant conditioning could increase the strength of jogging behavior, thus making it more resistant to extinction, she encouraged Mr. H. to continue his jogging in the same setting. As Mr. H. progressed in his Self-Modification program, he began fading the rewards by the following means: delaying them, rewarding himself only intermittently, and relying primarily on intrinsic rewards, such as self-praise and increased feelings of self-control and self-esteem.

Although it was concern over physical fitness that brought Mr. H. to the Nursing Center, he also became aware of other areas of lifestyle that needed to be altered to increase his level of health and prevent future illness. He began attending relaxation classes and enrolled in a discussion group on nutrition and health. The nurse continued to follow the progress of Mr. H., seeing him for lifestyle monitoring at regular intervals after the period of intensive work on self-modification. In addition, Mr. H.'s wife became a client at the Nursing Center in order to obtain professional assistance in changing her lifestyle. This provided peer support for Mr. H. in achieving and maintaining his health care goals.

Case Study 2

Another client, Ms. M., came to the Nursing Center and was also diagnosed as having a problem of health maintenance alteration. She needed assistance to stop smoking.

Realizing the addictive nature of such behavior, the nurse carefully explored with Ms. M. the importance of health as a personal value and her perceived control over her own health behavior. The nurse explained the importance of completing a comprehensive health assessment during the first two to three clinic visits in order to develop a health protection and promotion plan. The nurse described the nature of Self-Modification to Ms. M., who was intrigued with the intervention and willing to try it. Ms. H. indicated that she had tried several "quit smoking" programs that required immediate cessation of all smoking, and they had not worked for her; therefore, she wanted to try a more gradual approach with the hope of being successful. While Self-Modification was the intervention employed, two different strategies were used in working with Ms. M: operant conditioning (managing rewards and reinforcements) and stimulus control (cue restriction or elimination).

Realizing the dependence of smoking patterns on both time and place cues, Ms. M. was instructed in how to keep a self-observation sheet. On her coding sheet, which she carried with her at all times, she recorded the frequency of smoking in terms of time of day and setting in which it occurred. The nurse discussed with Ms. M. the development of a plan for cue restriction, because smoking had become an automatic behavior (habit) for her. She reported often lighting up before she realized it, and then, even though aware of her behavior, finishing the cigarette. Since Ms. M. worked in the inner city some distance from where she lived, she rode rapid transit transportation and ate lunch in the cafeteria of the corporation for which she worked.

Beginning approaches to cue restriction involved encouraging Ms. M. to sit in the section of the train marked "No Smoking" and to eat lunch in the "No Smoking" section of the cafeteria. This restricted the cues for smoking to which Ms. M. was exposed. She decided to continue to smoke at her desk at this time because this behavior would be the hardest to give up. At the end of three weeks, smoking behavior had decreased according to self-observation reports. Ms. M. contracted with the nurse for rewards following abstinence from smoking during each week of the first five weeks of her Self-Modification program. Rewards contracted for included a book on exercise, one-half hour of the nurse's time to talk about anything Ms. M. wished, and the opportunity to borrow a set of tapes on relaxation from the Nursing Center.

Ms. M. continued with her Self-Modification program by removing ashtrays from her kitchen table, avoiding smoking following her evening meal, and eventually omitting a cigarette during and after breakfast. Because of a relapse that occurred during the seventh week of the program, it appeared that more time was needed before cue restriction could progress further. Ms. M. stabilized her Self-Modification program for a week to ensure continuing success. An important step in her personal program to stop smoking was leaving cigarettes at home so that she no longer smoked at work. She removed the ashtrays from her desk, did not carry cigarettes or a lighter, and let her secretary know that she was not to be offered a cigarette. In addition, she asked her secretary to inform clients and others wishing to see her that they were to refrain from smoking during appointments with her.

Because addictive behavior is not well understood and is highly resistant to change, still other behavioral strategies were employed. Sipping herbal teas that did not contain caffeine was used as a replacement behavior for smoking. Ms. M. kept a variety of flavors of tea in her desk drawer at work. In addition, she was instructed in how to use "thought stopping." When she would think how good a cigarette would taste she would immediately say "Stop!" either out loud or to herself and focus her thoughts on the pleasant aromas of tea or another pleasing thought or sensation. These additional strategies enhanced the success of her smoking cessation program.

Self-Modification appeared to result in successful cessation of smoking after 13 weeks. The need for both short-term and long-term follow-up was discussed with Ms. M. She agreed that this was essential, given the addictive nature of the behavior that she was attempting to eliminate. The nurse explained to Mrs. M. that the more frequently she refrained from smoking in the presence of cues to smoke, the stronger the habit not to smoke in those situations would become as a result of associative learning.

Ms. M. was encouraged to consider other areas of self-change that would enhance personal health. The importance of developing a lifestyle that would promote higher levels of health and well-being and give Ms. M. increased personal control over health behaviors was discussed. The nurse continued to see Ms. M. monthly over the next 12 month period. Ms. M. then progressed to bimonthly and quarterly visits for lifestyle reassessment and monitoring.

DIRECTIONS FOR PRACTICE AND RESEARCH

Evidence indicates that personal behavior and lifestyle may account for 50 per cent or more of the factors that affect health and illness experience. The fact that health behaviors are not innate but learned indicates the as yet untapped potential of clients to unlearn health-damaging behaviors and adopt health-promoting lifestyles. Nurses, as key professionals in the delivery of health care, need to be skilled in assisting clients to make desired changes in those behaviors that impact on health. Self-Modification is a highly useful nursing intervention applicable to a number of different nursing diagnoses. Although the emphasis in this chapter has been on use of Self-Modification for illness prevention and health promotion, Self-Modification can also be used to alter illness and sick-role behavior.

The realities of the cost of health care, the limited impact of current health care technology on chronic health problems, and increased emphasis within society on the quality of life have resulted in renewed emphasis on personal responsibility for health. This does not negate the complementary responsibility of society for dealing with health issues of broader scope that impact on the quality of the environment in which people live. However, emphasis on self-responsibility in the area of health does mandate concerted efforts on the part of health scientists to investigate empirically the phenomenon of health and the nature of behaviors that are health-damaging or health-promoting.

The present state of knowledge about Self-Modification suggests the need for research in the following areas: factors affecting the initial acquisition of health behaviors; relationship of selected client characteristics, such as self-esteem, perceived control, and desire for competence to continue practice of health-promoting behaviors after initial acquisition; and health behavior patterns of groups with differing ethnic or racial and demographic backgrounds. In addition, strategies for Self-Modification must be tested clinically to determine their usefulness in changing various health behaviors. Further research is also needed to determine the potential of Self-Modification for ultimately changing the health behaviors not only of individuals but also of families and larger social groups.

EDITORS' COMMENTS AND QUESTIONS

Pender bases the intervention of Self-Modification on principles of learning that have been well developed and tested in educational psychology. This chapter illustrates how these principles can be applied in nursing situations. Assisting the client to learn the internal and external conditions for changing personal behavior is well illustrated in the two case studies.

Questions for Discussion

1. *What is the distinction between Behavior Modification and Self-Modification?*

2. *Pender describes the strategies for achieving Self-Modification with health behaviors. How can these strategies be utilized with illness behaviors and sick role behaviors?*

3. *How does this intervention facilitate self-responsibility for health?*

4. *Can Self-Modification be used with groups?*

References

Berni, R., and Fordyce, W. E. *Behavior modification and the nursing process.* St. Louis: C. V. Mosby Company, 1977.

Bircher, A. U. On the development and classification of nursing diagnoses. *Nursing Forum, 1975,* 14, 10–29.

Brailey, J. It takes more than will power: The use of behavioral self-control in weight reduction. *Occupational Health Nursing,* 1982, 30, 17–20.

Hunt, W. A., Matarazzo, J. D., Weiss, S. M., and Gentry, W. D. Associative learning, habit and health behavior. *Journal of Behavioral Medicine,* 1979, 2, 111–124.

Kanfer, F. H., and Karoly, P. Self-control: A behavioristic excursion into the lion's den. *Behavior Therapy,* 1972, 3, 398–416.

LeBow, M. D. *Behavior modification: A significant method in nursing practice.* Englewood Cliffs, N.J.: Prentice-Hall, 1973.

Martin, R. A., and Poland, E. Y. *Learning to change: A self-management approach to adjustment.* New York: McGraw-Hill Book Company, 1980.

Panyan, M. *How to use shaping.* Lawrence, Kan.: H. & H. Enterprises, 1980.

Pender, N. J. *Health promotion in nursing practice.* Norwalk, Conn.: Appleton-Century-Crofts, 1982.

Rottkamp, B. C. A behavior modification approach to nursing therapeutics in body positioning of spinal cord-injured patients. *Nursing Research,* 1976, 25, 181–186.

Swain, M. A., and Steckel, S. B. Influencing adherence among hypertensives. *Research in Nursing and Health,* 1981, 4, 213–222.

6

PATIENT CONTRACTING

DEBORAH PERRY JENSEN

DESCRIPTION OF INTERVENTION

Contracting is a fairly recent intervention concept in the health care field, first appearing in the health literature in the early 1970s and in the nursing literature in the late 1970s. Contracting has been used successfully for control of drug and alcohol abuse, for control of pain, and for increasing compliance among hypertensive subjects. Establishing a patient contract is a systematic method of increasing desirable patient behavior (Steckel, 1980). Other definitions of Contracting in health care include the following:

1. An agreement between two or more people in which a promise or commitment from one is given in exchange for something from the other (Vanicelli, 1979).

2. The systematic arrangement for granting a reinforcement in return for performance of a specific behavior (Steckel and Swain, 1977).

3. An agreement between health professional and patient; this is not a legal agreement and some prefer to call it setting goals or self-care activities (Herje, 1980).

4. A binding agreement between two or more persons (Hayes and Davis, 1980).

5. Two parties, one who desires to change behavior and another who will assist in the process, come to terms regarding the desired or targeted new behavior and the reinforcement in exchange for performance of that behavior (Swain and Steckel, 1981).

First and foremost, it is essential that the contract terms are mutually agreed upon by the patient and nurse (Blair, 1971; Langford, 1978; Herje, 1980; Steckel, 1980; Steckel and Swain, 1977). Vanicelli (1979) conducted a study that shows the importance of patient input when establishing a contract. In this study one hundred alcoholics were randomly assigned to one of four contract conditions.

No Contract. The patients were told by the coordinator (either a psychiatric nurse or mental health worker) to think about their problems and appropriate steps for resolving them.

Staff-Authored. The patients were asked to read the written guidelines about the contract format and then talk with their coordinator so that the coordinator could write the contract.

Mutually Authored. The patients were instructed to write the contract together with the coordinator.

Patient-Authored. The patients were instructed to write the contract and return it for the coordinator to sign.

In general the findings revealed that the greater the patient input in establishing the contract, the more likely the patient was to return to the clinic for aftercare, to remain in the same job, and maintain abstinence from drinking alcohol.

Guidelines for establishing a patient contract vary from general instructions to detailed specifications. Herje (1980) listed seven characteristics of a good patient contract:

1. Realistic (Does the goal seem possible?).
2. Measurable (How often can you do this? What will you do in the next week?).
3. Positive (What goals are you working toward? What strengths can you build on?).
4. Time-dated (When can you start this? What will you do in the next week?).
5. Written (Could I [or would you] write down these goals we are discussing?).
6. Rewardable (If you achieve this goal, what reward could you give yourself?).
7. Capable of being evaluated (How can I help you evaluate your goals?).

Steckel (1980) specifically stated that a contract must include: (a) the specific desired patient behavior, (b) the reinforcer (reward), (c) a written document, (d) the date, (e) the signature of both patient and nurse, and (f) a carbon copy (one for the patient and the other to remain in his or her chart or care plan).

Some authors have cited patient reinforcers as an important part of patient contracts (Herje, 1980; Steckel, 1980), whereas others have not.

REVIEW OF RESEARCH

Contracts have been used effectively in various health care situations. Boudin (1972) reported a case study that involved successful contracting to decelerate amphetamine use. A detailed contract was drawn up by the therapist and patient with the following terms:

1. Each knew the other's whereabouts at all times and the contract included check-in times for the patient.
2. The patient agreed to give up all drugs accessible to her.
3. The patient's money was deposited in a joint bank account. Any drug use or suspected drug use resulted in the loss of $50 to a specified organization the patient was opposed to supporting.

During a three-month period, there was only remission, and a two-year follow-up revealed no return to amphetamine use.

Another study by Bigelow and associates (1976) involved 20 male volunteers with histories of alcohol abuse. Written and signed contract terms included the patient's ingesting disulfiram daily under nurses' observation for the first 14 treatment days, then on alternate days. Patients were also required to place a monetary security deposit with the clinic as a guarantee of their participation. Any failure to report to the clinic and ingest the disulfiram would result in loss of part of the deposit. Of the 20 subjects, 80 per cent maintained abstinence for a longer time while enrolled in the contracting program than at any other time in the previous three years.

Simons and associates (1979) reported successful use of pain medication contracts at a burn treatment center in San Diego. The contract was established by the patient, the physician, and the head nurse. It included the total number of analgesic doses the patient was allowed in 24 hours and the maximum number of dosages that could be taken in any one hour. No doses could be saved for the following day and, in turn, the nurse complied with the patient's medication request. In another report, Swain and Steckel (1981) investigated 115 hypertensive outpatients who were randomly selected and randomly assigned to one of three groups; routine clinic care, routine care plus an educational component with Counseling, or routine care plus education and Contracting. The contract used in this study was written, dated, and signed by both the patient and clinic nurse. The patients in this group contracted to attain a specific score on a written hypertension test and to keep their clinic appointments as scheduled. The contract group was found to have a significantly higher level of knowledge about their hypertension (in terms of test scores) and a significantly higher return visit rate (i.e., keeping their follow-up appointments) than the other two groups.

Zangari and Duffy (1980) reported successful use of Contracting with a 64 year old woman with cancer of the spine. The patient initially required narcotic injections for pain every three hours and bedrest. A written contract was established by the patient and nurse to increase the patient's ambulation and amount of self-care. Through Contracting, the patient accomplished her long-range goal "to go home for Christmas in command of daily care."

STEPS OF THE INTERVENTION

How the nurse goes about establishing a patient contract is outlined by Hayes and Davis (1980) and can be divided into five steps:

Problem Identification and Priority Ranking. The client and clinician explore their individual perceptions about the client's health and develop a problem list.

Contract Development. This includes a description of the responsibilities and expected activities of the client and clinician.

Contract Implementation. The client and clinician focus on those tasks which each has accepted as a responsibility.

Contract Evaluation. Fulfillment of the contract is based on the achievement of the goals developed. Periodic renegotiation of the contract terms may be necessary.

Contract Termination. A target date for realization of the contract terms is important.

In 1982, Steckel wrote *Patient Contracting*, a comprehensive textbook that focused on the development of contracts within the nursing process. To utilize written contracts effectively, Steckel asserts that nursing must focus practice and education on its unique contribution to health care rather than being limited by the disease model. Steckel holds that the process of Contracting applies the principle of positive reinforcement: The performance of a behavior can be increased when it is followed by a favorable consequence. Steckel reported her own successful use of contracts to increase compliance among dialysis clients through diet adherence, and among hypertensive outpatients through appointment keeping, lowering blood pressure, and weight loss. Case studies were cited in each chapter to illustrate how Contracting is carried out step by step.

SELECTION OF CLIENTS

Possible nursing diagnoses for which Contracting may be appropriate are Noncompliance, Knowledge Deficit, Ineffective Coping, Alteration in Parenting, and Self-Care Deficit. Noncompliance, in particular, is a widespread problem and has been documented to involve an average of one third of the patients who are instructed to carry out a medical regimen (Davis, 1968).

Patients with severe organic brain syndrome (acute or chronic) and acute or chronic psychotic reactions are not considered likely candidates for Contracting because of an inability to understand or remember the contract. Very young children and the severely retarded are also poor candidates (Simons et al., 1979; Hayes and Davis, 1980). Herje (1980) suggested that because of denial, confusion, or grief, the patient may be unable to participate. Etzwiler (1974) described the patient who is uncooperative and recommended trying to negotiate and offering viable alternatives. The point, Etzwiler asserted, is to start somewhere to get patients involved in their own care; after building rapport, patients are often more willing to add to their responsibilities.

Case Study

The author utilized Patient Contracting with a group of adult diabetics to study the relationship between contracting and compliance. More specifically, the following question was addressed: Does the establishment of a contract between the adult diabetic patient and nurse increase the patient's compliance with a diabetic treatment program? For purposes of this pilot project, the following definitions were used:

Contract. A written, signed (by patient and nurse), and dated agreement between the patient and nurse. The contract includes the expectations for the patient, the reinforcement to be given if the expectation(s) are met, and the target date for those expectations to be achieved.

Adult Diabetic Patient. An inpatient 18 years of age or older.

Compliance. An increased score of at least one point from the pre- to post-knowledge test. Additionally, an affirmative response by the patient (just prior to taking the post-test) that he or she had read and studied the booklets as agreed upon in the contract.

Eight patients, four women and four men, completed the project. Seven of the patients were insulin-dependent diabetics and the eighth patient was taking an oral hypoglycemic agent. Four of the patients were newly diagnosed diabetics. The remainder of the patients had been diagnosed as having diabetes anywhere from one to thirty years ago. The patients ranged in age from 24 to 73 years with a mean age of 50.4 years. Mean educational level was 12.9 years ranging from 9 to 15 years. Six of the patients were married, one was widowed, and one was single.

This project took place at a large university hospital. The pre-test, Contracting, and post-test took place at the patient's bedside. Each patient was approached and informed about the knowledge test and contracting procedure. Demographic data were obtained from the patient and medical chart concerning the patient's age, sex, educational background, medical diagnosis, and date of diagnosis. The patient completed a pre-test to measure knowledge of diabetes. Knowledge was assumed to be a necessary condition for patient compliance. Patients who do not have an understanding of diabetes and its management cannot be expected to follow a prescribed program correctly (Swain and Steckel, 1981). The 22 question multiple-choice test was adapted from a test developed by Teske (1971). The test contained questions about the disease process and its management, insulin administration, exercise, hygiene, and foot care. Three judges (staff physician, nurse clinician, and registered nurse who worked in the diabetic clinic) agreed that the test was a valid indicator of the patient's knowledge of diabetes. Reliability was established by split-half examination, and a .91 Spearman-Brown score was obtained by Teske. The pre-test was scored, and the score was shared with the patient. A contract was then established between the patient and nurse whereby the patient would read and study four diabetes booklets; the contract also specified a target post-test score and date on which to take the post-test and identified the reinforcer for attaining that score. Table 6–1 shows a sample contract. Before administering the post-test, each patient was asked, "Did you read and study the booklets as we agreed?" This question was used to compare the response with the patient's pre- and post-test scores, realizing such self-reported information is susceptible to the patient's distortion in a desire to please the nurse or be viewed favorably (McSweeney, 1981). On the target date, the reinforcer was given, if earned. The nurse then clarified any questions answered incorrectly on the test and offered to answer any other questions.

Five of the patients' post-test results were in the predicted direction, with an increase from their pre-test to post-test scores. One patient's score remained unchanged, and one patient's score decreased. Three of the five patients with increased scores reached their targeted score and received the agreed-upon reinforcer. Six patients responded "yes" to the self-report question, and the one patient who answered "no" was the patient whose score decreased on post-testing. These results, presented in Table 6–2, suggest that the increased compliance may have been due to the Contracting.

Several recommendations can be made as a result of this project. Patients often had difficulty identifying a desired reinforcer when asked what they wanted in return for meeting the written expectations. Therefore, a written list of possible reinforcers could have been helpful for the patients. The

Table 6–1. SAMPLE CONTRACT

I, _____, will

1) Read and study the following booklets about diabetes given to me:
   a. "You and Diabetes"
   b. "Urine Testing"
   c. "How To Take Insulin"
   d. "Site Selection and Rotation"

2) On _____, I will take a written test and earn a score of _____ or more out of a possible _____.

In return for:

Signatures _____

_____

Date _____

Table 6–2. TEST RESULTS AND SELF-REPORT RESPONSES OF INSULIN-DEPENDENT DIABETICS

Patient	Pre-test Scores (x)	Post-test Scores (y)	Difference Scores (y-x)	Self-Report
1	18	20	+2	yes
2	18	21	+3	yes
3	12	18	+6	yes
4	19	18	−1	no
5	20	20	0	yes
6	19	21	+2	yes
7	21	22	+1	yes

reinforcers requested by patients were reasonable and easily obtainable; examples were a pad of writing paper, one dollar, a pocket notebook, and a bar of soap.

For future research, a larger sample size is desirable with the use of a control group and randomized assignment. Another recommendation for further investigation would be the use of an alternate form of post-test with a longer time interval—perhaps two to four weeks—between tests.

For purposes of this project, the contract used was basically a nurse-authored contract. The nurse established that the contract would include a pre-test, reading and studying four diabetes booklets, and a post-test to be carried out by the patient. What was left open to negotiation was the time interval between the tests, the target score, the target date, and the reinforcer. The nurse encountered no reluctance by any of the patients to sign the contract. Contract negotiation time ranged from 4 to 10 minutes (mean time, 6.25 minutes). Hence, the use of contracts may well prove to be an economical use of the nurse's time.

RECOMMENDATIONS

Given the importance of the patient's active involvement and compliance with the plan of treatment, Contracting as a nursing intervention should be further studied. This will necessitate the collaboration of the nurse researcher and the nurse involved in direct patient care. Lewis and Michnich (1977) concluded that contracts could be of great value to health care, but the authors went on to say that there have been no well-designed experimental studies to assess the impact of the intervention. Written and verbal contracts could be compared and their effectiveness evaluated. In addition, specific populations for which Contracting would be useful is another area for nursing research.

SUMMARY

The concept of Contracting as a nursing intervention has received increasing attention in the literature. Contracting is a written and signed agreement between a patient and a nurse whereby the patient agrees to do something by a specific time in return for a reinforcer provided by the nurse. To date, Steckel and Swain have conducted the bulk of nursing research regarding Contracting, studying the nursing diagnoses of Noncompliance and Knowledge Deficit among adult hypertensive patients. The author's personal experience with Contracting with diabetic patients was reported and suggestions for future nursing research were proposed. The impact of Contracting on health care could be considerable. Contracting holds promise as a step in the right direction toward enhancing patient compliance and knowledge.

EDITORS' COMMENTS AND QUESTIONS

This chapter reviews the process of Contracting to assist the client to increase desirable behavior. The bulk of the work on this nursing intervention has been done by Steckel and associates. The essential components of the intervention appear to be (1) client input into goal setting, and (2) provision of positive reinforcement when the goal is achieved.

Questions for Discussion

1. *Have you used Contracting with a client? How effective was it?*
2. *Name several reinforcers that would be appropriate for a nurse to provide.*
3. *What are the pros and cons of using verbal contracts? Written contracts?*
4. *Have you ever used Contracting for self-learning?*

References

Bigelow, G., Strickler, D., Liebson, I., and Griffiths, R. Maintaining disulfiram ingestion among outpatient alcoholics: A security-deposit contingency contracting procedure. *Behavior Research and Therapy*, 1976, *14*(4), 378–380.

Blair, K. It's the patient's problem—and decision. *Nursing Outlook*, 1971, *19*(9), 587–589.

Boudin, M. Contingency contracting as a therapeutic tool in the deceleration of amphetamine use. *Behavior Therapy*, 1972, *3*, 604–608.

Davis, S. Variations in patients' compliance with doctors' advice: An empirical analysis of patterns of communication. *American Journal of Public Health*, 1968, *58*(2), 274–288.

Etzwiler, D. D. The contract for health care. *Journal of the American Medical Association*, 1973, *224*(7), 1034.

Etzwiler, D. D. Why not put your patient under contract? *PRISM*, 1974, *2*(1), 26–28.

Gustafson, M. B. Let's broaden our horizon about the use of contracts. *International Nursing Review*, 1977, *24*(1), 18–19, 24.

Hayes, W. S. and Davis, L. What is a health care contract? *Health Values*, 1980, *4*(2), 82–89.

Herje, P. A. Hows and whys of patient contracting. *Nursing Educator*, January-February 1980, 30–34.

Krosnick, A. Self-management, patient compliance and the physician. *Diabetes Care*, 1980, *3*(1), 124–126.

Langford, T. Establishing a nursing contract. *Nursing Outlook*, 1978, *26*(6), 386–388.

Lewis, C. E., and Michnich, M. Contracts as a means of improving patient compliance. In Barofsky, I. (Ed.), *Medication compliance*. Thorofare, N.J.: Charles B. Slack, 1977.

McSweeney, M. Measuring the effect of patient teaching. Diabetes Educator, Fall 1981, 9–15.

Planned patient education system used in three hospital settings. *Cross-Reference*, 1977, *7*(4), 10–11.

Rosen, B. Contract therapy. *Nursing Times*, 1978, *74*, 119–121.

Schulman, B. A. and Swain, M. A. Active patient orientation. *Patient Counselling and Health Education*, 1980, *2*(1), 32–37.

Simons, R. D., Morris, J. L., Frank, H. A., Green. L. C., and Malin, R. M. Pain medication contracts for problem patients. *Psychosomatics*, 1979, *20*(2), 122–123, 127.

Steckel, S. B. Contracting with patient-selected reinforcers. *American Journal of Nursing*, 1980, *80*(9), 1596–1599.

Steckel, S. B. and Swain, M. A. Contracting with patients to improve compliance. *Hospitals*, 1977, *51*, 81–84.

Steckel, S. B. *Patient Contracting*. Norwalk: Appleton-Century-Crofts, 1982.

Swain, M. A. and Steckel, S. B. Influencing adherence among hypertensives. *Research in Nursing and Health*, 1981, *4*(1), 213–222.

Teske, A. E. Comparison of teaching methodology: The traditional tutorial method and programmed instruction. Iowa City: University of Iowa: 1971.

Vanicelli, M. Treatment contracts in an inpatient alcoholism treatment setting. *Journal of Studies on Alcohol*, 1979, *40*(5), 457–471.

Zangari, M. E., and Duffy, P. Contracting with patients in day-to-day practice. *American Journal of Nursing*, 1980, *80*(3), 451–455.

COUNSELING

Counseling, as a nursing activity, has only recently been addressed in nursing literature. This is true despite the widely accepted assumption that nursing is a helping, caring process based on a personal relationship between a nurse and a patient.

RELATED LITERATURE

Drawing heavily from various social and psychological theorists, nursing leaders have repeatedly sought to define the unique quality of the nurse-patient relationship. A landmark contribution was made by Peplau in 1952 when she described nursing as a "significant therapeutic, interpersonal process." She further suggested that the nurse may fulfill a variety of roles, such as teacher, technical expert, or counselor in order to promote patient growth and personality development in the direction of maturity. Orlando (1961), reflecting her strong background in mental health and psychiatric nursing, coined the term the "dynamic nurse-patient relationship." Orlando emphasized that the nurse-patient relationship constantly changes in response to the status of the patient's immediate unmet needs. As early as 1956 Orem introduced the concept of self-care as the focus of nursing. Later, in 1971 and again in 1980, Orem further developed her view of nursing as the provision and management of systems of self-care for individuals or multiperson units. Orem identified five general methods by which the nurse can act to promote client self-care. Two of Orem's general methods of assistance, that of guiding another and that of supporting another physically or psychologically, spoke to the art of nursing or the complementary nature of the nurse-patient relationship. King (1971) emphasized the interpersonal relationship in nursing, describing it as goal-directed activity based on a process of action, reaction, interaction, and transaction. Finally, Paterson and Zderad (1976) developed the concept of humanistic nursing. They believed that the crux of nursing was the existence of an authentic or genuine dialogue between the nurse and patient, and they viewed the goal of this dialogue as promoting and nurturing human potential through an intersubjective or interdependent transaction.

99

Recognizing that these nursing writers have adopted much of their concept of Counseling from classic psychosocial literature, it is important to understand the basic tenents of the major Counseling approaches. Although there are numerous approaches to counseling theory, all of these can be somewhat arbitrarily distinguished as having either a predominantly cognitive or predominantly affective approach. The major cognitive approaches include the trait and factor, rational-emotive, eclectic, psychotherapy by reciprocal inhibition, and behavioral viewpoints (Sherzer and Stone, 1974). The affective approaches include the psychoanalytic, client-centered, existential, and Gestalt viewpoints (Shertzer and Stone, 1974). The lists are not exhaustive of all approaches since they omit such new ideas as reality therapy and transactional analysis. Nevertheless, the division proposed by Shertzer and Stone does serve to organize the classic approaches as to the basic focus of the counseling activity. Proponents of the cognitive approach have emphasized the importance of factual knowledge and increased awareness by the client, whereas those who claim a more affective approach have focused more on the exploration of the client's attitudes, emotions, and feelings.

For the purpose of comparison, two affective approaches (client-centered and existential) and two cognitive approaches (behavioral and eclectic) are examined by identification of the antecedents and behaviors of counseling (Table 7–1). Specifically, each counseling approach is compared on its assumptions about the nature of man, the client's anxiety, the goal of the counselor, and the technique used by the counselor. A brief summary of the strengths and limitations of each approach is included below.

CLIENT-CENTERED COUNSELING

Although various authors support the client-centered approach to Counseling, Rogers is most often cited as the originator of this viewpoint. Rogers (1961) viewed the person as a basically positive, socialized, rational being moving toward self-actualization. The person's self-concept acts as a regulator of behavior. Client anxiety exists when there is incongruence between an individual's self-concept and experience (Patterson, 1969). This situation occurs when conditions of worth are violated and needs for self-respect are frustrated. The goal of client-centered counseling is the facilitation of a relationship between the client and counselor that promotes client congruency, self-direction, and full functioning. The task of the counselor is a sharing of self, thus creating a relationship characterized by behaviors of genuineness, transparency of real feelings, acceptance, and prizing of the individuality and worth of the client (Rogers, 1951, 1961; Rogers and Stevens, 1967). In contrast, techniques of tests and appraisal, history-taking, or formulation of diagnosis and prognosis are seldom used and are generally perceived as antagonistic to the counseling process.

This approach has obvious strengths and limitations. A major strength is the establishment of the client as the central focus of Counseling. Correspondingly, the counselor's attitudes rather than techniques are believed to have the greatest effect on the counseling relationship.

EXISTENTIAL COUNSELING

Existentialism, which originated in the late nineteenth century, closely parallels psychoanalytic theory while actually predating Freud's analytical views. Contributors to existential thought include such philosophers, theologians,

Table 7–1. COUNSELING APPROACHES

	Nature of Man/Personality Constructs	Nature of Client Anxiety	Goal of Counseling	Role of Counselor/Major Counseling Techniques
Affective Orientation:				
Client-centered	Rational, positive, forward moving toward self-actualization Self-concept acts as a regulator of behavior	Incongruence between individual's self-concept and experience	Promote client congruency and full functioning	Creation of active relationship Counselor expression of genuineness, transparency of real feelings, and acceptance and prizing of client Limited use of tests, questioning and diagnosis
Existential	Lives in three worlds: "world around," "own-world," "with-world" Searches for meaning of life and freedom	Conflict between being and nonbeing	Use anxiety as opportunity for client growth and experience of existence as real so client can develop commitment	Direct involvement with client Therapy a partnership Counselor risks his own being with client Uses psychoanalytic techniques but not tests and appraisal devices
Cognitive Orientation:				
Behavioral	A reactive being Behavior is an interaction of heredity and environment	Learned responses to cues in certain situations, which operate as secondary or acquired drives	Within ethical limits, solutions of whatever problems the client brings to the counselor Three criteria for goal: individual to client, observable/measurable, compatible with values of counselor	Highly active role techniques Techniques of conditioning, extinction, generalization, counterconditioning, reinforcement, social modeling and desensitization.
Eclectic	Both rational and irrational but having asocial tendencies Has self-regulatory abilities Personality is the changing state of coping with environment	Not explicitly stated	Independent self-regulation To assist the individual to learn to adapt more efficiently	Role from active to passive depending on nature of client problems and resources Techniques vary, e.g., empathy, warmth, genuineness, history taking, and diagnosis Counseling process consists of overlapping stages: relationship establishment, working period, and resolution and closure.

Adapted from *Shertzer, B., and Stone, S. Fundamentals of counseling* (3rd ed.). Boston: Houghton Mifflin Company, copyright © 1980. Adapted with permission.

psychologists, and writers as Kierkegaard, Tillich, Heidegger, Sartre, Minkowski, Binswanger, May, Frankel, Landsman, Arbuckle, and Kemp. The core of existentialistic thought is identified as freedom, which is closely related to the concept of reality (Arbuckle, 1965). Existentialistic Counseling is an endeavor to understand a rational, whole person's being by relating to one's own totality. Being is described as a real, continuous state of becoming, which is not concerned with contrasting one's aspects of subjectivity or objectivity. Human beings are considered to live in three modes of the environment, generally referred to as the "world around," "world of interpersonal relationships" or "with-world," and the "own world" (Kemp, 1971). The underlying concept of being-in-the-world emphasizes each person's unique structure of meaningful relationships and the environment in which that person relates to others. Human beings are considered to move in directions of growth, self-realization, independence, and autonomy. The nature of human anxiety is considered to be the conflict between being and nonbeing rather than a focus on normal or neurotic anxiety, which existentialists view as limiting.

In contrast to other counseling approaches, the existentialist does not engage in trying to free human beings from the anxiety of "being" versus "nonbeing." Rather this conflict is seen as presenting an opportunity for client growth and experience of existence as real so that the individual can act upon self-potentialities and develop a commitment to self-growth and change. The existentialist counselor engages in a relationship of direct involvement with the client, since therapy is viewed as a partnership. While being mindful not to impose personal ideas or feelings on the client, the counselor risks his or her own self as a means of stimulating the client's becoming. Emphasizing the counselor's presence and the client's being, the counselor uses such psychoanalytic techniques as free association and interpretation while generally avoiding tests and appraisal devices.

Landsman (1965) addresses the issue of whether existentialism can be considered a science, noting that seldom will two proponents of this approach agree on the meaning of words or even share a commitment to limiting the obvious vagueness of existentialistic thought. Traditionally, existentialists seem to abhor operational definitions, believing they obscure thought process and limit meaning. In contrast, the greatest value of existentialistic counseling rests on the use of the counselor's self-being in enrichment of the helping relationship rather than the mechanics of technique.

BEHAVIORAL COUNSELING

Behavioral theory (Hosford, 1969) states that a person's behavior is learned as a function of his or her environment. Although the interaction of both heredity and environment account for human behavior, environmental manipulation is believed to be the key to altering behavior. Human personality and behavior are shaped as a result of reacting to environmental stimuli. Client anxiety, then, is described as a pattern of unadaptive, learned behavioral responses to cues that may be operating as secondary or acquired drives or as a response to an originally neutral stimulus (Goldstein, 1973; Shertzer and Stone, 1974).

The counseling goal in behaviorism is defined as the solution of whatever problems within ethical limits that the client brings to the counselor. Goal setting is considered complete with the statement of an individual and measurable client goal. In addition, the counselor must be willing to help the client achieve this goal (Hosford, 1969). The counselor engages in a highly active but friendly role with the client, using various desensitizing, social modeling, and reinforcement techniques. Although behavioral theory is based in part on work by Pavlov, Skinner (1938, 1953, 1963) is generally credited with the development of the behavioral modification concepts of conditioning, extinction, generalization, and counterconditioning commonly employed with this approach.

Behaviorist techniques are often highly criticized (Hosford, 1969; Shertzer and Stone, 1974). A pertinent issue is whether a counselor has the right to manipulate or control client behavior. Another factor often debated is whether the techniques used are impersonal, cold, or immoral by not allowing unique, specific treatment of each client's problems. In contrast, behaviorists are generally considered to have advanced Counseling as a science by placing emphasis on measurable counseling outcomes that suggest how environmental limitations can be removed or reduced.

ECLECTIC COUNSELING

Eclecticism, as a distinct viewpoint in modern psychology, can be traced to the 1950s, when it emerged in response to the then growing disillusionment with existing counseling approaches. Thorne, who in 1945 founded the *Journal of Clinical Psychology* and compared Counseling to the learning process, is considered the leading proponent of eclecticism (Shertzer and Stone, 1974). In its essence, eclecticism involves the selection and application of various clinical methods to the needs of each specific counseling situation. The task of the eclectic counselor is to match elements from compatible and diverse theories and combine them into a mutually consistent whole-system approach, which is left open to constant revision and inclusion of new discoveries.

From the perspective of eclecticism, each person is considered to be both rational and irrational but to have asocial tendencies. Through use of intellectual resources and training, human beings acquire self-regulatory abilities. Personality is defined as the changing states of coping with environment, maintaining stability, integrating opposing functions, and maximizing self in order to satisfy needs and cope with reality (Shertzer and Stone, 1974, p. 242). The nature of human anxiety generally is not explicitly stated.

Counseling goals are set that are specific and realistically attainable for the client and which promote independent self-regulation and acquisition of self-enhancing behaviors (Dyer and Vriend, 1975). These authors also described the counseling process as composed of overlapping stages. The counselor's role varies on the active-passive continuum depending upon the nature of the client's problems and resources. The semantic description of core qualities of the counseling encounter differs depending on the authors cited. Tyler (1969) discussed counselor acceptance, understanding and sincerity. Truax and Carkhuff (1967) used the terms "nonpossessive warmth," "empathetic understanding," and "genuineness." Carkhuff (1973) proposed a simple, practical framework for the art of helping, comprising four behavioral dimensions of attending, responding, initiating, and communicating.

Eclectic practitioners are sometimes viewed as escapists whose methods are incapable of supporting meaningful research and whose stance is too unsystematic to permit identification of the most appropriate techniques and methods based on the immediate client reaction (Carkhuff, 1966). Speaking in support of eclecticism as an emergent viewpoint that offers the counselor flexibility and openness to new theory and methods, Brammer (1969) related the importance of the counselor's developing his or her own unique style of Counseling while ultimately striving for a general theory of personality structures and behavior change.

COUNSELING VERSUS OTHER HELPING STRATEGIES

Before discussing the general applicability of Counseling as a viable nursing intervention, it is helpful to identify how Counseling differs from other helping strategies. Citing the analysis of the word Counseling by Vaughan in 1976, Ashton (1979, p. 1340) offered the following definition of Counseling.

> The person-to-person form of communication, marked by the development of a subtle emotional understanding often technically described as "empathy" or "rapport"; this centered on one or more of the problems of the client and was free of authoritarian judgements and coercive pressures by the counselor.

One critical aspect of Counseling is that it is a process of shared therapeutic communication based on an attitude of respect for others. Philosophically, the concept of Counseling is further refined if the belief held by Litwack, Litwack, and Ballou (1980) are accepted. They hold that the terms Counseling and Health Counseling is synonymous, since the shared focus of activity is the promotion of the client's well-being or health. Well-being is defined as having a multiple dimension with emotional, intellectual, physical, social, and spiritual aspects.

Hopson (1978) offered a differentiation between four common types of helping strategies utilized by nurses: direct action, giving advice, teaching, and counseling. He suggested that the first three types of activities focus on what the helper does for another person whereas in Counseling the helper engages in a person-to-person relationship in which the responsibility for the outcome rests primarily with the client. Ideally, the counselor and the client are co-workers in this process. The goal, then is that the client will achieve more self-understanding and self-direction with a potential for greater self-management than existed when help was sought.

Hochbaum (1980) directly addressed the appropriateness of Patient Counseling versus Patient Teaching, especially when noncompliance is a factor. He suggested that nurses' efforts at Patient Teaching often fail due to a lack of understanding of the client's motivations and reasons for the noncompliant behavior, such as failure to follow a therapy regimen. Hochbaum believed nurses should see themselves less as educators and more as counselors to patients.

A distinction also needs to be made between Counseling and Psychotherapy. Counseling is most appropriate when a client exhibits normative behavior and the goal is focused on enhancing coping behaviors. Psychotherapy is indicated when the client has severe personality disorders and exhibits pathological behavior. In addition, the practice of therapy is reserved for the highly skilled practitioner who has both the legal right and educational preparation to intervene in a patient situation, which frequently necessitates the use of multiple therapies (e.g., prescription of medications).

In addition to differentiating between the types of helping strategies, it is also important for the nurse to recognize the ethical implications inherent in the counselor role. A fundamental obligation of the counselor is to respect the integrity and right to self-determination of each client. In various situations, it is appropriate for the counselor to act in a manner that guides, supports, or directs the client in coping or decision-making activities. However, it is generally considered unethical for the counselor to manipulate client behavior in a manner that results in diminished freedom of choice. It is also unethical for the nurse-counselor to attempt to provide counseling services beyond experiential qualifications and level of competency indicated by the nature of the specific counseling situation. Lastly, information obtained through the nurse-client relationship is appropriately discussed only within the professional setting and, when necessary, with other health professionals who are directly involved in the client's care. When professional collaboration is indicated, it is also the counselor's responsibility to explain to the client the reason and nature of the information shared.

DEFINITION AND PROCESS OF COUNSELING

Since nurses interact with such a broad population and in a variety of human relationships, I prefer the eclectic approach and offer the following definition of Counseling. *Counseling is an interactive helping process between a counselor and a client characterized by the core elements of acceptance, empathy, genuineness, and congruency. This relationship consists of a series of interactions over time in which the counselor, through variety of active and passive techniques, focuses on the needs, problems, or feelings of the client which have interfered with the client's usual adaptive behavior.*

The core elements of Counseling that shape the counseling relationship have been well described by Rogers (1951) Carkhuff (1969), and Truax and Carkhuff (1967). Acceptance or unconditional positive regard (Rogers, 1951) implies that the counselor truly has an interest in and concern for the client as a human being with intrinsic worth and dignity. Empathy involves experiencing or sensing another's feelings and behaviors—"world"—as if it were your own. When the counselor is able to communicate empathy, the client feels acceptance and freedom to disclose more personal information. The client frequently responds verbally in a manner that indicates this such as "you really do understand what I mean." The last core element, referred to as congruency by Rogers and as genuineness by Truax and Carkhuff, implies that the counselor is a natural, relaxed, and honest member of the counseling relationship. It is imperative that the nurse counselor first be in touch with personal feelings and behaviors before attempting to intervene in a meaningful way with the client through the intervention of Counseling. Thus, Counseling activity is directed at the facilitation of the client's personal development or growth.

The process of Counseling consists of three overlapping stages: (1) initial phase, (2) working or maintenance phase, and (3) closure and termination. The initial phase consists of the establishmemt of a therapeutic relationship between the counselor and client that is based on trust and respect. It is during this phase that the length of the counseling relationship is determined and goal setting occurs. In the working or maintenance phase, the counselor helps the client move toward greater self-understanding and self-regulation and to experiment with alternate behaviors. Counseling activity in this phase frequently includes a variety of both active and passive techniques, such as active listening, questioning, reflecting, clarifying, interpreting, confrontation, tests and appraisal tools, and self-disclosure. Table 7–2 displays a summary of the strategies most commonly used in Counseling and their intended uses. In the closure and termination phase, the client actually begins to apply and

Table 7–2. COMMON COUNSELING STRATEGIES

Strategies	Description	Uses
Active listening	An attitude of total attentiveness focusing on the client's expression of both verbal and nonverbal behavior	Most effective tool to communicate counselor empathy with the client To provide cues to the client's inner experience To minimize the counselor's tendency to make premature judgement
Questioning	Inquiring or asking for more information in the form of a question	To clarify a matter which is open to discussion; to minimize doubt or uncertainty To facilitate client exploration of a problem or situation
Reflecting	Restating or rephrasing the content or feeling of a client's statement (one type of active listening)	To understand the meaning of what the client is trying to express in either behavior or speech
Clarifying or interpreting	Stating the client's message with additional feedback or explanation	To increase the clearness of communication between counselor and client
Providing information or feedback	Using professional expertise to transmit pertinent information into facts, data, responses	To add to current knowledge or relate new knowledge to prior understanding
Selecting or weighing alternatives	Assisting the client to list and prioritize all possible alternatives to a problem	To aid in expanding options and narrowing choices May facilitate the client's experimentation with unfamiliar options in a nonthreatening setting
Confrontation	Verbalizing the discrepancy between the client's feelings and behaviors (between real and ideal self)	To focus the client's awareness on actions that are incongruent with self-image and actual behavior
Tests and appraisal tools	Using psychological paper and pencil tests or other appraisal tools which the counselor can administer and interpret	To help increase client self-awareness To add to the counselor's data base about the client (Examples: self-inventory of cardiac risk factors or the Holmes and Rahe Social Readjustment Rating Scales)
Self-disclosure	Revealing selected aspects of one's own experiences or personality	To foster genuineness and trust in the counseling situation when used appropriately

incorporate new thinking and new behaviors into his or her personal world. Termination of Counseling may be initiated by either the counselor or client, but ideally should be mutually agreed upon.

APPLICATION OF COUNSELING

Based on this discussion of both the nature and the process of Counseling, I suggest that Counseling as a nursing intervention is particularly appropriate for the individual client or client group experiencing a problem in coping with situations or developmental concerns. Those diagnoses presented by the Fifth National Conference Group for Classification of Nursing Diagnosis that seem especially relevant include the following:

○ Coping, Ineffective Individual or Family
○ Grieving

○ Fear
○ Family Processes, Alterations in
○ Knowledge Deficit
○ Noncompliance
○ Parenting, Alterations in
○ Rape-Trauma Syndrome
○ Spiritual Distress
○ Sexual Dysfunction
○ Self-Concept, Disturbance in
○ Self-Care Deficit
○ Violence, Potential for

It is important to recognize that those nurse-patient relationships for which Counseling is an effective intervention are identified through an accurate assessment of client needs as an ongoing part of the nursing process.

As state codes of nursing are revised and reflect the guidelines in *Nursing—A Social Policy Statement* of the American Nurses' Association (1980), which defines nursing as "diagnosis and treatment of human responses," independent nursing interventions are being expanded and more carefully documented. For example, the Iowa Code lists Health Counseling as a function of a professional nurse. A 10 year review of the nursing literature revealed that nurses have indeed recognized the need for and employed counseling-type activities in relation to a wide variety of patient problems and nursing diagnoses. One difficulty that is apparent, however, is that these behaviors often were not formally labeled as Counseling.

For example, Billings (1980) discussed the important role of the medical-surgical nurse in responding to the "psychosocial aspects" of patient care. She proposed the "emotional first aid" model based on Hagerman's work related to approach, avoidance, and aggressive behavior and the need-based theories. Billings stated that the nurse needs to intervene when the patient's behavior becomes so extreme it is counterproductive or interferes with the nurse's ability to implement the treatment plan. She discussed the application of her model through presentation of three case studies: a quadriplegic patient exhibiting dependency needs; a postsurgical patient exhibiting reluctance to participate in self-care of his temporary colostomy; and the spouse of a terminal cancer patient who was exhibiting anger and aggression. Using the terminology proposed by the National Nursing Diagnosis Conference Group, these patient problems could be restated as Ineffective Individual Coping; Self-Care Deficit, Alteration in Fecal Elimination; Disturbance in Self-Concept; and Anticipatory Grieving.

Several authors have emphasized the specialized needs of spouses of terminally or critically ill patients in relation to coping with the grieving process. Breu and Dracup (1978) focused on the needs of spouses of coronary care unit patients who were dealing with the phenomenon of anticipatory grief. Based on work done at UCLA with spouses of patients admitted to the coronary care unit, they developed a nursing care plan for the grieving spouse. One of the needs specifically addressed in this plan was the spouse's need for support and ventilation. Consistent with a counseling approach, one of the interventions suggested was the establishment of a consistent one-to-one relationship with a primary nurse.

Rogers and Mengel (1979) addressed the communication needs of families of terminal cancer patients engulfed in the grieving process. In this comprehensive article, the authors not only included guidelines for assessing the family's ability to deal with the impending death but also outlined corresponding nursing interventions. The stated goal of these interventions was to facilitate an open communication system among and between the patient, family, and nurse. Although the specific term Counseling was never used by them, Rogers and Mengel have made a major contribution in identifying specific counseling strategies appropriate for the nursing diagnosis of Anticipatory Grieving, including listening, encouraging, role modeling, providing and reinforcing information, identifying family strengths, involving patient and family in the decision-making process, and promoting autonomy through manipulation of the physical environment.

Addressing the validity of Counseling as a nursing intervention more directly, Jeter (1978) adopted Glasser's reality therapy approach to Counseling in the rehabilitation of the ostomy client deprived of fecal or urinary control. Jeter proposed that it is the responsibility of both the staff nurse and the specialized enterostomal therapist to assist the patient in moving from feelings of loss, denial, and invasion of privacy toward an attitude of self-confidence, acceptance, and independence in self-care. Her model outlined eight steps for assisting the client to make a positive psychological adjustment to the impact of ostomy surgery.

The literature also supports the use of counseling strategies by the nurse when intervening with specialized client groups. White (1978) was one of the early authors who specifically referred to Counseling as a nursing intervention. However, it should be noted that she discussed Counseling from the perspective of a psychiatric nurse specialist. She outlined her use of a maladaption-adaption model through the therapeutic approach of the interpersonal nurse-client relationship in working with depressed clients. Lichtenstein (1981) offered a guideline for effective nursing intervention with abused women. She emphasized the nurse's role in establishing a relationship with the client based on trust, provision of information, clarification of misconceptions, support in decision making, and referral. Strang (1982) suggested how the nurse can incorporate selected psychotherapy techniques into the nursing process in developing a therapeutic relationship with the client under treatment for drug dependence. The role of the nurse in providing Sexual Counseling for patients, such as those with a spinal cord injury or following myocardial infarction, was supported by Scalzi (1982) and Istre (1979), again based on the nature of the interpersonal relationship that develops between the nurse and the patient.

IMPLICATIONS FOR NURSING AS A PROFESSION

In addition to the use of Counseling in any given nurse-client relationship, Counseling as a nursing intervention also has implications for the development of nursing as a profession and for nursing research. One of the issues facing the nursing profession today is the need to delineate the role and function of the nurse who practices as a clinical specialist or nurse practitioner. In this regard, Streff and Streff (1982) offered an excellent discussion of the Counseling dimension of the pediatric nurse practitioner's role. They saw the pediatric nurse practitioner (PNP) as one who, by virtue of educational preparation and clinical expertise, was able to provide comprehensive health care for children and adolescents in relation to the situational and developmental concerns. A four-step counseling model reflecting Peplau's interpersonal process of nursing (1952) was presented as a framework for the counseling process. The authors suggested that this model allows the nurse to intervene in an independent manner with the child and family to provide didactic information, anticipatory guidance, and assistance in adapting to stressful situations, such as an obese adolescent who feels isolated from her peers. In short, Streff and Streff offered a beginning approach to clarifying the "expanded" nursing role by analysis of the manner in which the PNP practitioner incorporates and utilizes Counseling as an independent nursing intervention in the practice setting.

In the past, social science literature has mainly examined the effects of Counseling on client behavior of physically well subjects, such as college students; very few research studies were done in which the subjects were actually classified as patients. One study reported in recent nursing literature (Watson, 1983) did examine the effects of postoperative Counseling on the self-concept of cancer patients following ostomy surgery. The results supported the hypothesis that the patients who received the Counseling intervention demonstrated more positive measures of self-concept or self-esteem than did the patients in the control group. Whereas age, sex, and type of ostomy surgery were not found to be significant variables, Watson recommended that these factors in addition to the effect of the time interval between the intervention and the measurement of self-concept be considered in future studies.

The study by Lane and Liss-Levinson (1980) described an approach combining Education and Counseling, which was developed for use with cancer patients and their families. A wide variety of Counseling services, ranging from one-time Individual Counseling to supportive Group Counseling, was provided by the project team, composed of a nurse patient educator and a psychologist. The evaluative data revealed numerous positive effects of this combination approach, such as greater comfort with self-care (e.g., ostomy management), improved communication between patient and family members, and decreased anxiety behavior. One significant contribution of this project was the generation of a representative list of major informational, educational, and psychosocial needs of cancer patients and their families. This list may serve as stimulus for further nursing research in the study of the effects of Counseling on patient coping methods.

Case Study

The following case study describes my own experiences with a rehabilitation client and illustrates some of the key elements of Counseling. The discussion is limited to one aspect of the total patient situation, since the purpose is simply to demonstrate application of the counseling process. The specific approach reflects an orientation to Orem's theory of nursing and Eclectic Counseling.

Lisa was a 24 year old single woman who had suffered a closed head injury as a result of a bicycle-automobile accident. At the time of the counseling intervention, Lisa was three months post trauma and had just been transferred from an acute care setting to the rehabilitation unit.

Lisa's initial symptoms of acute brain stem involvement and coma had subsided, but right-sided ataxia and left spastic hemiparesis were present. The ataxia made it particularly difficult for Lisa to perform such basic activities of daily living as eating, dressing, or toileting in a conventional manner, leading to self-care deficits in these areas. For example, Lisa's efforts at self-feeding even finger foods nearly always resulted in most of the food ending up in her hair, or her lap, or on the floor.

This difficulty in eating was especially disturbing to Lisa's parents, one of whom stayed with her during nearly all her waking hours. They gave verbal and nonverbal expression to many feelings about Lisa's self-care limitations, including embarassment, frustration, anxiety, hopelessness, and anger, as well as deep concern. Basically, they responded to these feelings with ineffective coping measures of overprotectiveness and projection onto the staff. For example, they continually thwarted the treatment plan, especially in the area of activities of daily living, by feeding and dressing Lisa themselves. Only with great insistence by the staff would they allow Lisa to attempt these tasks on her own. Thus, while Lisa's parents were attempting to function as care agents, the efforts were frequently not therapeutic in reducing Lisa's dependence behavior or in increasing her self-care abilities. Several diagnoses were readily apparent: Self-Care Deficits in feeding and dressing, Dependent Coping Mode (Lisa), and Ineffective Family Coping. Recognizing the complexity and interrelatedness of these patient-family problems, I selected the intervention of Counseling in addition to other direct care nursing activies.

Since a beginning therapeutic relationship already existed between the nurse and Lisa and her parents based on the provision of direct personal care, the next major task was identification of the overall counseling goal. The goal agreed on implicitly by Lisa and explicitly by her parents was to promote Lisa's maximal physical recovery and independent functions and to assist her to learn ways of coping with the functional limitations remaining.

Following identification of the mutually accepted goal statement, the working phase of Counseling began. The specific Counseling activities employed corresponded in general to Orem's five methods of helping. For example, the nurse provided Lisa's parents with clear, factual information regarding the treatment regimen and her progress in each of the therapies ordered. This helped them examine their own fears and anxieties regarding Lisa's ultimate recovery more realistically. Psychological support was provided through the use of active listening, reflection, and clarification of their expressed feelings and underlying concerns. A caring environment was conveyed through demonstration of the counselor characteristics of empathy, warmth, and genuinenes. Based in part on Lisa's initial problem with choking at mealtime, the parents were quite reluctant to allow her to attempt self-feeding. The nurse provided reassurance for the parents by not only supervising Lisa at mealtimes but also by sharing with the parents on a regular basis any progress Lisa made in mastering self-feeding. These behaviors served to build up the parent's trust level so that by the fourth week of care they were more receptive to Lisa's use of various adaptive feeding devices and agreed to remain out of the dining area at mealtimes. As still another means of promoting independence, the nurse provided Lisa with various opportunities to make beginning choices affecting her daily care—e.g., where she wanted to sit in the dining room, type of finger foods, and so forth.

Plans for termination of Counseling actually began during the first week when the nurse discussed the length of time she would be working with Lisa and her parents as a nurse clinician (total of 12 weeks). In the termination phase, the nurse summarized Lisa's progress to date and offered praise and reinforcement of the new skills she was exhibiting; her parents were also praised for increasing behaviors and attitude of support rather than overprotectiveness. In addition, the nurse counselor reviewed, as she had been doing on a weekly basis with the floor nursing staff, the client's progress to date in order to facilitate continuity of care.

As nursing responds to the challenge to further define its domain, it is imperative that independent nursing interventions be integrated into practice in accordance with nursing diagnoses. Indeed, Counseling has broad applicability to many aspects of health promotion and health maintenance.

EDITORS' COMMENTS AND QUESTIONS
Nursing curricula have included content on the interpersonal relationship of nurse and client since the 1960s. Individual nurses have
used counseling techniques for many years. This chapter emphasizes the theory from which these techniques are drawn. Although
all nurses are taught and use counseling techniques, most nurses
lack the theoretical base, which is described here.

Questions for Discussion
1. *Which approach to Counseling do you prefer?*
2. *Is Counseling an intervention, a theory of nursing, or the
philosophical basis of nursing?*
3. *Distinguish between Counseling and Psychotherapy.*

References

American Nurses' Association. Nursing—a social policy statement. Kansas City, Mo.: American Nurses' Association, 1980.
Arbuckle, D. Existentialism in counseling: The humanistic view. Personnel and Guidance Journal, 1965, 43, 558–573.
Ashton, K., Sharing the burden. Nursing Times, August 9, 1979.
Billings, C. Emotional first aid. American Journal of Nursing, 1980, 80, 2506–2509.
Brammer, L. Eclecticism revisited. Personnel and Guidance Journal, 1969, 48, 192–197.
Breu, C., and Dracup, K. Helping the spouses of critically ill patients. American Journal of Nursing, 1978, 78, 51–53.
Carkhuff, R. Counseling research, theory and practice—1965. Journal of Counseling Psychology, 1966, 13(4), 467–480.
Carkhuff, R. Helping and human relations. New York: Holt, Rinehart and Winston, 1969.
Carkhuff, R. The art of helping. Amherst, Mass.: Human Resource Development Press, 1973.
Dyer, W., and Vriend, J. Counseling techniques that work. Washington, D.C.: American Personnel Guidance Association Press, 1975.
Eldred, A. All nurses should be counselors. American Association of Industrial Nurses Journal, 1967, 15(3), 43–48.
Glasser, W. Reality therapy. New York: Harper and Row, 1965.
Goldstein, A. Behavior therapy. In R. Corsini (Ed.), Current psychotherapies. Itasca, Ill.: F. E. Peacock Publishers, 1973.
Hochbaum, G. Patient counseling vs. patient teaching. Topics in Clinical Nursing, 1980, 2(2), 1–7.
Hopson, B. Counseling—a case for demystifying and deprofessionalising. Nursing Times, January 12, 1978.
Hosford, R. Behavioral counseling—a contemporary overview. The Counseling Psychologist, 1969, 1(4), 1–33.
Istre, S. The physical aspects of counseling for patients with congenital or acquired spinal cord injury. Orthopedic Nurses' Association Journal, 1979, 6(12), 468–483.
Jeter, K. A realistic approach to enterostomy rehabilitation. Nursing Forum 1978, 17(1), 73–83.
Kemp, C. Major contribution: Existential counseling. Counseling Psychologist, 1971, 2(3), 2–30.
King, I. Toward a theory of nursing: General concepts of human behavior. New York: John Wiley and Sons, 1971.
Landsman, T. Existentialism in counseling: the scientific view. Personnel and Guidance Journal, 1965, 43, 568–573.
Lane, D., and Liss-Levinson, W. Education and counseling for cancer patients—lifting the shroud of silence. Patient Counseling and Health Education, 1980, 2(4), 154–160.
Lichtenstein, V. The battered woman: Guidelines for effective nursing intervention. Issues in Mental Health Nursing, 1981, 3, 236–250.
Litwack, L., Litwack, J., and Ballou, M. Health Counseling. New York: Appleton-Century-Crofts, 1980.

Orem, D. Nursing: Concepts of practice (2nd ed.). New York: McGraw-Hill Book Company, 1980.

Orem, D. Nursing: Concepts of practice. New York, McGraw Hill Book Company, 1971.

Orem, D. The art of nursing (Chapter 8, p. 85). Division of Hospital and Institutional Services of the Indiana State Board of Health, October 1956.

Orlando, I. The dynamic nurse-patient relationship. New York: G. P. Putnam's Sons, 1961.

Paterson, J., and Zderad, L. Humanistic nursing. New York: John Wiley and Sons, 1976.

Patterson, C. A current view of client-centered or relationship therapy. Counseling Psychologist, 1969, 1(2), 2–25.

Peplau, H. Interpersonal relations in nursing. New York: G. P. Putnam's Sons, 1952.

Rogers, B., and Mengel, A. Communicating with families of terminal cancer patients. Topics in Clinical Nursing, 1979, 1(3), 55–61.

Rogers, C. Client-centered therapy—implications and theory. Boston: Houghton Mifflin Company, 1951.

Rogers, C. On becoming a person. Boston: Houghton Mifflin Company, 1961.

Rogers, C., and Stevens, B. Person to person: The problem of being human. Walnut Creek, Calif.: Real People Press, 1967.

Scalzi, C. Sexual counseling and sexual therapy for patients after myocardial infarction. Cardiovascular Nursing, 1982, 18(3), 13–17.

Shertzer, B., and Stone, S. Fundamentals of counseling (2nd ed.). Boston: Houghton Mifflin Company, 1974.

Skinner, B. The behavior of organisms. New York: Appleton, 1938.

Skinner, B. Science and human behavior. New York: Macmillan, 1953.

Skinner, B. Behaviorism at fifty. Science, 1963, 140, 951–958.

Strang, J. Psychotherapy by nurses—some special characteristics. Journal of Advanced Nursing, 1982, 7:167–171.

Streff, M., and Streff, C. The counseling dimension of the nurse practitioner. Pediatric Nursing, 1982, 8, 9–13.

Truax, C., and Carkhuff, R. Toward effective counseling and psychotherapy. Chicago: Aldine, 1967.

Tyler, L. The work of the counselor (3rd ed.). New York: Appleton-Century-Crofts, 1969.

Watson, P. The effects of short-term postoperative counseling on cancer/ostomy patients. Cancer Nursing, 1983, 6(1), 21–29.

White, C. Nurse counseling with a depressed patient. American Journal of Nursing, 1978, 78, 436–439.

8

NUTRITIONAL COUNSELING

GERALDINE BUSSE

All persons have some knowledge and experience in nutrition. For example, common generalizations include (1) food is necessary for life and survival; (2) food and people's eating patterns influence their social interactions and lifestyle; (3) food is often regarded as a status symbol; and (4) the belief or value of a particular food reflects the culture of the people. It is apparent from these few generalizations that the nurse should have some knowledge about nutrition and the resources relating to it if the nurse is to fulfill the expected role as a health team member.

DEFINITIONS

Nutrition, as we know it today, is "the science that interprets the relationship of food to the functioning organism" (Howard and Herbold, 1978, p. 5). It has been recognized as an independent field of study since 1926 with the appointment of Mary Swartz Rose as a professor of nutrition at Columbia University. The nutritional state of an individual at the time of an acute illness or injury may determine the rate of recovery and rehabilitation. Every nursing curriculum has courses in nutrition. In an integrated curriculum, there is a constant reference to the relationship of the client's health status and nutrition. This is reflected in the nursing diagnoses that are made after a careful assessment of the client's responses to his or her condition.

Pender (1982) states that "adequate nutrition is a critical element in the nurturance of health.... Dietary inadequacies (malnutrition), in the guise of overnutrition or undernutrition, plague 30 to 50 percent of Americans and are found at all socioeconomic levels .... The overconsumption of saturated fats, cholesterol, sugar, and salt has been linked to a number of chronic illnesses that are major causes of death and disability in the United States" (p. 275).

The role of nutrition in prevention of pellagra, scurvy, rickets, and kwashiorkor is well known. The Framingham (Massachusetts) heart study further documents the influence of dietary patterns on health. This longitudinal research study analyzed the eating and activity patterns of a selected group of men and their incidence of heart disease. The findings of this study have influenced the amount of red meat and animal fats consumed by Americans. The American Heart Association's advice about dietary habits for the prevention of heart disease has been influenced by this research. Likewise, the counseling and teaching of clients with heart attacks regarding their diet, with the goal to prevent recurrence of another heart attack, is based on some of the findings of this study. Other longitudinal studies also demonstrate the relationship of family dietary patterns with incidence of cardiovascular disease. For example, the University of Iowa College of Medicine is engaged in such a research study in Muscatine, Iowa. The school-aged persons in this community have their blood pressure monitored at regular intervals. The families of children with high blood pressure readings are studied carefully, and an extensive analysis is done of the family's diet pattern.

Counseling is one dimension of a nurse's role. Counseling is a helping process between the nurse, the client, and family that requires a relationship of openness and respect. It is a method for assisting persons to identify feelings and to clarify beliefs and values in order to make appropriate decisions (Leahy, Cobb, and Jones, 1982). Counseling may be described as a helping or educational process in which individuals define their needs and explore alternative solutions. Change occurs when the person not only identifies the problem but owns it and makes a plan and acts upon it (Eagan, 1981). The intervention of Counseling is described in Chapter 7.

Mason and Burness (1977) view the nutritional counselor as having the skills of a communicator, facilitator, and manager. To be effective, the nutritional counselor must be knowledgeable about nutrition and human behavior.

Nutritional Counseling is an intervention frequently shared by several members of the health team. Freeman and Heinrich (1982) note that the way the health team works may take several forms. There may be no more than systematic exchange of information between the members. The team may have a more formal organization, with a designated leader who exercises general control, and with each member having defined roles and limits. It may be that roles are blurred, and leadership is shared or rotated to adapt to the particular situation. For the team approach to be successful, the members must respect and trust each other; goals must be explicit and stated in such a way that their intent is clear to all; there is clear allocation of responsibility for action agreed upon; adaptive role interchange should be possible, if indicated; and team planning efforts must be economical in terms of time and cost.

REFERENCES AND RESOURCES ON NUTRITION

The public is bombarded daily with nutrition information by radio, television, and the press. For example, in a local newspaper, Flannery's article, "A diet for every foible—but the best diet is nutritious, sensible, changes behavior" took up only a small part of a six page section devoted to food. Dozens of magazines carry information or advertisements about food and nutrition. Hence, one may assume that all clients have some knowledge about food and its properties. Beliefs are influenced by a person's experience, and there are people who believe any printed word as an absolute fact. This is understandable, as often the articles in the lay press quote studies from respected research centers. It is also true that many researchers and sponsors of research utilize the press and other media to inform the public about their activities, as this is one method of obtaining public support for further research. Sometimes, however, the results of these studies are not reported accurately and the limitations of the study are not fully explained. The nurse must evaluate this information on nutrition in terms of its applicability to the needs and concerns of the client.

How does the nurse evaluate nutrition information? The knowledge explosion may make some facts learned in the basic educational program obsolete. The nurse who feels completely knowledgeable in all areas of health care, including nutrition, is not exhibiting the expected professional behavior of a qualified health team member. If the person has this attitude the client is denied the expertise of a nutritionist or dietitian. The mark of a well-educated professional is the ability to say "I don't know, but I'll try to find out." The nurse working in a hospital has a resource readily available—the dietary department and its dietitians can assist with solving the client's nutritional problems. Either the dietitian may work directly with the client and share the goals with the nurse so that the nurse may reinforce the suggested behavior changes, or the dietitian may consult with the nurse, suggesting strategies to improve the nutrition of the client. Many small hospitals only have a part-time dietitian, who has limited time available to counsel the patient directly. The dietitian may also give the nurse a list of references that might help increase the understanding of the nutritional counselor. The appendix at the end of this chapter is an example of such a reference list, developed for my use by the Dietary Department of University of Iowa Hospitals and Clinics.

The nurse working in the community setting, be it home, school, or industry, can similarly obtain nutrition information. The larger health departments, community health nursing agencies, and social services departments and agencies employ nutritionists and dietitians. If the local agency or department does not have a nutritional consultant, the nurse may request the help of the State Health Department or Department of Social Services, which in some states is known as the Department of Human Services. In some states these departments are combined and known as the Department of Health and Social Services. At the state level there are also the Department of Agriculture and the State Extension Services. All of these agencies are able to provide information on nutrition. For example, in Iowa each county has an Extension Service office, which offers nutritional consultation through the Iowa State University Extension Service. The Extension Service offers consultation in many areas, such as gardening, preserving of food, home making, and parenting. It sponsors group meetings and provides newsletters and pamphlets on various topics. The nurse may find State Extension Services to be valuable resources in helping clients to meet their nutritional concerns.

Some state agencies also have national counterparts, such as the Department of Health and Human Services and the Department of Agriculture. Voluntary and private agencies also supply nutrition information, such as the National Dairy Council (6300 N. Riverside, Rosemont, IL 60018) and National Livestock and Meat Board (444 N. Michigan, Chicago, IL 60611). Various voluntary health-related organizations also are resources. For example, the American Heart Association publishes a cookbook as well as much information on the appropriate dietary pattern for persons with heart disease. This association is also concerned about the influence diet has on the prevention of heart disease. Many other voluntary health organizations offer similar educational services on nutrition.

Professional organizations that may be utilized for obtaining nutrition information include the American Dietetic Association, American Medical

Association, and American Public Health Association. Many nursing periodicals frequently have articles relating to nutrition.

In addition to the resources described, local school systems can be excellent resources. Home economics teachers have access to the latest nutrition information and may influence the cooking and eating patterns of many families. As nurses work with clients in promoting good nutrition it often becomes apparent that choice of food is the issue. Sometimes suggesting that the client explore ideas with a local expert who is familiar with local practices, such as the home economics teacher or the county home economist, is helpful. These persons may be the client's friend or neighbor and may help the client change a harmful diet and cooking pattern.

NURSING RESEARCH

Few nurses have conducted research in the area of nutrition. The tube feedings studies by Walike and associates (1973, 1975, 1977) are a major contribution to nursing knowledge. The CURN Project selected a lactose-free diet as one of 10 protocols to design and test (Horsley, Crane, Haller, 1981). This protocol recommends the elimination of lactose from the formulas of tube feeding diets of adult patients to minimize diarrhea, distention, flatulence, fullness, and rejection of feedings.

More nursing research in the area of nutrition is definitely needed. It would appear that this research should focus upon two areas: (1) assisting the client with changes in nutritional lifestyle, and (2) feeding problems that result from disturbances of food intake.

APPLICATION OF THE NURSING PROCESS IN NUTRITIONAL COUNSELING

In the delivery of nursing care there are several phases: assessment, making of a nursing diagnosis, planning, implementation of the plan, and evaluation. This is a continuous process. The evaluation of the outcomes in light of the nursing diagnosis begins the assessment phase again, and the cycle repeats itself.

The nursing diagnosis is a statement of the client's response to a situation or condition. This response may be seen as actually or potentially unhealthy for the client; nursing intervention can help change the client's behavior in the direction of health. When Nutritional Counseling is done, the nursing diagnosis is usually one of three: (1) Alterations in Nutrition, Less than Body Requirements; (2) Alterations in Nutrition, More than Body Requirements; (3) Potential Alterations in Nutrition.

Nutritional Counseling: Assessment

In the assessment phase of the nursing process the nurse should be aware of certain accepted standards that are utilized in the evaluation of the client's nutritional status. Age, weight, and activities influence the nutritional requirements of an individual. The recommended dietary allowance (RDA) represents the nutritional standards for assessing and planning dietary intake. They are defined by the Food and Nutrition Board of the National Research Council (NRC). Since their development in 1943, the allowances have continually been updated in accordance with the most current scientific research. Every five years new data are reviewed and both the RDA and background information on nutrients and their functions are revised. Countries other than the United States (e.g., Canada) and the Food and Agriculture Organization (FAO) have also issued standards on nutrient needs (Howard and Herbold, 1978). The U.S. Department of Agriculture publishes a bulletin "Nutritive Value of Foods" (1972), which contains tables that list the nutrients in 615 foods commonly used in the United States. The tables are easy to comprehend as the foods are listed in measures commonly used, such as cups, ounces, pounds, or pieces a certain size. These two technical sources can serve as a data source for assessing and evaluating the adequacy of a client's dietary intake.

In evaluating the nutrition of the client the nurse must be aware not only of the function of the various nutrients but also of the stage of the growth and development of the individual. For instance, in childhood the demand for calories is relatively high compared with adulthood. The NRC recently reduced the caloric recommendations for children, since children in an industrialized society have reduced general activity and require fewer calories (Williams, 1977).

The client's age, stage of growth and development, past eating experiences, injury, and disease are some of the factors the nurse must consider as he or she assists the client to meet the nutritional requirements in a manner that is acceptable and appropriate. The following illustrations demonstrate the typical nutritional counseling situations nurses are likely to encounter. The pregnant woman has an increased need for protein, calcium, and iron because of the developing fetus. The premature infant unable to breast-feed with an intolerance to fat requires a specific formula alteration. The four-year-old child who has had only milk and other liquids will require nutritional supplement. The motorcycle accident victim with head and facial fractures may require many alterations in nutrition, including the manner in which the food is presented for ingestion. The diabetic client may need assistance in controlling carbohydrate intake. The client receiving chemotherapy may be unable to tolerate many foods because of nausea and yet has an increased need for protein and other essential nutrients. An elderly client with a chronic illness may have very limited interest in food because of cost and difficulty of preparation.

Growth is most rapid in the first year of life. It is expected that an infant will double its birth weight by six months and triple it by the age of one year. After that the rate of growth appears to occur in spurts. Hence the parent of the two year old may seem distressed because the child almost stops eating by the parent's assessment. The child's rate of growth is slower than the first part of its life so the child has need for fewer calories. Also at this age, in many American families this is the time when food is utilized as a reward for "good" behavior. Unfortunately, the food that is used for "being good" or "a nice boy or girl" is a piece of candy or similar concentrated carbohydrate. This learned behavior carries over into adult life. If we have had a "bad day" at work or at home with the kids we reward ourselves to a special food. To some that treat may be a fudge sundae, a piece of cake, or maybe a sweet alcoholic beverage. This indulgence may then keep the person from eating essential nutrients.

When the child enters school he or she may be introduced to many changes in eating patterns. The school lunch is a very different situation from eating at home. There may be pressures to play or join the group so that there isn't time to eat. This pattern often is repeated in the adult professional world. Students and teachers sometimes schedule classes or activities over the usual meal time so that lunch or dinner may be missed. The hospital environment too may be so busy that there is no time to eat. Pender (1982) estimates that convenience foods constitute 60 per cent of the American diet. It takes time to prepare food and it takes time to eat. It appears that many persons do not give these factors a very high priority. This fact has given rise to a fast food industry. The foods available are often high in fat, carbohydrates, and salt, and low in fiber. To the young these foods are status foods, because "all the kids eat them." Adolescence is a period of rapid growth and change and there is a need for increased amounts of food. The American fashion of "thinness is beautiful" influences the eating patterns of many adolescent girls, as well as many adults.

The older adult, because of limited activity, requires fewer calories. Often the elderly adult has less interest in preparing food and so may fall into the habit of a tea and toast diet. Not only is this easy to prepare but it is also easier to eat, as many older adults are edentulous.

As stated earlier in this chapter, clients have some exposure to nutrition information. It is commonly known that a balanced diet means eating daily the basic four food groups: cereals and bread products, meat and protein foods, dairy products, fruits and vegetables. This grouping of foods is easy to understand; however, the nurse must discover how the client perceives the fulfilling of the "basic four" in his or her eating pattern. For example, the client may think that a Danish pastry with a half teaspoon of strawberry jam constitutes both a bread product and fruit. The nurse's perception would be different. In helping clients to modify their eating patterns because of a disease process, such as diabetes or hypertension, the nurse must know the clients' perceptions of the basic four food groups as well as their perceptions of the disease.

The assessment of the client's nutritional status begins by observing his or her general appearance and response to food. In gathering and analyzing nutritional data, the nurse would observe the skin, posture, muscle tone, state of alertness, and mobility. The physical assessment and health history would include the client's elimination patterns, and information about prior eating and drinking patterns. It is important that the nurse learn how the client perceives his or her nutritional needs now and how these were met in the past. For example, breakfast may consist of leftovers from the evening meal, such as cold spaghetti; alternatively a family may have a five meal pattern rather than the expected three meal pattern. Some people have favorite foods and eat these daily. "Breakfast isn't breakfast unless there is oatmeal." Noting what foods the client chooses from the selected menu provided by many institutions will give the nurse clues about the client's food likes and dislikes. In addition, observing which foods are left on the tray will assist the nurse in assessing the client's dietary habits. The nurse may find it helpful to ask the client or family member to record what has been eaten in a 24 hour period. Veninga (1982) includes a tool that can be used when gathering data of a client's dietary intake. Veninga's form has two set of headings: a horizontal and vertical. The horizontal headings are milk and milk products; meat and milk alternatives; fruits and vegetables; breads and cereals; beverages; snacks. To clarify these headings there is a list of specific food items identified for each food group. The vertical headings are breakfast, lunch, dinner, and snacks. This tool would provide the nurse much data about the client's dietary habits.

It may be helpful for the nurse working with families to observe their food buying habits. The author worked with a group of community health nurses who were concerned that many of their clients appeared obese and had dental caries. In gathering data about their eating habits the nurses reported that many clients indicated they were eating according to "the basic food pattern." Clients often answer questions according to what they think the nurse expects. To obtain accurate information the consultant nutritionist suggested that the nurses ask the clients what the clients had on their shopping lists for the current week. Coffee, carbonated beverages, and bread and cereal were on most lists, and a small number included dairy products and fresh vegetables and fruits. This data helped nurses to revise their goals for health promotion with these clients.

When assessing the client the nurse should note the dental condition. If the client has no teeth or missing teeth, an inquiry about favorite foods may indicate a dietary pattern of soft foods. In this instance it could be that the client avoids meats and fresh fruit and vegetables. Likewise questioning about favorite foods may reveal that the client avoids certain foods because of past illness, such as an episode with a gastric ulcer or colitis. Questioning may also reveal that certain favorite foods are eaten infrequently because of cost or because of the difficulty the client has in preparing food.

In assessing the dietary pattern of clients the nurse should be aware of the client's ethnic background. Often, by asking how the family celebrates special days, such as birthdays and holidays, data can be gathered about the client's feelings about food. This may also give the nurse information about the client's taste for sweets, salt, and other spices. Assumptions are frequently made about ethnic groups—for example, that a person with a German background is fond of sauerkraut and beer, or that Hispanic individuals always have a taste for certain "hot" spices. Further questions about clients' eating patterns may reveal their knowledge and beliefs about various nutrients, such as vitamins, minerals, salt, and sugar.

Finally, the nurse must understand what food means to the person. Each ethnic group has special foods, and certain foods are status symbols of age, wealth or prestige. It has been said that "by the time a person can afford to eat a sirloin steak every day his arteries cannot tolerate it." Nutritional Counseling requires the nurse to have a holistic approach, encompassing the environment, the culture, past experiences, age, weight, and the disease process.

Nutritional Counseling: Diagnosis

An analysis of the data assembled through careful assessment of the client's nutritional status results in a nursing diagnosis. If the data reveals that the client is obese, the nursing diagnosis would be Alteration in Nutrition, More than Body Requirements. The 4 year old child who has never eaten solid food and has a secondary anemia would have a nursing diagnosis of Alteration in Nutrition, Less than Body Requirements. If the client had difficulty eating and drinking as in the case of the cancer client receiving chemotherapy with symptoms of nausea and distention, the nursing diagnoses would be Fluid Deficit and Potential Alteration in Nutrition, Less than Body Requirements. The elderly client with a chronic illness who has diet limited in fiber content would have the diagnosis of Alterations in Bowel Elimination, Constipation.

Nutritional Counseling: Planning

After making a nursing diagnosis the nurse should plan with the client and establish achievable goals. In the beginning of the nurse-client relationship not all of the goals desired by nurse and client may be the same. Mutually agreed upon goals are the result of a trusting relationship that is built on respect and the keeping of promises, as well as careful listening to what is being said and allowing of sufficient time. Mutual goals are developed by considering the assessment data and the client's perceptions. Sometimes the client may state his or her goals or expectations very simply by saying "Help me to get well, so I can work again, or help me to be rid of this pain, or help me to die." In setting goals for change in the nutritional status the nurse begins where the client is, and explores with the client how he or she perceives diet may affect his or her goal for wellness, relief of pain, or death. For the goal to be achieved the client must identify the diet modification and take responsibility for change. Egan (1981) states the client must own the problem before goals are achieved.

The client and nurse should agree on what is a realistic goal. The obese client may want to lose 50 pounds in two weeks. The client should be counseled that this is not a realistic or a safe expectation for this length of time. The nurse can help the client to set both long-term and short-term goals. For example, a realistic short-term goal for the obese client might be a 1 to 2 pound loss of weight per week, the long-term goal being a 12 pound loss in six weeks. The child or adult who had agreed that he or she would increase the protein intake over the next two weeks might begin with the goal of always eating three bites of meat with each meal, and having a half of a meat sandwich as an evening snack this week. Next week the client eats half of the serving of meat at each meal.

The modifications in a diet should be specific, reasonable, and clear; the desired outcome must be valued by the client.

Nutritional Counseling: Implementation

In the implementation of the plan the client should feel that he or she is involved and can control the outcome. In Nutritional Counseling often the choices are limited. With diabetes, there are certain dietary restrictions. This may mean that certain foods will need to be eliminated. The nurse should encourage the client to discover how old food patterns fit into the diabetic regime. The diabetic who is addicted to eating pie could continue to eat pie by counting the pie crust as part of the fat and bread exchange and the fruit filling as a fruit exchange in one of his meals. Likewise the client with hypertension can be given a choice of other condiments and flavorings when the sodium intake must be limited. The nurse may help the client to look upon this as an adventure or experiment that might also prove helpful to others who also may have the problem of limiting their salt intake. The client who takes pride in being a gourmet cook may enjoy searching for different recipes or may even develop original recipes and cook books to share.

Certain physical limitations may make the implementation of the goal of adequate nutrition difficult. The nurse must be very aware of the words that are used in presenting a change in the diet. For example, the client who is on a soft diet may refuse to eat if the food looks like and is labeled "baby food." It may be possible for a family member or nurse to mash the food or cut it into small pieces in the presence of the client so the food initially appears in the same form to which the client has always been accustomed. Possibly the client would be able to manage "finger foods." Implementing these changes may mean that the nurse and dietitian will need to consult with the client.

Dependent clients who must be fed by someone should be allowed to control the rate at which they are fed and given a choice of what foods to eat first. One older man, for example, who had two arm casts always wanted the nurse to start with the ice cream so it would not melt. It is important that food be presented in an attractive manner, and that hot foods be hot and cold foods cold. The environment at meal time also affects how the client responds to food. Ask yourself, is the bedside table in a good position so the client can reach the tray? Is the client ready to eat (hands washed, in proper position, etc.)? Can the client manage to lift the lids and open the boxes with only one hand when the other has an IV in it?

The attitudes and beliefs of the significant others also influence how well a plan for dietary changes is implemented. Family members may deny that the client has a condition that requires alterations in the dietary pattern; or they may bring gifts of foods that should not be included in the client's diet. The client may feel intimidated in this situation. For example, the diabetic patient may eat a piece of candy because it is a gift from his best friend. The nurse should attempt to involve the family in the planning of appropriate goals and include them in the implementation of the goals. Change is difficult and takes time. Nothing succeeds like success, so complimenting the client and family upon the accomplishment of each goal may help in achieving the desired changes in dietary patterns.

In the implementation of the goals clients must be involved and allowed to carry them out in their own styles. An elderly retired physician was hospitalized. He had always eaten three eggs and two servings of cereal for breakfast, a combination of fruit and vegetables for lunch, and his evening meal had been a repeat of breakfast. He became very upset because the hospital menu did not accommodate his desire for cereal in the evening, and he ate very little at the evening meal. The nurse talked with him about his nutritional goal of increasing his protein and fiber intake. Together with assistance from the dietitian the menu was modified, so every evening his supper tray had two boxes of cereal with milk plus the usual evening meal. Not only did his dietary intake improve, but also his relationships with the staff became better. He was involved and in control and this helped him to feel that he was a significant person and that the staff cared about him and respected his ideas and life style.

Nutritional Counseling: Evaluation

The client and nurse constantly evaluate the diet and its effects. The client may express his or her feelings about the goals. The nurse may have some very concrete measurements of evaluation, such as the ratio of fluid intake and output, hemoglobin values, blood pressure readings, or weight gains and losses. Sharing of these specific measurements with the client is helpful in evaluating mutual goals and in the teaching and counseling of the client about the disease process as well as a diet modification to achieve the desired outcomes.

It is important that the goals be evaluated when the client is ready and has time. The client in a hospital often is very busy, attending to own personal care, which may be very time-consuming because of energy limitations; having many diagnostic tests and procedures; visiting with family and friends; resting; thinking and worrying about future decisions; and adapting to the many hospital staff members involved in the care giving. The client at home or in a school, industry, and long-term care facility may have similar activities and concerns. Therefore, the nurse should contract with the client for an appropriate time to talk about the goals of dietary modifications. Even though the client may agree to a specific time (e.g., after lunch or after talking with the physician), he or she may not be ready at that time to evaluate progress in the goal of dietary modification. In Nutritional Counseling the nurse should listen to the present concerns and help relate these to the established goals. It may be that the nurse may need to restate the purpose of the contract, which was to evaluate the goals related to diet modification. The feeling tones are important to evaluate. The client may feel that he or she has failed in reaching the desired goal or that now it appears to be impossible. Sometimes the nurse may have to express these feelings for the client and review the accomplishments that have been achieved. It is possible also that at this point that the client feels that these dietary changes will be too difficult for the family as they conflict with their usual diets. It may mean a new way of cooking for just one person.

In evaluating the feelings and concerns about goal achievement in diet modification, assessment begins again, and goals may be changed as both the client and nurse have more data about the situation. Clients may request consultation with other team members so they and their families may understand the desired outcomes. Or the nurse may suggest a conference with family members so that possible nutrition resources may be explored. Owing to the pressure of early discharge from hospitals, the nurse must anticipate which goals may be most difficult and share the fact with the client that change is difficult.

Evaluation takes time and is an ongoing process. Both the nurse and client should share in measuring goal achievement. Some nurses review the care plan with the client daily; others have checklists that they use when they make client rounds. Some community agencies have record forms for specific conditions that enable nurses to evaluate goals with the client.

Many persons influence the nutritional status of the client and family. Hence, it may benefit all to have an evaluation conference. This could allow for the analysis of common goals, shared leadership, the merging of resources, and the establishing of collaborative relationships in which roles are interchangeable (Freeman and Heinrich, 1981). As a result, the dietitian may instruct the client in the hospital to determine how to improve the palatability of the diet, or the nurse may instruct the client and family in specific alterations in diet. The health team may make referrals to each other or to appropriate agencies and consultants for after discharge.

CASE STUDIES
Case Study 1

Jane, a 23 year old secretary, is pregnant; her husband Bill, age 25 years, is a graduate student. Their income is limited and their work schedules have helped them develop a habit of skipping meals, especially breakfast. Jane's lunch is often a diet drink and a snack such as cheese and crackers from the vending machines.

On Jane's visit to the prenatal clinic her blood pressure was 170/90 and her hemoglobin was 10 g/dl, weight was 135 pounds, and height 72 inches. She told the nurse "this baby was a surprise." On the second clinic visit Jane had lost 10 pounds. The other laboratory values were the same as on the first visit. The clinic nurse in reviewing the eating pattern of the family, learned they did not like to drink milk.

You are the clinic nurse with these available data. What is your nursing diagnosis? How would you implement and evaluate the following nursing care plan?

Nursing Diagnoses

○ Alteration in Nutrition, Less than Body Requirements: low iron and calcium intake and weight loss.

○ Ineffective Family Coping: unplanned pregnancy.

Nutritional Counseling

1. Explore with Jane and Bill their daily living routines and how they spend their time.

Goals. (a) Jane will go to bed by 11:00 P.M. and set the alarm for 6:30 A.M. so there will be time to eat breakfast. (b) Jane will pack lunch in the evening while Bill washes the dishes. (c) They will spend at least 30 minutes each evening talking to each other about their plans so both short-term and long-term goals may be clarified.

2. Explore their eating habits: food likes and dislikes of both Jane and Bill; when and how grocery shopping is done; discuss the selections of food in the vending machine with Jane.

Goals. (a) Bill and Jane will keep a 24 hour food diary for one week, noting all snacks. (b) Jane will eat at least one food high in calcium each day. (c) Jane will eat at least one iron-rich food each day (a list of these foods to be supplied). (d) Jane and Bill will plan a menu for one week, making sure that all of the basic food groups are included. (e) Jane and Bill will shop after dinner on Friday night utilizing the grocery list based on the menus for the week. (f) Jane and Bill will shop for groceries only once a week. (g) Jane will limit her use of the vending machine to once a day, and will choose a food that is high in calcium (yogurt) or iron (raisins).

3. Discuss and inform them about resources: financial, nutrition, parenting groups.

Goals. (1) Jane and Bill will develop a food budget. (b) They will talk with a nutritionist at the clinic so nutrition resources such as supplemental programs for women, infants, and children (WIC) can be evaluated. (c) They will review the pamphlets on nutrition given them at the clinic before the next clinic visit. (d) They will telephone the Health Department to obtain information about prenatal classes. (e) Jane will ask her friends at work about their Lamaze experience and call the instructor for information about the class, etc. (f) Bill will explore the health benefits of their health insurance regarding clinic visits, hospitalization, and home visits by community health nurses. (g) Bill and Jane will determine if they desire a referral to the consultants available, such as the social worker, family counselor, or other professional persons.

Case Study 2

Blanche is a 62 year old widow with 14 living children. The youngest is a 21 year old son who lives at home and is unemployed. Blanche was a cook in the local nursing home until deteriorating vision limited her reading of recipes. She is a diabetic who is insulin-dependent and weighs 200 pounds. Her height is 62 inches. She was hospitalized for five days for cataract extraction. During this time she worried about how she would manage on discharge and how her youngest son was managing at home.

From these data what are the possible nursing diagnoses? Identify possible goals Blanche would desire. Identify goals the nurse in the hospital might have. Identify mutual goals that Blanche and the community health nurse might reach.

Nursing Diagnosis

○ Alterations in Nutrition, More than Body Requirements
○ Sensory Deficit due to cataracts
○ Self-Care Deficit due to vision limitation and limited mobility due to obesity
○ Knowledge Deficit of disease process of diabetes
○ Alteration in Parenting
○ Home Maintenance Management Impaired

Nutritional Counseling

Blanche's Goals:
1. Be able to read again.
2. Lose 50 pounds so she could move about better.
3. Be able to go to work again.
4. Help her children with their problems.

Hospital Nurse's Goals for Blanche:
1. Be able to do self-care.
2. Be able to instill own eye drops.
3. Improve understanding of her diabetic regimens demonstrated by
   (a) Proper filling of syringe.
   (b) Using appropriate injection technique.
   (c) Rotating sites of injection.
   (d) Checking urine each morning.
   (e) Wearing shoes when walking around room.
   (f) Evaluating her menu by using the ADA materials.
   (g) Talking with the diabetic nurse specialist and dietitian.
   (h) Attending the group sessions on diabetes.
4. Discuss her worries and concerns about her family.
5. Accept a referral to the community health nurse upon discharge.

Mutual Goals of Blanche and Community Health Nurse:
1. Be able to manage her daily living activities in her home.
2. Be able to control her diabetes and infections by following the foot care recommendations and wearing shoes.
3. Be able to cope with family crises.
4. Follow a weight reduction regime.
5. Follow the cataract care regimen by keeping appointments with optician and physician.
6. Be able to cope with the financial needs.
7. Participate in the Diabetic Association monthly meetings.
8. Utilize transportation resources.

The attainment of nursing goals depends on the nurse-client relationship and will take time. Therefore, a nurse should contract with the client about a convenient time for visits or conferences. The nurse should assess the readiness of the client to modify past dietary habits; he or she should also be aware of the client's past experiences and respect the client's knowledge. For example, Blanche has much knowledge of cooking for large groups and her work experience would have given her knowledge of modifying menus to meet specific alterations. In evaluating and assessing the nursing care goals, the strengths of the clients should be emphasized and the weaknesses identified. When the client accepts these areas of weakness and wants to change, mutual goals are the result. The client controls the rate of change, but the nurse should help to remove those barriers that negate change. Some of the modifications of the diet may be the attitudes and feelings of other family members; therefore, the nurse might involve the family members in helping the client with shopping and food preparation. The dietary change may be a costly one, so the client should have the benefit of consultation with appropriate resource persons. The assistance of a home maker might be helpful. From these examples it is apparent that nutritional counseling is very complex. The nurse must be knowledgeable about nutrition and human behavior, for each client is unique and different.

EDITORS' COMMENTS AND QUESTIONS

Nutritional Counseling has long been a role of the nurse. In the past the nurse was directly involved in selection and preparation of food for clients. Today, the nurse is involved primarily in feeding problems and in assisting the client to make good decisions concerning nutritional intake. Busse emphasizes that the assessment of nutritional problems is a complex process because of the importance of food and personal appearance in our culture. As Nutritional Counseling is a basic intervention appropriate for the beginning student, this chapter is written in a manner appropriate for the undergraduate nursing student.

Questions for Discussion

1. *How does the role of the nurse differ from that of the dietitian in Nutritional Counseling?*

2. *Discuss the importance of team planning in Nutritional Counseling.*

3. *How can the family be included in Nutritional Counseling?*

4. *How can nursing contribute to research in this area?*

References

Egan, G. *The skilled helper.* Monterey, Calif.: Brook/Cole Publishing Company, 1981.

Flanney, C. *A diet for every foible.* Iowa City, Iowa: *Press Citizen* (newspaper), April 27, 1983.

Freeman R., and Heinrich, J. *Community health nursing practice.* Philadelphia: W. B. Saunders Company, 1981.

Goodhart, T., and Shils, M.: *Modern nutrition in health and disease,* (6th Ed.). Philadelphia: Lea and Febiger, 1980.

Horsley. J., Crane J., and Haller, K. B. *Reducing diarrhea in tube-fed patients: CURN project.* New York, Grune & Stratton, 1981.

Howard, R. B., and Herbold, N. H. *Nutrition in clinical care.* New York: McGraw-Hill Book Company, 1978.

Leahy, K., Cobb, M., and Jones M. *Community health nursing.* New York: McGraw-Hill Book Company, 1982.

Mason, M., and Wenberg, B. G. and Welsh, P. K. *The dynamics of clinical dietetics.* New York: John Wiley and Sons, 1977.

Pender, N. J. *Health promotion in nursing practice.* Norwalk, Conn.: Appleton-Century-Crofts, 1982.

Robinson, C., and Lawler, M. *Normal and therapeutic nutrition.* New York: Macmillan, 1977.

Strauss, A. *Chronic illness and quality of life.* St. Louis: C. V. Mosby, 1975.

Spradley, B. (Ed.) *Readings in community health nursing.* Boston: Little, Brown and Company, 1982.

U.S. Department of Agriculture. *Nutritive value of foods,* Bulletin 72, Home and Garden. Washington, D.C.: U.S. Printing Office, 1972.

Veninga, K. S. Nutrition assessment: A guide for community nurses. In B. Spradley (Ed.), *Readings in community health nursing*. Boston: Little, Brown and Company, 1982.

Walike, B. C., and Walike, J. W. Lactose content of tube feeding diets as a cause of diarrhea. *Laryngoscope*, 1973, *83*:1109–1115.

Walike, B. C., and Walike, J. W. Relative lactose intolerance. *Journal of the American Medical Association*, 1977, *238*:948–951.

Walike, B. C., Padilla, G., Bergstrom, N., Hanson, R. L., Kubo, W., Grant, M., and Wong, H. L. Patient problems related to tube feeding. In M. V. Batey (Ed.). *Communicating nursing research* (vol. 7). Boulder, Colo.: WICHE, 1975.

Williams, S. R. *Nutrition and diet therapy*. St. Louis: C. V. Mosby, 1977.

Yen, P. K. *How to Cook for One or Two . . . and Enjoy It. Geriatric Nursing*, March/April 1983, pp. 115–118.

Zifferblatt, S. M., and Wilbur, C. S.: Dietary counseling: Some realistic expectations and guidelines. *Journal of the American Dietetic Association*, 1977, *70*, 591.

Appendix 8–1. NUTRITIONAL COUNSELING REFERENCES*

Andrew, B. J. Interviewing and counseling skills. *Journal of the American Dietetic Association*, 1975, *66*, 576.

Beaton, G. H. Evaluation of nutrition intervention: Methodologic considerations. *American Journal Clinical Nutrition*, 1982, *35*, 1280.

Becker, M. H., and Maiman, L. A.: Sociobehavioral determinants of compliance with health and medical care recommendations. *Medical Care*, 1975, *8*, 10.

Becker, M. H., Maiman, L. A., Kirscht, J. P., Haefner, D. P., and Drachman, R. H. The health belief model and prediction of dietary compliance: A field experiment. *Journal Health and Social Behavior*, 1977, *18*, 348.

Danish, S. J. Developing helping relationships in dietetic counseling. *Journal of the American Dietetic Association*, 175, *67*, 107.

Danish, S. J., Ginsberg, M. R., Terrell, A., Hammond, M. I., and Adams, S. O. The anatomy of a dietetic counseling interview. *Journal of the American Dietetic Association*, 1979, *75*, 626.

Dunbar, J. M., and Stunkard, A. J. Adherence to diet and drug regimen. *In* R. Levy, B. Rifkind, B. Dennis, and N. Ernest (Eds.), *Nutrition, lipids, and coronary heart disease*. New York: Raven Press, 1979.

Evans, R. J., and Hall, Y. Social-psychologic perspective in motivating changes in eating behavior. *Journal of the American Dietetic Association*, 1978, *72*, 378.

Ferguson, J. Dietitians as behavior-change agents. *Journal of the American Dietetic Association*, 1978, *72*, 231.

Fiedler, K. M., Beach, B. L., and Hayman, J. Dietetic performance evaluation: Establishment of validity and reliability. *Journal of the American Dietetic Association*, 1981, *78*, 149.

Glanz, K. Strategies for nutrition counseling. *Journal of the American Dietetic Association*, 1979, *74*, 431.

Glanz, K. Dietitians' effectiveness and patient compliance with dietary regimens. *Journal of the American Dietetic Association*, 1979, *75*, 631.

Glanz, K. Compliance with dietary regimens: Its magnitude, measurements and determinants. *Preventive Medicine*, 1980, *9*, 787.

Haefner, D. P., and Kirscht, J. P. Motivational and behavioral effects of modifying health beliefs. *Public Health Reports*, 1970, *85*, 478.

Hirsch, E. Z., Benassi, R., Liddle, L., and Rogers, P. An interdisciplinary clinical training program for dietitians. *Journal of the American Dietetic Association*, 1977, *70*, 149.

Laquatra, I., and Danish, S. J. Effect of helping skills transfer program on dietitians' helping behavior. *Journal of the American Dietetic Association*, 1981, *78*, 22.

Ling, L., Spragg, D., Stein, P., and Myers, M. L. Guidelines for diet counseling. *Journal of the American Dietetic Association*, 1975, *66*, 571.

Mahoney, M. J., and Caggiula, A. W. Applying behavioral methods to nutritional counseling. *Journal of the American Dietetic Association*, 1978, *73*, 372.

Mason, M., Wenberg, B. G., and Welsh, P. K. *The dynamics of clinical dietetics*. New York: John Wiley & Sons, 1982.

Model workshop on nutrition counseling in hyperlipidemia. NIH Publication No. 80-1666. Washington, D.C.: U.S. Government Printing Office, 1980.

Rosenstock, I. M. The health belief model and nutrition education. *Journal of the Canadian Dietetic Association*, 1982, *43*, 184.

Wylie, J., and Singer, J. Growth process in nutrition counseling. *Journal of the American Association*, 1976, *69*, 505.

Zifferblatt, S. M. Increasing patient compliance through the applied analysis of behavior. *Preventive Medicine*, 1975, *4*, 173.

*Developed by Dietary Department, at University of Iowa Hospitals and Clinics, Iowa City, Iowa 52242.

9

SEXUAL COUNSELING

KARLENE M. KERFOOT
KATHLEEN C. BUCKWALTER

Historically, nurses have not had the right or ability to use sexual counseling as an intervention when working with clients. Nurses were not taught sexual content or even information about the reproductive functioning of males and females in schools of nursing. Nurses lived cloistered lives in nursing dormitories under the close supervision of matrons and were admonished from wearing any apparel or jewelry that hinted of sexuality. They were to create a chaste, modest, and asexual image of the profession.

The publication of Masters and Johnson's work in the late 1960s contributed to legitimizing counseling in the area of sexuality. Masters and Johnson's work (1966) provided the first valid and well-researched information about sexuality on which to build clinical practice. Their publications made sexuality an appropriate area of research for health professionals. It was not until the early 1970s, however, that the first substantial publications on sexuality appeared in the nursing literature.

In addition to Masters and Johnson's work, the changing role of women also affirmed sexuality as an area of study and practice for nurses. Prior to the women's movement of the 1970s, the predominant cultural beliefs were that women were to be naive about sexuality and that information about sexuality was to be vested in the men of the culture. Consequently, male physicians could discuss sexuality with the patient, but female nurses could not. The women's movement has made significant strides in allowing both men and women access to information about sexuality. Virginia Johnson was a pioneer among women researching in the field of sexuality.

Schools of nursing began to add specific material in the area of human sexuality in the 1970s, although this content varied greatly. Most schools presented content on reproductive biology, and some included lectures on various aspects of sexuality, whereas a few others added electives in sexuality. Still others with integrated curriculums threaded content on sexuality throughout the various educational levels. However, very few schools of nursing offered a broadly based curriculum with sufficient depth to prepare their graduates to function effectively as sexual counselors.

Practice settings also vary in the latitude they provide nurses to intervene with clients having sexual problems. Whether or not Sexual Counseling is a valid nursing intervention is often controversial. In some settings, if nurses make a commitment to holistic care of clients and become involved in obtaining sexual histories and providing sex education and counseling, they are stigmatized as being sexually immoral or overinterested in sexuality to the exclusion of other aspects of patient care.

In many practice settings defining who has the right to discuss sexuality with patients is an issue. In settings where nurses act as handmaidens of physicians, they cannot discuss sexuality with clients without the express permission of the physician. In settings where a more collaborative model is practiced, counseling about sexuality is seen as something that is shared among health professionals. The easiest solution to this problem is allowing the person who is the best prepared in sexual counseling and best able to establish therapeutic relationships with patients to be responsible for meeting the client's needs for sexual information.

The 1980s have thus far been a period of economic retrenchment that has affected schools of nursing and practice settings. Just when counseling about sexuality was coming to be an accepted part of nursing practice, economic considerations have dictated shorter working weeks and even layoffs for nurses in some parts of the country. In some cases, schools of nursing have eliminated course content in sexuality. Consequently, sexual counseling frequently is seen as a luxury that the school cannot afford to teach and the practice setting cannot support. This development is unfortunate, because without adequate sexual counseling many people will be troubled or uncomfortable and suffer great disruption to their self-esteem.

This chapter will discuss Sexual Counseling by briefly reviewing nursing assessment as it pertains to sexuality and will provide an overview of the nurse's role in sexual counseling.

NURSING ASSESSMENTS OF SEXUALITY

It is often difficult for professionals to ask the probing questions that are necessary to obtain accurate data about sexual functioning on which to base nursing interventions. There are many reasons for this. The ones commonly expressed by health professionals are: (1) feeling uncomfortable invading a very private portion of people's lives, (2) lack of knowledge of the techniques of asking questions about sexuality, and (3) lack of knowledge of the sexual consequences of many drugs and illnesses. These three areas will be discussed briefly in this section.

The first problem, invasion of the sexual privacy of clients, can be a concern for clients, but in many instances is more the nurse's problem. Many clients expect that health professionals will ask questions about sexuality and are surprised when the nurse does not. For example, a 59 year old man with depression was being interviewed by a nurse in a mental health center. When she initiated a discussion about sexuality and depression he responded by saying:

> I was wondering when you would ask me questions about sexuality. I didn't know how to start talking about it, but I knew that you would get around to it. It's a good thing you people are trained to talk about sex. It sure makes it easier for me.

If nurses actually believe that sexuality is a natural, everyday part of life, they will accept the fact that in order to provide appropriate nursing care, they must put as much emphasis on sexuality as on nutrition, activities of daily living, and other facets of a client's existence. Workshops on sexuality and sexual reassessment can help the nurse overcome feelings of unease about asking personal questions (de Lemos, 1977).

The second problem, lack of knowledge about the techniques of interviewing, can be overcome by education. Workshops that provide the learner with an opportunity for role-playing can be very helpful. A few techniques can aid the nurse when obtaining a sexual assessment. Green (1975) has suggested some practices to assist in discussions of sexuality with clients. We have modified these to be specific for nursing interventions, as follows:

1. When the counseling relationship is initiated, the nurse needs to tell the client that sexuality is an important part of life and that illness, medications, and stress (or whatever other problems the client is experiencing) often alter sexual functioning.

2. As the interview proceeds, tell the client that questions about sexual functioning will be asked and the interviewer will be prepared to answer any questions that come to mind about sexuality.

3. Preface questions about sexuality with a statement that tells the client that many people experience what you are about to discuss with them. For example:

> "Many people feel uncomfortable discussing sexuality. . . ."
> "Many people with colostomies wonder about how this operation will affect sexual functioning."
> "Many people using hypertensive medication have questions about the effect of this drug on potency."
> "Most people have some sexual difficulties sometime during their marital relationship."

The interviewer can then go on to ask questions about sexuality because he or she has clearly indicated that sexual problems in response to illness are common, and that the interviewer is prepared to discuss these.

4. Begin with the least sensitive topics and proceed to the more sensitive. Most clients will discuss highly personal sexual matters with the nurse only after a trust relationship has been established and after the nurse has proved herself or himself as a competent professional. The nurse interviewer can earn this respect by starting with nonthreatening information and then proceeding to more difficult topics. Both the interviewer and the client can remain more comfortable if this rule is maintained.

5. Summarize the interview at the conclusion to help the client to learn from the summary. It is also the time to ask if the client has further questions and to set the stage for later interviews by stating that the counselor will be glad to answer any questions and will be discussing other aspects of sexuality in future encounters.

The third problem, lack of knowledge of the ways illness and drugs may affect sexuality, has recently become easier to solve. Masters and Johnson's monumental work on the human sexual response cycle (1966) is the best place for nurses to begin acquiring cognitive skills. When knowledge of the anatomy and physiology of the normal sexual response has been mastered, nurses are then ready to become familiar with the deviations in sexuality that frequently affect clients in their particular nursing specialty. Textbooks are not the best source. Specialty journals, however, often have articles on specific illnesses and sexual functioning. For example, the journals *Sexuality and Disability* and *Medical Aspects of Human Sexuality* are excellent sources of articles on specific sexually related topics. It should be noted that more information is available about male sexual functioning than female with regard to specific alterations, as to date more research has been done with males than with females.

Information about sexuality and drugs is sometimes more difficult to find. The *Physician's Desk Reference* will often include a notation that a particular drug has been associated with male sexual problems and more rarely will include information about the effects of medication on the sexual functioning of females. Pharmacology textbooks are another source of information, as are practitioners in the field.

In addition to the professional literature, nurses should be aware of information in the lay literature. Clients often inquire about articles in popular magazines that discuss sexuality; if the nurse is aware of this information, he or she is in an excellent position to confirm the accuracy of the information or discredit a highly sensationalized or misinformed article.

Although the techniques of managing a sexual assessment can be learned fairly easily, the problem frequently lies in deciding what questions to ask in a sexual assessment. This decision rests largely with factors in the professional environment that determine what should and should not be included in the assessment. However, at a minimum, information about the following areas should be included and obtained from the assessment: (1) effect of illness on sexuality, (2) effect of medication on sexuality, (3) effect of changes in sexuality on significant others, and (4) knowledge level of the client about sexuality in general.

NURSING DIAGNOSES AND INTERVENTIONS IN SEXUALITY

Of the nursing diagnoses accepted by the Fourth National Conference, almost all have implications for changes in sexuality. Several diagnoses have obvious sexual implications, such as Rape-Trauma Syndrome and Sexual Dysfunction; both of these diagnoses have specific interventions that have been identified and are being researched at the present time (Burgess and Holmstrom, 1974; Masters and Johnson, 1966). However, the application of sexual counseling to other diagnoses is more subtle. In order to begin conceptualizing how sexuality relates to nursing diagnoses, let us first discuss the sequelae of these diagnoses and their effects on sexuality.

Many of the accepted diagnoses on the National Conference List imply hospitalization of the client. Hospitalization in and of itself can alter sexuality and cause either transient or permanent changes. Hospitalization for something as simple as an appendectomy has been implicated in changes in sexuality. Whenever there is a cessation of usual patterns of sexual activity for a period of time, problems with sexual functioning can appear. For example, after the death of a spouse, sexual activities normally are interrupted for a period of time while grieving is completed. When the widow (widower) chooses to resume sexual activities, he or she may find that nothing works as well as it did previously and anxiety or depression may develop. It is very normal for a period of adjustment to occur following interruption of sexual activities before the usual pattern can be resumed. Men may have transitory problems with impotence or premature ejaculation and women can experience problems with lubrication or achieving orgasm. This adjustment period is normal and nothing to be alarmed about. However, some clients become unduly anxious, which further damages their chances of reestablishing usual sexual practices. Clients need to know that even transitory bouts of illness, such as the reactivation of an ulcer, gallbladder problems, or life changes, such as divorce or the birth of a baby, can affect sexual functioning. The client can be reassured that these changes will be transitory unless they choose to allow themselves to become overly alarmed.

Clients who have experienced severe, even life-threatening diagnoses, such as Alterations in Cardiac Output, often become fearful that the resumption of sexual activities following the acute phase of the illness will precipitate further complications and perhaps death. Persons who have had a heart attack or a cerebrovascular accident often believe that (1) sexual activities might have caused their problems, or (2) that resumption of sexual activities will cause further harm to their conditions. Significant others often share similar beliefs and will therefore fail to initiate sexual activities or will refuse to participate if initiated by the partner. These clients are often left with lowered sexual self-esteem because of their physical condition, and it is important for the nurse to give them factual information about resumption of sexual activities. The nurse must not only clarify with the client what is and is not allowed, but he or she must also discuss this matter with the client's significant others so that both the clients and their partners have some understanding of the situation.

Other nursing diagnoses imply permanent changes in established sexual activities. For example, Self-Care Deficits that can accompany the onset of multiple sclerosis, arthritis, low-back pain, spinal cord trauma, and morbid obesity, to name a few conditions, suggest that there will probably be actual physical changes in sexual expression necessitated by the illness itself. For these types of problems, clients and their significant others need to find alternative forms of sexual expression that are acceptable to their sexual lifestyle.

Finally, some clients use illness or change in some part of their life as a reason to alter their sexual behaviors. These people have usually been uncomfortable with their sexuality and find that surgery or illness is an excuse they can use to cease their former activities. For example, clients who have had hysterectomies or prostate surgery may tell their spouses that the doctor informed them that further sexual activities might be harmful, and that they are forbidden to have sexual intercourse. The nursing diagnosis of Coping, Ineffectual Individual might be applied to clients in this situation. The problems of these clients are deep-seated and complicated. A highly skilled nurse therapist with advanced preparation in the areas of sexuality and psychotherapy would be appropriate for intervening with this kind of coping problem.

SEXUAL COUNSELING

Sexual Counseling needs to be differentiated from Sexual Therapy as a nursing intervention. Sexual Counseling is defined as the assessment and use of techniques that the graduate professional nurse should be able to use competently with clients, such as active listening, encouraging effective coping mechanisms, use of humor, early intervention, reinforcement of healthy sexual practices, permission giving, including significant others, and the identification of medications and health deviations that may affect sexuality and body image. Sexual Therapy is defined as activities requiring specialized training that focus on specific sexual disorders, such as impotence and orgasmic dysfunction, or on complicated client problems involving sexuality. The issue of who is qualified to do these interventions is a very difficult problem because the nursing profession has not delineated levels of practice either generally or specifically for sexual interventions.

Watts (1979) proposes two levels of interventions that would correspond to this chapter's definitions of Sexual Counseling and Sexual Therapy. According to Watts, a registered nurse should be able to screen for sexual functioning and to use limited Sexual Counseling, which consists of information about sexual feelings, behaviors, and myths. Only registered nurses with advanced training in sex education and counseling should provide Sexual Therapy, and nurses working at the level of Sexual Counseling need to know when it is appropriate to refer clients to more specialized and highly trained practitioners.

Types of Counseling

Nurses have accepted responsibility for the counseling of clients in a variety of settings and with a variety of health promotion and illness topics. However, counseling about sexuality has been a more recent function within the nursing profession. There are two types of counseling that nurses can use: (1) counseling about sexuality that focuses on the normal activities of everyday living, and (2) counseling about the specific alterations in health that the client is experiencing and their effect on sexuality.

Most nurses would agree that health professionals have an obligation to prevent future problems. This obligation should also apply to the sexual health of clients. If clients can be knowledgeable about healthy sexual practices, many sexual dysfunctions and psychological traumas would be avoided. As an example of counseling about healthy sexuality, one can cite sexual myths that remain common in our society. These myths often contribute to a lack of understanding of healthy sexuality and prevent clients from realizing their full potential. For example, there are many myths about masturbation in our culture. Whereas other cultures accept it as a healthy sexual response, it is not uncommon for clients to feel guilty about this sexual practice and to fear that masturbation may have brought their present problem. Many clients who are having urological surgery, for example, have discussed the possibility that masturbation had contributed to their illness.

Sexual activities are probably one of the greatest sources of guilt in our culture. Because our society is relatively conservative in what we sanction sexually, many clients experience sexual guilt. Sexual practices have, in the minds of some clients, been responsible for everything from acne (masturbation as the causative factor) to cervical or prostatic cancer (extramarital affairs or refusal to participate in sexual activities with a partner). Many clients see illness as punishment for sexual sins. It is, therefore, imperative to assess the amount of sexual guilt associated with a client's perception of the causative factors of his or her illness.

Sexual Counseling often serves to alleviate sexual guilt, but nurses can clear up misconceptions only after clients disclose their beliefs. Some clients need referrals to clergy for help in dealing with guilt, and still others require referrals to psychotherapists to help solve the problem. The nurse needs to make an accurate assessment of the depth of the client's guilt feelings and of her own skills in this area.

One thing the nurse should not do in situations of sexual guilt is to offer premature reassurance. Although the client's sexual guilt might seem unreasonable to the nurse, it is very real to the client. It is imperative that the nurse not prematurely terminate discussion of these feelings by lightly brushing it aside with comments such as: "But it wasn't your fault. You couldn't help it. I don't believe you did anything wrong, and neither should you."

Nurses can reinforce healthy sexual practices by (1) determining the particular developmental age of the client and (2) discussing concerns that are common to that developmental stage. For example, when working with elderly clients, the nurse might suspect concerns about sexual functioning as related to the aging process. The nurse could approach the elderly client in a manner similar to this:

> Many people I have worked with have some concerns about sexuality as they grow older. They believe that additional years signal an end to their sexual activities. Unfortunately many myths are prevalent in our culture about the aging process and sexuality. How have the passing years affected your sexuality?

From that broad opening statement, the nurse can go on to gather and provide information that is accurate and research-based whenever the client identifies myths and misinformation.

This approach can be used with any age group. The basic concept is that the nurse makes an assessment about the client's understanding of the normal developmental tasks expected at their level, and then provides additional information as needed in an effort to counter any myths and misinformation the client holds. It must be recognized that some people cling to beliefs that are necessary to maintain themselves in their particular lifestyle or culture. The framework from which myths evolve must also be considered.

The second type of counseling is that associated with altered sexuality as a result of health deviations. The effect of medication and the effect of the illness on sexuality are two areas in which the nurse can intervene.

Many medications have side effects that alter sexuality. Clients react in a variety of ways to this problem. If clients do not know that the medication is responsible for the alteration, they will personalize the experience and feel that there is something wrong with them. Failure experiences can often lead to permanent sexual dysfunctions. The psychological damage from such a situation can be devastating. If the client suspects that the medication is responsible for sexual alterations, one recourse might be to avoid taking the medication altogether. It is very difficult for many clients to admit to the nurse that they have discontinued taking their medication because of its side-effects on sexual function. Consequently, more commonly clients simply do not reveal that they have discontinued the medication. If the nurse is not aware of this problem and fails to make an assessment of noncompliance as a result of sexual side-effects, the treatment regimen often appears to be failing for unknown reasons.

Nurses can effectively discuss the possible sexual side-effects of medications with clients and make accurate assessments of the effect of drugs on the client. If the sexual side-effects are intolerable, often another drug can be substituted or a different administration schedule arranged. Usually some alternative drug is available so the client can tolerate medication.

Counseling about the effects of illness on sexuality needs to be included with any plan of nursing care. If this responsibility is not met, several things can occur:

1. If clients do not realize that the alteration is a product of their illness, they might personalize the problem and blame themselves for the sexual alteration, which can be psychologically damaging.

2. If clients are not educated about alternative forms of sexual expression, they are denied a part of life that many people with various forms of illness have learned to enjoy.

3. Relationships are often disturbed if clients cannot work out suitable sexual arrangements after an injury or illness. This can lead to divorce, extramarital relationships, and failure to communicate, which could be avoided in many instances if nurses would take the responsibility of intervening with educational content appropriate to the client's health state.

For example, a newly diagnosed male diabetic client had been experiencing problems with impotence for six months before his diagnosis was made. During the medical and nursing assessments, no one questioned him about the possible sexual consequences of diabetes. Therefore, he continued to feel inadequate about his sexual performance and became very depressed that he could no longer satisfy his wife sexually. She also felt sexually inadequate and thought that her husband no longer found her attractive. It wasn't until they moved to another town and were seen by a nurse practitioner in practice with internists that the client discovered that his impotence was part of the disease process associated with diabetes. With the help of the nurse practitioner, he and his wife learned new ways of giving each other sexual pleasure, and the marriage survived. Potentially destructive situations such as this can be avoided if nurses use the intervention of sexual counseling with their clients.

Techniques of Counseling

The following section describes several techniques nurses may use in the process of counseling.

Listening is probably one of the most undervalued aspects of Sexual Counseling. Often clients can work through many problems if they have access to an empathetic listener, one who can, simply through being there, help the client explore their difficulties and to develop their own interventions. Empathetic listening does not mean that the nurse sits in silence. Rather, he or she is an active listener who guides the client through the steps of problem-solving as it becomes appropriate. With the use of empathetic listening, clients can become comfortable with discussions of sexuality, and learn how to discuss their particular sexual needs with significant others.

Sexual counseling *with significant others* also involves giving information. This consists of making sure that the family member has been exposed to the same amount of sexual information as the client. There are many examples of situations in which the client was given information about sexuality and the family member was not. For example, wives of clients with cardiac disorders who have been excluded from sexual counseling have often been reluctant to initiate intercourse because of fear of precipitating another heart attack (Harding and Morefield, 1976). Consequently, because of ignorance, a family member cannot reinforce the new information learned by the client. In another example, a male client with impotence caused by the peripheral neuropathy of diabetes was given information about satisfying his wife by means other than intercourse. His wife was not included in this discussion and totally misunderstood her husband's insistence on participating in sexual activities she considered inappropriate. Clients need to be given sexual information within the context of what is appropriate for them. Therefore, it is imperative that the spouse or sexual partner be included in this type of counseling.

Changes in sexuality due to developmental processes, medications, surgeries, divorce, and a variety of other experiences can cause a *change in body image*. It is virtually impossible to experience a change in body image without also experiencing a change in perception of oneself as a sexual person. Just as with any loss, alterations in body image may be accompanied by mourning and grief. Nurses can assist clients who are experiencing alterations in sexuality based on changes in body image by helping them to express their grief and anger. Positive role models of other clients who have successfully conquered similar problems are effective when the client is ready for this kind of help. Nurses can also intervene by dispelling myths and misconceptions about what changes in body image actually mean. For example, many women have a distorted image of the changes they will experience after a hysterectomy. With correct information, many clients can come to better accept their alterations in body functioning. It is important that the nurse does not reinforce the client's lowered self-esteem. If the nurse nonverbally displays aversion to the sight of a burn, for example, the client may feel that perhaps he or she can never be accepted sexually. Counseling with significant others is critical in helping the client overcome problems with body image. The sexual partner may also need help in dispelling myths and misconceptions, and perhaps also in determining alternative expressions of sexuality. If a loss or mutilation of a body part is involved, the nurse needs to intervene so that the sexual partner does not display aversion to the change. The following case history illustrates a typical response to loss of a body part.

Case History

In a farm accident, a 45 year old male store owner experienced an amputation of his arm just below the right shoulder joint. Six months later, he spoke of the frustrations of meeting physical demands and his depression while adjusting to using his nondominant hand for all activities: "We did not resume sexual activity for about two to three weeks after I was discharged to home and at first I had some problem with impotence. I had been told by the nurse at the hospital that it might be normal to lose interest in sexuality and sexual intercourse for quite some time after the accident and not to be concerned about it. The impotence did concern me for a while but we were able to resume sexual relationships and as the nurse told me, my problems with impotence have ceased. I was very protective of my arm at first and there was some pain, both phantom and real, at the incision because of pressure, and I know that my wife had a very hard time adjusting to the fact that the arm was gone. There were times when I know she was trying to keep from crying when we were hugging and caressing and it has taken her many months to get over those feelings. As far as sexual intercourse we used the female dominant position for many months after resuming sexual activity. The nurse had suggested we try some positions that might be more comfortable than the traditional male dominant one. Once in a while we would have sexual relationships facing each other on our sides but because I'm a bit overweight, this was difficult to do sometimes." (Buckwalter, Wernimont, and Buckwalter, 1982, p. 204)

Whenever a person suffers a significant assault to physical or emotional health, he or she can better survive to lead a productive and satisfying life if able to make sense out of the event and utilize *effective coping mechanisms* that will place the event in proper perspective. Through active listening and discussions, nurses can help clients learn useful coping strategies.

Much of health care focuses on client problems, illnesses, and weaknesses. In order to develop effective coping strategies, clients need help in identifying their strengths and in using whatever behavior patterns helped them adjust to past problems. Family members can also help in identifying those strengths and successful strategies that have been used in the past.

The key to successful client adjustment is the acceptance that things will change but will not necessarily be worse than before. If the client can adopt this attitude, then chances of success in coping with sexual impairment are enhanced. This belief allows clients the freedom to experiment and try new behaviors that their "normal" functioning did not permit them to try in the past. Clients must believe that although their old style of sexual functioning was good, new behaviors can be just as satisfying and acceptable.

Although initially clients may not see anything funny in their condition, *humor* is a tool that can be very helpful when used appropriately. In our culture, sexuality is often approached with extreme seriousness and is not seen as a joyful event. Consequently, this solemn attitude prevails when sexual functioning is disrupted. Humor can be used to release anxiety, can help the client anticipate potential embarrassing problems, and can teach the client to help people laugh with him or her as a way of relieving tension associated with changes in sexual functioning. The following case study illustrates this.

Case History

Sarah was 22 years old when she underwent surgery for an ileostomy for life-threatening bowel disease. The nurse who worked with her before and after surgery was credited by Sarah with helping her cope effectively with the impact of surgery on her sexuality. Prior to her ileostomy, Sarah had been sexually active with several partners. The nurse helped Sarah to see that she could remain sexually active if she so chose. They laughed about the passage of flatus at inopportune times. They enjoyed making a covering for her stoma that said "Make love not war." Sarah adjusted well to her ileostomy, and went on to work with self-help groups of people undergoing similar surgeries.

Humor does not have to be slapstick, joke-telling humor. Quiet laughter and humorous anecdotes are sufficient. Most clients respond well to this, although some, of course, are too afflicted with the gravity of their situation at a particular time to see any humor in the event. The nurse should use good judgment in this regard to determine if humor is appropriate.

The nurse is usually seen as an authority figure with valuable knowledge and training. Clients often look to nurses for validation and reassurance about particular sexual practices. Annon (1976) describes *permission-giving* as a part of Sexual Counseling. Permission-giving can take two forms: (1) permission and reassurance that the sexual practices the client is currently engaged in are appropriate and healthy, and (2) permission to experiment with new forms of sexual expression for sexual enhancement, or to cope with alterations in sexual patterns because of illness or injury.

Given the opportunity, clients will often wish to confirm with the nurse that a particular sexual practice is alright and will cause no harm. Practices such as masturbation, oral-genital sex, and anal intercourse are guilt-provoking for some people and they wish to know if any harm will come to them if they persist in these practices. Nurses need to provide answers to clients based on their sexual lifestyle and needs. Clients who are freed from guilt because they have been provided with appropriate information in a tolerant manner can be helped enormously.

Clients who have experienced alterations in their sexuality because of illness, injury, or drugs respond well if the nurse can provide reassurance and permission to experiment with alternative forms of sexual expression. For example, male patients with spinal cord injuries can be sexually active, but often must utilize alternative forms of sexual stimulation, such as oral-genital sex, to satisfy a partner. If this practice had not been within the sexual lifestyle of the couple, permission to experiment with this form of expression is often useful in helping the couple obtain sexual satisfaction.

Most nurses think of Sexual Counseling in terms of one-to-one situations. However the *use of groups* can often be effective in working with clients about matters of sexuality. Two types of groups can be used. The first is composed of clients who have new changes in sexuality and clients who had previously experienced the same alteration but who have developed positive coping strategies to handle the problems. It can be inspiring when newly impaired clients can see that the injury can be resolved and effective sexual expression developed. The second group is composed of clients who are at similar stages of diagnoses or adjustment. For example, clients with new colostomies can be placed in a group for sexual education and support. This type of group helps the individuals learn to verbalize their problems to people with whom they feel safe. This group is ideal for utilizing techniques of role-playing and self-disclosure as methods to confront problems clients will encounter in the future. Audiovisual aids are particularly useful in group settings. Films and didactic material can be combined effectively with slides and devices appropriate to particular clients, such as vibrators, artificial phalluses, and anatomical models of the reproductive organs (Eisenberg and Rustad, 1976).

Intervening before certain surgeries and procedures can help alleviate the threat to self-esteem that lack of knowledge and lack of control can precipitate. Clients almost always do better if they know what to expect and what options they have to choose from before they are confronted with a crisis situation. For example, Suzie, a 27 year old graduate student, was faced with the decision of having a colostomy because of severe colitis. She adjusted to the surgery well because her primary nurse did a variety of things that allowed Suzie to maintain control throughout the hospitalization and afterward. The nurse discussed what Suzie could expect sexually after the surgery, presented Suzie with hypothetical situations of having to explain to a potential sexual partner about her colostomy, and arranged for Suzie to talk with a former patient who had similar surgery about how she had coped sexually. All of these activities helped Suzie anticipate the surgical process and to feel as if she had options available from which to choose.

Nurses can more effectively intervene if they can anticipate what the client's concerns will be at the onset of an illness or change in lifestyle. Similarly, clients can become more active participants in their care if the nurse can help them to anticipate their future and to develop options that are congruent with their lifestyle.

Much of the work of adjustment to illness or injury occurs following hospitalization. Although not often conceptualized as an intervention, discharge planning and monitoring represent a very important part of nursing care and Sexual Counseling. Problems frequently become more acute after discharge, when the person attempts to return to work and to resume the roles of lover and spouse. If appropriate assessments have been made and realistic family-centered discharge planning attempted, the client can continue to progress at home. Nurses working in hospitals need to know the community well enough to provide appropriate referral sources for the client. Discharge planning forms the basis for future care and effective adjustment.

CONCLUSION

Sexuality is a minimally researched field, and there has been very little nursing research on Sexual Counseling. Sexual Therapy has been better investigated as a result of the work of Masters and Johnson's and others who followed them. Despite the paucity of research, nursing can play a vital role in changing this area. One advantage of examining common practices of nurses with regard to the sexual counseling of clients is that valid research questions can evolve from this type of discussion. For example, what kinds of anticipatory guidance are appropriate for clients undergoing tubal ligations? What is the best way to present educational information about sexuality to a client undergoing coronary artery bypass surgery? Questions like these need to be studied. The future of nursing research in the area of sexuality is an exciting one.

Sexual Counseling as a nursing intervention has been reviewed in this chapter from the perspective of specific assessments and techniques to use with clients who are experiencing potential or actual changes in sexuality. Sexual Counseling is not a luxury—it is a necessity. Many problems can be prevented if nurses can anticipate the sexual sequel of medications and illnesses and help the client cope effectively with these changes.

EDITORS' COMMENTS AND QUESTIONS

Masters and Johnson have legitimized the topic of sexuality for both the public and health professionals. Today's client expects satisfaction from sexual experiences. Two types of Sexual Counseling appear to be appropriate in this relatively new area of nursing practice: (1) counseling about normal sexual patterns, and (2) counseling about specific alterations in sexuality due to an alteration in health. Accurate information in these two areas can alleviate many problems and guilt feelings in clients.

Questions for Discussion

1. Do nurses have adequate sexual knowledge to do Sexual Counseling?

2. Distinguish between Sexual Counseling and Sexual Therapy. Can all nurses do both?

3. What is the role of the family in Sexual Counseling?

4. Do you routinely assess the client's sexual functioning? Why or why not?

5. What diseases and drugs affect sexual functioning?

References

Annon, J. S.: The PLISSIT model: A proposed conceptual scheme for the behavioral treatment of sexual problems. *Journal of Sex Education and Therapy*, 1976, *2*, 1–15.
Buckwalter, K., Wernimont, T., and Buckwalter, J.: Musculo-skeletal conditions and sexuality (part II). *Journal of Sexual Disability*, 1982, *5*, 195–207.
Burgess, A. W., and Holmstrom, L. L.: Crisis and counseling requests of rape victims. *Nursing Research*, 1974, *23*, 196–202.
de Lemos, H.: Changes in helping professionals' knowledge and attitudes following a human sexuality workshop led by a nurse. *Journal of Psychiatric Nursing*, 1977, *15*, 11–21.
Eisenberg, M., and Rustad, L.: Sex education and counseling program on a spinal cord injury service. *Archives of Physical Medicine Rehabilitation*, 1976, *57*, 136–140.
Green, R.: *Human sexuality: A health practitioner's text.* Baltimore, Williams & Wilkins, 1975.
Harding, A., and Morefield, M.: Group intervention for wives of myocardial infarction patients. *Nursing Clinics of North America*, 1976, *11*, 339–347.
Masters, W. H., and Johnson, V. E.: *Human sexual response.* Boston: Little, Brown and Company, 1966.
Watts, R. J.: Dimensions of sexual health. *American Journal of Nursing*, 1979, *79*, 1972.

10

REMINISCENCE THERAPY

DIANE BRONKEMA HAMILTON

DEFINITION OF INTERVENTION

Reminiscence is thinking about or relating past experiences, especially those personally significant (McMahon and Rhudick, 1961). The widespread occurrence of reminiscence in aged persons was perhaps first noted by literary critics familiar with the practice of writing toward the end of the life cycle. Thomas Jefferson, Somerset Maugham, and Flannery O'Connor serve as examples for this viewpoint. Jefferson's friends expected him to begin writing his memoirs when he first retired. Repeatedly he refused. At age 77 Jefferson began his autobiography so information could be passed on to his family (Brodie, 1974). Letters written to John Adams reveal that as Jefferson reminisced he came to believe the pleasures of his life outweighed the pains (Brodie, 1974).

Reminiscence can be oral, written, or silent musings of the past. However, when considering reminiscence as a nursing intervention, the nurse taps the silent memories and stimulates verbal or written memories to assist the client to meet objectives that have been set forth in the nursing care plan.

Reminiscence can be conceptualized as having three components: memory, experiencing, and social interaction. Much of the memory research in the last decade has been of a neurophysiological nature or relates to learning in the aged. The exact mechanisms involved in memory are still unclear and will not be discussed in this chapter. However, the purpose of memory is of particular interest to the nurse using Reminiscence Therapy.

All memory implies a time lapse. A person must be able to perceive time to remember. Remembering also implies that an event is grounded in experience but that there must be *recall* of the event for it to be a "remembrance." Long-term memory studies suggest that it is the importance of the event to the person that determines whether a memory can be recalled (Botwinick and, Torandt, 1974). Memory in all stages of life has the function of organizing past experiences to satisfy personality needs. It also provides a sense of

139

continuity from the past to the present (Lewis, 1971). Remembrances occur within the individual and are affected by present experiences, hopes, and values. As the individual evolves, the memories may alter. Reflections of an adult on his or her personal past lends an understanding of a person's development over time (Leiberman and Falk, 1971).

Experiencing refers to a process whereby individuals engage in an introspective examination of their feelings (Gendlin, 1962). Gendlin contends that when an individual focuses on a felt experience, symbolizes the feelings, and draws meaning from the sensation, he or she is "experiencing." Gorney (1968) studied the presence of experiencing in aged clients as related to patterns of reminiscing. He studied 172 aged persons (60 to 90 years of age) in the community and in institutions. He devised an "experiencing scale" that measured the degree to which an individual manifested introspection from verbalizations. He found that virtually all subjects who possess a high level of experiencing are engaged in a reminiscence process. Thus, he provided support for the notion that introspection on feelings is a component of reminiscence activity.

Memory and experiencing by themselves are only a part of the quality of reminiscence. Perhaps equally important is the idea that these chronologies unfold before another person. Social interaction and human gestures of touch, caring, and listening do much to help a person increase feelings of comfort and feeling of expression (Burnside, 1975, 1980). The nurse can provide the social interaction for individuals, couples, or a group therapy setting.

In a clinical setting the nurse will observe these three components of reminiscence. The client will recall a remembrance and share the memory, as well as the feelings of the experience, with the nurse. Reminiscence Therapy involves the nurse's tapping the ongoing memories and utilizing the phenomena of reminiscence with clients in order to achieve a higher level of wellness.

REVIEW OF LITERATURE

The history of psychotherapeutic interventions indicates that utilizing the life history of a client for assessment and treatment is not a new idea. Martin (1944) describes a therapeutic approach in which she asked the client to relate his life history in detail from his earliest memory to the present. After analyzing these data combined with psychological testing, she provided the client with a list of corrective slogans to assist him in changing his life. Other authors (Grotjahn, 1951; Linden, 1953; Meerlo, 1961) describe various approaches in which support and listening to life histories played a part in the therapy of the aged client. However, one of the strongest proponents of utilizing reminiscence for treatment of the aged is Butler (1960, 1973, 1974, 1975), who coined the phrase "the life review." Basing his hypothesis on Erikson's epigenetic theory, Butler (1963) maintains that the last crises that humans face (ego integrity versus despair) may be resolved while the aged review and weigh their past. He says that the life review process is a universal phenomenon that is precipitated by an awareness of death.

McMahon and Rhudick (1961) investigated what value reminiscence may hold for the aged. They studied 25 noninstitutionalized male Spanish-American War veterans between the ages of 78 and 90 years. Using an hour-long nondirective interview, they classified each subject's responses according to time orientation (past, present, or future). The statements of the past were labeled as reminiscences. The subjects were also scored on degree of depression by evaluating the tone of their statements. One year later McMahon and

Rhudick found that the nondepressed group who reminiscenced more had a higher survival rate. They concluded that reminiscence was positively correlated with adaptation to aging.

Following McMahon and Rhudick's classic study (1961), several other investigators searched for empirical support for the value of reminiscence in helping the aged cope with stress and the aging process. Leiberman and Falk (1971) studied 180 aged (average age, 78 years) and 25 middle-aged (average age, 49 years) individuals. One group lived in the community, a second group was awaiting nursing home placement, and a third group lived in a nursing home. Using a structured interview they measured the type, consistency, and selection of memories, as well as whether the memories served as a problem-solving mechanism or as an emotional gratifier. They found that the group of aged in an unstable life situation (awaiting nursing home placement) did reminisce more. However, the data did not support the relationship between reminiscence and successful adaptation to aging.

Havighurst and Glasser (1972) explored the relationship between frequency and affective quality of reminiscence and adaptive value. Because of weak correlations between variables, they concluded that the relationship between how much time people give to reminiscence and its affective quality are probably "overdetermined" by professionals. They noted that reminiscence is caused by many factors, implying that the aged do not reminisce in order to adapt.

Despite these inconclusive findings on the question of adaptational significance of reminiscing, Lewis (1971) proposed that memories help the aged work through losses and maintain their self-esteem. He suggested that consistency of the self was one characteristic that assisted the aged in healthy adaptation (Lewis, 1973). With the loss of roles, relationships, and worldly possessions the aged may find their self-esteem threatened. Lewis (1971) studied 24 men over the age of 65 years who resided in their own communities. Each subject was interviewed in two 1 hour sessions. In the first session, the subject's self-concept was measured and a structured interview was used to stimulate reminiscence. In a second interview two weeks later, an experimental threat was presented to each subject. A 30 minute interview followed the threat to determine if there was a change in the amount of reminiscing. The findings showed that certain aged persons may deny the implications of threat to self by linking past to present and thereby maintaining the integrity of the self (Lewis, 1971).

Many of the reminiscence studies revolved around the idea that reminiscence would increase ego integrity. Boylin, Gordon, and Nehrke (1976) searched for empirical support of that notion. They studied 41 men over the age of 60 years in a domiciliary setting. Using a structed questionnaire they measured the frequency of the reminiscing, the affect associated with the reminiscing, and the time period each subject related. Ego development was assessed using a scale that reflected behaviors specific to each of Erikson's stages of development. A positive relationship was observed between ego integrity and reminiscing.

Other investigators have searched for a typology of reminiscence. It was first observed by McMahon and Rudick (1961) that not all aged persons reminisce in the same manner. They described three reminiscence types. The "halo effect" reminiscers are those persons whose remembrances deprecate the present and glorify the past. The client who demonstrates the halo effect will tell the listener of great displays of strength, courage, and invulnerability. The second type, the "justifiers," talk of unrealized goals, failures, and wishes to relive their lives. The justifiers have a judgmental and evaluative tone to the memories of their lives. The third type, the "story tellers," tend to be very entertaining as they relate their escapades and exploits with great relish. These clients provide knowledge of a bygone era to listeners and preserve their own self-esteem. They usually neither deny nor justify their past.

Postema (1970) observed four types of reminiscence. "Well-adjusted" reminiscers have achieved a large degree of acceptance of their lives as well as the changes in society. "Defensive" reminiscers are guarded about sharing memories. When they relate their memories, they present those aspects of the past that are complimentary to their self-esteem. "Avoiders" make every effort to talk of present or future life events, and will not talk about the past. Both "defensive" reminiscers and "avoiders" seem to have learned adequate defense mechanisms to deflect troubling aspects of their lives. "Conflictual" reminiscers have neither the acceptance nor the defenses to deal with dissatisfactions of their past. When the self-concept of these four groups was measured, the "conflictual" reminiscers had the lowest scores.

Tobin (1972) explored the themes of the elderly's earliest memory. After interviewing 120 subjects, he observed that content of memories fell into loss and nonloss themes. Nonloss themes may include memories about family or school, although feelings of anxiety, aggressiveness, and wish fulfillment may surface. Loss themes may be memories that deal with interpersonal losses, such as separation from friends and family, injury to self, or death in the family.

Coleman (1974) delineated categories that correspond with different functions of reminiscence. The aged who find the past a source of strength he called "simple reminiscers," whereas those who analyze the past to achieve ego integrity were labeled "life reviewers." "Informers" are the aged who utilize the past to teach valued lessons to others.

Although these social scientists have studied different aspects of reminiscence, the accumulation of knowledge can be used by nurses in clinical practice and research. The exact nature and value of reminiscence are still being explored, but findings thus far would suggest that reminiscence is of value to the aged and should be encouraged rather than dismissed as a symptom of dementia. The nurse can expect that the aged client's style of relating the past will be individualistic and can provide important subject and objective data significant to his or her care.

REMINISCENCE AS A NURSING INTERVENTION

Nurses have identified Reminiscence Therapy as an independent nursing intervention. Burnside (1980) was one of the first nurses to use Reminiscence Therapy to meet the psychosocial needs of the elderly. She maintained that older persons who have survived 70 or 80 years of human history have a need to be listened to while they share their thoughts of the past.

Nursing research on reminiscence differs from the social science research in that nurses looked for the *effects* of Reminiscence Therapy on the client. Instead of holding one or two time interviews with the client to view the phenomenon of reminiscence, nurses have encouraged reminiscence for a period of time (eight weeks to two years) in order to understand the outcome of the intervention.

Hibel (1971) suggested that Reminiscence Therapy may be a nursing intervention that decreases depression in the aged institutionalized client. She designed an experimental study in which 15 depressed subjects were treated for eight weeks with individual Reminiscence Therapy.

In her control group, which consisted of the same number of subjects, she used Reality Therapy as the intervention. She found no statistically significant decrease in depression measurement. However, the nursing staff working with the clients observed that the group of clients receiving Reminiscence Therapy demonstrated an increased desire to socialize, increased memory ability, increased self-care activities, and increased interest in life. These behavioral observations led the nursing staff to believe that the group of clients who had received Reminiscence Therapy were less depressed after the intervention.

Desirable behavior changes have been observed by Hala (1975) when Reminiscence Therapy was used over a two year period. The behaviors observed included an increase in socialization and hygiene efforts, a decreased need for tranquilizers, and a decreased automated compliance with staff. In a community setting, Chennelly (1979) studied aged persons who had recently moved to a senior apartment complex and assessed the effect of reminiscence on adjustment to life change. She spent four 1 hour sessions with each of eight subjects doing Reminiscence Therapy. With the eight subjects of her control group she conversed about random topics. She found the subjects receiving the Reminiscence Therapy had a significantly higher rate of satisfaction with their new environment.

Reminiscence Therapy can be conducted with groups or individually. The nurse's decision will be guided by the setting, the nursing diagnosis, and the goals set with the client. The quality of community health nursing practice often lends itself to using an individual's or a couple's reminiscence, as groups are not accessible. In the acute care setting, when the client is medically ill, individual reminiscence may be easily worked into bathing time. In long-term care facilities, geriatric day care centers, halfway houses, and clinics for the elderly, group reminiscence is effective and has the advantage of allowing resocialization.

Individual Reminiscence Therapy

Individual reminiscence demands active listening, presence, and caring from the nurse. She or he will want to set aside adequate time for the client so as not to appear hurried. It is possible to use 15 or 20 minute intervals throughout the day, but it is not helpful to try to attempt Reminiscence Therapy "on the run."

Butler (1974) suggests several methods that may stimulate the process of reminiscing:

1. Encourage writing of past events.
2. Tape the reminiscence and play it back to the client.
3. Ask the family to bring in photo albums.
4. Help the client organize memorabilia in a scrapbook.
5. Have the client start a family tree.
6. Encourage the client to write to old friends.

The nurse can encourage the client to draw pictures of memorable events with chalk, crayons, or watercolors. Objects in the environment may stimulate the aged to reminisce. For example, a nurse observed that Mrs. S. had many flowers in her room. The nurse asked, "Have you always enjoyed flowers, Mrs. S.?" This question stimulated a review of gardens that Mrs. S. had cared for in past homes, as well as the life events that necessitated frequent relocation

Table 10–1. TASKS TO STIMULATE INDIVIDUAL REMINISCENCE

Writing life memories	Writing to old friends
Taped memories with playback to client	Writing down family trees of known rela-
Photograph viewing	tives
Artwork demonstrating past events	Genealogy study of unknown relatives
Poetry reading and writing related to past life	Studying historical events and relating them
Collecting old objects in environment	to personal past
Cooking foods related to the past	Walking in garden or potting plants
Playing records related to the past	

of her family. Poetry, artwork, current events, and sounds and smells may stimulate a deluge of old memories. Encouraging small assignments (Table 10–1) will often get the aged involved in the reminiscence process.

The nurse will begin where the older person is emotionally and proceed sensibly. Poor timing and inappropriate interpretations will be met with defenses such as hostility and denial. Drawing the client out in a supportive manner and using basic communication skills, such as focusing, reflecting, and restating, will help develop the relationship. Although a catharsis of feelings and memories may occur, often the aged will share a portion of a memorable event and reflect on its impact for days. The topic may resurface slightly altered as reflection can add or subtract portions of the memory.

The emotions accompanying reminiscence vary, but an element of pain often arises as memories surface. Joy and laughter also are a part of the reminiscence process, as most lifetimes are a combination of peaks and valleys. It is important to comment on the affective quality accompanying the memories in an empathetic manner in order to validate the feelings of the older person. Occasionally a client digresses in thought associations. Thought patterns seem unconnected, and numerous details make the central idea unclear to the listener. Usually direct questions refocus the person back on life events: Tell me how you met your husband. What was the happiest day of your life? What color was your wedding dress?

Individual reminiscence is an opportunity for nurses to help the aged view their uniqueness and value, establish a relationship with a long-lived survivor, and learn about the challenging process of living.

Group Reminiscence Therapy

Group reminiscence offers the advantages of helping a greater number of clients as well as increasing interaction with others (Butler, 1974; McMordie and Blom, 1979). Small groups with six to ten members are best for this type of therapy (Ebersole, 1976; King, 1982). A small group allows for group stages to proceed but gives each person sufficient time to talk. Members are usually chosen utilizing multiple criteria: (1) does the client have a nursing diagnosis amenable to Reminiscence Therapy? (2) is the client over 65 years? (3) can the client hear? (4) if the client cannot hear, will he or she gain from or enjoy the group environment, or simply be frustrated? (5) is the client interested in attending? However, the nurse must decide the selection of group members based on judgment, not on a rigid set of rules. For example, many aged clients initially indicate they are not interested in attending a group. However, often after one or two sessions they find the experience enjoyable. Or the nurse may find that a heterogeneous age group (ages 45 to 80 years) proves to be a therapeutic endeavor. Creativity and flexibility are important attributes in the nurse when dealing with any nursing intervention.

Table 10–2. TOPICS FOR DISCUSSION IN GROUP REMINISCENCE

Early childhood memories	Presidents, politics, elections
"Most favorites" (Christmas, birth- days, siblings, dress, etc.)	Termination (funerals, old friends)
	Relationships (pets, spouses, relatives)
Transportation	Travel
Medical care	Wars
Occupation, skills, hobbies	Fashions
Food preparation	Cost of living
"Firsts" (car, telephone, dress, televi- sion, job, child)	

It is wise to choose a room which is large and comfortable. Arrange the chairs in a circle in close proximity so the people can hear each other as well as respond to nonverbal cues.

The therapist takes a strong leadership role with a group of aged persons providing a high degree of structure. A consistent meeting time and place are important. Reminders can be placed on wall calendars or staff members can remind the group members prior to each meeting. A reminiscence group is usually scheduled to last one hour. This allows enough time for all members to talk, but discourages long recitations. Although there is social interaction in heterogeneous age groups, it appears that many elderly take turns in speaking to the audience. When this occurs, the leader can ask other members' views to spark interaction.

The group leader often introduces varied topics to stimulate memory and interaction (Table 10–2). The nurse may want to assess the interests of the members and choose a topic for the first session that seems to interest the group. For example, "most favorites" is a topic that is nonthreatening and holds the interest of most aged clients. As the group sessions continue the nurse will persist in assessing appropriate topics and may want to elicit topics from group members. Topics generally relate to the past life of group members. For example, "farm days" would not be included in a reminiscence group whose members had lived their entire lives in central city New York! Music, snacks, or more creative endeavors may be added to the group's activities. Berger (1978) added brief body exercises to a reminiscence group. She had the members raise their arms and asked them to share what was being reached for. Responses varied: "I'm reaching for the moon," "I'm reaching for good health" (Berger, 1978, p. 64). She also used round robin story-telling. She began the story with "Once upon a time . . ." and each member added a thought or an event. The associations of aged people are a reflection of their own life experiences.

Objects brought by the leader also stimulate memories (Table 10–3). Mason jars, antique telephones, high buttoned shoes, and quilts can be coordinated with the introduced topic. The smells and tastes of the past can be recalled with foods, flowers, or extracts. In one group an aged woman commented on the perfume the leader was wearing. This stimulated recollections of special evenings when she wore her favorite scent, "Evening in Paris."

Old movie clips and music are effective in bringing back recall of the

Table 10–3. OBJECTS TO STIMULATE GROUP REMINISCENCE

Photo albums	Plants
Records	Movies
Maps	Newspapers, magazines
Antiques (china, Mason jars, toy model cars)	Hand work (quilts, crochet)
	Family coat of arms
Food	Memorabilia

Table 10–4. ACTIVITIES TO STIMULATE GROUP REMINISCENCE

Family reunions	Reminiscence diaries
Old dances	Exercise
Old popular movies or family slides	Round robin story-telling
Plant growing	Taped sounds (rain, machinery, birds,
Painting	railroad cars)
Writing poems, stories	Fashion shows of old clothes

events of that era. These sessions become very lively and close any hint of a generation gap beween members and leaders. At times events of the present will relate to the past. At the time of one group meeting an intense snow had engulfed the town. Although another topic had been planned, the snow sparked a discussion of weather in "olden days." Sometimes group members will generate their own topics and bring personal memorabilia to share with the group. Often the members will demonstrate a skill such as rope tying or quilting to the "young" leaders (Table 10–4).

Silent periods also occur in reminiscence groups. Some topics stimulate old private memories and the aged will take time to reflect or may rehearse the thought silently before sharing it with the group. The nurse can wait through the silence or may want to ask, "What thoughts did that trigger in you?"

At times group members will become uncomfortable with a topic. They may state they do not want to talk about a certain topic, but more often, they will ignore it and create a stream of conversation around what they perceive to be of interest. The nurse's action will depend on the objectives (short-term or long-term). He or she may want to guide the conversation back to the chosen topic. On the other hand, if fear, boredom, or high anxiety is perceived in group members, it may be judged best to focus on the topic the group has introduced.

The elderly are living historical novels who have written and acted out their past. Reminiscence provides the aged with an inner source of continuity through memory, introspection of feelings, and sharing. Their willingness to share their past provides the nurse with a powerful intervention tool.

IDENTIFICATION OF NURSING DIAGNOSES

To determine if reminiscence is the intervention of choice, the nurse begins with an assessment of the client. Reminiscence may be useful as an assessment tool (Ebersole, 1981; Pincus, 1970); the theme of the memories may reflect the priority need of the client. For example, a client who focuses on past experiences with family traditions, rituals, and holidays may be revealing a high need for love and belonging (Maslow, 1970). A client who talks at length about his professional life may be telling the nurse of his need for self-esteem. The content of memories, what subjects are avoided, and past conflicts will give important subjective data to the assessment.

As the nurse observes and listens to the aged client the collection of subjective and objective data continues. This process will lead the nurse to a conclusion concerning the problem(s), which will be the focus of the nursing care. The problem, the cause of the problem, and the signs and symptoms are often called the nursing diagnosis. The nursing diagnosis and subsequent goals set with the client must be considered when selecting Reminiscence Therapy as an appropriate intervention.

Nursing diagnoses listed by the National Conference Group on Nursing

Table 10–5. NURSING DIAGNOSES COMPATIBLE WITH REMINISCENCE THERAPY

Ineffective individual coping	Disturbances in self-concept
Ineffective family coping	Sensory perceptual alteration
Diversional activity deficit	Self-care deficits
Fear	Spiritual distress
Grieving (anticipatory and dysfunc- tional)	Alterations in thought process
	Social isolation

Diagnoses (Gordon, 1982) that may be amenable to Reminiscence Therapy are given in Table 10–5. Nurses have described clinical observations and nursing research results that suggest that patients with these nursing diagnoses respond favorably to Reminiscence Therapy (Chenelly, 1976; Ebersole, 1976; Hala, 1975; Hamilton, 1980; Hibel, 1971; King, 1982; Rosenthal, 1982). It may be appropriate to utilize Reminiscence Therapy with other nursing diagnoses not listed in Table 10–5 (e.g., depression, memory deficit, powerlessness, alterations in comfort). Because reminiscence is a powerful intervention, the nurse must utilize good judgment in choosing reminiscence as an intervention. He or she must remember that not all aged people respond to reminiscence in the same manner (e.g., "justifiers" or "defensive" reminiscers) (McMahon and Rhudick, 1961; Postema, 1970). If the nurse detects extreme defensiveness about the past from the aged client, he or she may want to reassess the nursing care plan. In fact, some elderly find their past memories very painful and avoid reminiscence altogether. There is some indication that reminiscence is contraindicated with acutely psychotic patients. (Butler, 1963, 1974).

OUTCOMES OF REMINISCENCE THERAPY

The nursing diagnoses listed in Table 10–5 center on a theme of loss. The nurse who uses Reminiscence Therapy to decrease the patient's sense of loss may see multiple outcomes during treatment (Table 10–6). The losses that often accompany old age—loss of physiological integrity, loss of friends, role change, and threats to security—make the aged vulnerable to feelings of fear, grief, hopelessness, and helplessness. Remembering what one has been and what was accomplished, how one looked, and how one has been loved and appreciated can reduce the sense of loss and restore a sense of meaning to old times. How well the blizzard of '35, the dust storm, and the floods are remembered by these people! Recognizing old skills of survival may lead to drawing on past accomplishments to cope with present life. Those aged individuals who reminisce effectively are often highly functional (McMahon and Rhudick, 1961).

Many aged persons experience long days with few diversional activities. Once their recollections are prodded, they discover it is fun to sit down with others and "remember when." A certain hunger is satisfied in a hearty, healthy, and often humorous way. Looking back provides diversional activity,

Table 10–6. POSSIBLE OUTCOMES OF REMINSCENCE THERAPY

Increased socialization	Increased memory
Decreased loneliness	Increased interest in life
Increased coping patterns	Increased attention span
Awareness of conflicts and feelings	Increased adaptation to crises
Increased self-care activities	Decreased depression
Increased sensory perception	Increased self-esteem

increases socialization skills, and allows a reawakening of other diversional interests (Lewis, 1973).

The elderly may demonstrate a decreased self-concept by behaviors of overcompliance, noncompliance, or lack of self-care activities (Hala, 1975). Reminiscence allows them to review a lifetime of data about themselves, enabling them to see their abilities, achievements, and uniqueness. Group reminiscence seems to be particularly effective in increasing the self-esteem of the aged (Boylin, Gordon, and Nehrke, 1976; Hamilton, 1980; King, 1982; Lewis, 1971).

The objects and activities of Reminiscence Therapy provide a useful means of stimulating the senses. Sight, sounds, touch, and smell may be heightened by various methods. In one group, the memories of harvest time combined with the sights and smells of autumn provided members with a nostalgic journey to a productive time in their lives.

The group reminiscence process allows the cognitively impaired to bring latent memories to the surface (Ebersole and Hess, 1981; Kiernat, 1979). Even very confused participants are able to respond to familiar objects and events. The psychologically disturbed, particularly depressed clients, benefit from reminiscence as they share conflicts and recognize feelings. They affirm themselves and others as caring develops between group members.

CASE STUDY

Mr. H. H., a 78 year old white man, had been followed by S. P., a public health nurse, for four months. He was recovering from an aortic valve replacement, which had been the first major illness in his lifetime. The public health nurse believed that Mr. H.'s health had improved, but he was feeling discouraged and depressed due to a decreased appetite, intolerance to cold air, decreased mobility, and a loss of vigor. Because of the cold winter and rural living, social contacts with cohorts had decreased during his post-hospital recovery period. Since Mr. H.'s illness, his role as head of the extended family and business had shifted to his eldest son. Mr. H.'s wife was worried about her husband's tendency to "be down in the dumps." She felt that he had too much time to "think about everything."

After assessing the situation S. P. decided that Mr. H. was experiencing several nursing diagnoses related to the concept of loss (social isolation, deficit in diversional activity, disturbances in self-concept, grieving). She contacted M.S., a geriatric clinical specialist, who agreed to consult with Mr. and Mrs. H.

M. S. visited with them the following day and collected more assessment data. Mr. and Mrs. H. shared with the nurse that their awareness of death was "brought home" to them beginning with Mr. H.'s heart surgery. Furthermore, Mr. H. had been reading the obituaries daily and often commented that his friends were "dying off." He expressed a sense of regret that he was no longer able to run the farm and keep busy with the activities in the community. After much discussion, the couple and M. S. agreed that visits from the nurse may help to decrease his depressive feelings, increase his interest in life, and increase his ability to cope with the fear of "being a heart patient." Ten 1 hour home visits were planned over a period of three months.

Based on the nursing assessement and nursing diagnoses, M. S. decided that Reminiscence Therapy was an appropriate nursing intervention. The simple questioning and sharing of the past began to trigger memories of conflict, concerns, and accomplishments for both Mr. and Mrs. H. They spoke spontaneously about the past 70 years, covering joyful and sad experiences. Some sessions were sad and nostalgic as they had lost two sons in World War II. Other visits were filled with laughter, photo viewing, and long stories about various memorabilia in the house. Mr. and Mrs. H. began reminiscing together between M. S.'s visits. They completed a family history notebook and dictated oral history of their lives on tape. As the weather warmed they began to participate in social events and visit old friends. Mr. H. developed a sense of trust and regard for M. S. and on walks to the barn would express deeper feelings. He was able to share his feelings about aging and his satisfaction with his accomplishments in his lifetime. Both spouses were both able to verbalize regarding the impact of Mr. H.'s illness on their life. When the end of the three month period approached, they agreed that they felt better able to cope with the implications of "being a heart patient." M. S. had completed her intervention regime: presence, health teaching, and Reminiscence Therapy. The long-term objectives of this client had been met as a result of careful assessment, nursing intervention, and a great deal of sharing and caring.

RECOMMENDATIONS FOR PRACTICE AND RESEARCH

No therapy modality can fulfill the wants, needs, and hopes of all clients (King, 1982). However, Reminiscence Therapy is a psychologically sound nursing intervention that can be used to treat a multitude of nursing diagnoses.

The nurse must be flexible, warm, and caring and display the ability to listen while guiding the memories of the aged. The most positive results will occur when the nurse allows the therapy to continue for some time. Patience, tenaciousness, and creativity from the therapist will be more effective than probing and attempting instant insight.

Preparing materials for reminiscence group therapy can be quite time-consuming. Locating books, music, pictures, and antique objects requires "thinking time" and many trips to the library or flea markets. Local librarians, genealogists, and local historians can be of tremendous help.

Most often Reminiscence Therapy has been used with the aged population. However, because reminiscence is a universal phenomenon after the age of 10 years (Havighurst and Glasser, 1972), it is possible that reminiscence would be useful with persons of any age over 10. This topic has many possibilities for further research. Because the awareness of death stimulates the life review (Butler, 1974), nursing research on the effects of reminiscence on client groups experiencing life-threatening illness would be useful. Comparing the effects of oral, silent, and group reminiscing on the self-esteem of the aged would help nurses further delineate the most effective nursing intervention for clients.

Although empirical research is encouraged by most nurse researchers, Remininscence Therapy is a nursing intervention that may be amenable to a qualitative approach of study. It may be possible to document behavioral changes that occur in clients during Reminiscence Therapy which cannot be measured quantitatively. The essence of reminiscence may be more accurately described using a qualitative research methodology. Qualitative or descriptive studies (Hala, 1975; Hibel, 1971), yield a wealth of information, which may help nurses to comprehend reminiscence more fully.

CONCLUSION

The tendency of older persons to reminisce has often been viewed derogatorily as living in the past or senility, or somewhat more sympathetically as an expression of loneliness. Nurses are in a position to help aged people deal with crises and loss. The aged can glean positive outcomes from reminiscence intervention. Old age need not be a stage of alienation from society or from one's earlier life; it can be instead a continuation of the process of life, growth, and experience.

EDITORS' COMMENTS AND QUESTIONS
The aim of Reminiscence Therapy is to enhance wellness in the elderly through relating of personally significant past experiences.

Several favorable outcomes have been documented through nursing research. Hamilton gives good practical suggestions for application of the intervention.

Questions for Discussion

1. Discuss the advantages of using Reminiscence Therapy in group settings.

2. Compare structured versus nonstructured Reminiscence Therapy. Should clients always be encouraged to talk about the past?

3. How would you design a study to test the effectiveness of Reminiscence Therapy?

References

Berger, L. Activating a psychogeriatric group. *Psychiatric Quarterly*, 1978, *50*(1), 63–67.

Botwinick, J., and Torandt, M. *Memory, related functions and age*. Springfield, Ill.: Charles C Thomas, 1974.

Boylin, W., Gordon, S. K., and Nehrke, S. Reminiscing and ego integrity in institutionalized elderly males. *Gerontologist*, 1976, *16*, 118–124.

Brodie, F. *Thomas Jefferson: An intimate history*. Toronto: Bantam Books, 1974.

Burnside, I. M. Listen to the aged. *American Journal of Nursing*, 1975, *75*(1), 1800–1803.

Burnside, I. M. *Psychosocial nursing care of the aged*. New York: McGraw-Hill Book Company, 1980.

Butler, R. N. Intensive psychotherapy for the hospitalized aged. *Geriatrics*, 1960, *15*(9), 644–653.

Butler, R. N. A life review. *Psychiatry*, 1963, *26*(2), 65–76.

Butler, R. N. Mental health and aging. *Geriatrics*, 1974, *29*, 53–54.

Butler, R. N. *Why survive?* New York: Harper and Row, 1975.

Chennelly, S. *Reminiscing: A coping skill for the elderly* (unpublished master's thesis). Rochester, N.Y.: University of Rochester, 1979.

Coleman, P. G. Measuring reminiscence characteristics from conversation as an adaptive feature of old age. *International Journal of Aging and Human Development*, 1974, *5*(4), 281–294.

Ebersole, P. Reminiscing. *American Journal of Nursing*, 1976, *76*(8), 1304–1305.

Ebersole, P., and Hess, P. *Toward healthy aging*. St. Louis: C. V. Mosby, 1981.

Gendlin, E. T. *Experiencing and the creation of meaning*. Glencoe, Ill.: The Free Press, 1962.

Gordon, M. *Nursing diagnosis: Process and application*. New York: McGraw-Hill Book Company, 1982.

Gorney, J. *Experiencing and age patterns of reminiscence among the elderly* (unpublished doctoral dissertation). Chicago: University of Chicago, 1968.

Grotjahn, M. Some analytical observations about the process of growing old. In G. Roheim (Ed.), *Psychoanalysis and the social science*. New York: International University Press, 1951.

Hala, M. Reminiscence group therapy project. *Journal of Gerontological Nursing*, 1975, *1*(3), 34–41.

Hamilton, D. *The effects of reminiscence group therapy on the self esteem of aged institutionalized clients* (unpublished master's thesis). Iowa City, University of Iowa, 1980.

Havighurst, R., and Glasser, R. An explanatory study of reminiscence. *Journal of Gerontology*, 1972, *27*(2), 245–253.

Hibel, D. The relationship between reminiscence and depression among institutionalized aged males (doctoral dissertation, Boston University, 1971). *Dissertation Abstracts International*, 1971, *32*, 2253-B (University Microfilms No. 71–26, 667).

Kiernat, J. The use of life review activity with confused nursing home residents. *American Journal of Occupational Therapists*, 1979, *33*(5), 306–310.

King, K. Reminiscing psychotherapy with aged people. *Journal of Psychosocial Nursing*, 1982, *20*(2), 21–25.

Lewis, C. Reminiscing and self: Concept in old age. *Journal of Gerontology*, 1971, *26*(2), 240–243.

Lewis, C. The adaptive value of reminiscing in old age. *Journal of Geriatric Psychology*, 1973, *7*(1), 112–21.

Lieberman, M., and Falk, J. The remembered past as a source of data for research on the life cycle. *Human Development*, 1971, *14*(2), 132–141.

Linden, M. Group psychotherapy with institutionalized senile women. *International Journal of Group Psychotherapists*, 1953, *3*(2), 150–170.

Martin, L. *A handbook for old age counselors*. San Francisco: Geertz Printing Company, 1944.

Maslow, A. *Motivation and personality*, 2nd ed. New York: Harper & Row, 1970.

McMahon, A., and Rhudick, P. Reminiscing. *Archives of General Psychiatry*, 1961, *10*(3), 292–298.

McMordie, W., and Blom, S. Life review therapy. *Perspectives in Psychiatric Care*, 1979, *17*(4), 162–166.

Meerlo, J. Modes of psychotherapy in the aged. *Journal of American Geriatric Society*, 1961, *9*(3), 225–234.

Pincus, S. Reminiscence in aging and its implications for social work. *Social Work*, 1970, *15*(7), 47–53.

Postema, L. J. Reminiscing, time orientation and self-concept in aged men (doctoral dissertation, Michigan State University, 1970). *Dissertation Abstracts International*, 1970, *31*, 6880-B (University Microfilms No. 12–21, 332).

Rosenthal, T. Implementing a reminiscent discussion group. *Virginia Nurse*, 1982, Summer, 57–60.

Tobin, S. S. The earliest memory as data for research in aging. In D. P. Kent, R. Kastenbaum, and S. Sherwood (Eds.), *Research planning and action for the elderly: The power and potential of social science*. New York: Behavioral Publications, 1972.

11

ROLE SUPPLEMENTATION

SUE ANN MOORHEAD

To live means to experience role changes, and nurses frequently care for clients experiencing role changes. Role Supplementation is an intervention nurses can use to improve the client's transition between roles. The transition from one role to another is not always a pleasant experience and may produce stress for the individuals involved. In order to change their behavior, individuals must be aware of the rights and obligations of the new role. This requires that family and friends (significant others) recognize the role changes and modify their behavior accordingly (Banton, 1965). By using Role Supplementation as an intervention during these periods of transition, nurses can better prepare their clients and their families for new roles in life.

ROLE SUPPLEMENTATION

Role Supplementation is an intervention that facilitates role changes. Role Supplementation was first identified as an intervention by Meleis (1975), who discussed it as a means of improving role transitions and preventing role insufficiency.

> Role supplementation is defined as any deliberative process whereby role insufficiency or potential role insufficiency is identified by the role incumbent and significant others, and the conditions and strategies of role clarification and role taking are used to develop a preventative or therapeutic intervention to decrease, ameliorate, or prevent role insufficiency. Role supplementation is further defined as the conveying of information or experience necessary to bring the role incumbent and significant others to full awareness of the anticipated behavior patterns, units, sentiments, sensations, and goals involved in each role and its complement. It includes necessary knowledge and experience that emphasizes heightened awareness of one's own roles and other's roles and the dynamics of the interrelationships. (Meleis, 1975, p. 265)

As the definition suggests, Role Supplementation can be either preventive or therapeutic in nature. As a preventive intervention, Role Supplementation may clarify role insufficiency. As a therapeutic intervention, Role Supplementation may be utilized with individuals experiencing signs of insufficiency in role behaviors (Meleis, 1975).

ROLE TRANSITION AND ROLE INSUFFICIENCY

Role transition implies a change in role relationships, expectations, or abilities. During a role transition individuals are forced to assimilate new knowledge, change behaviors, and redefine their self-concepts (Meleis, 1975). Role transition as a concept is credited to Cottrell (1942) and is defined as the moving in and out of roles. In the transition, roles may be added or dropped. New roles may replace old roles or be added to old roles (Burr, 1972).

Three types of role transitions have been identified by Meleis (1975). The first considers role transitions from a developmental framework. Beginning with birth and ending at death, individuals encounter role transitions as a result of aging. For example, adolescents struggle with their identity and separate from their parents as they enter into adulthood. At the other end of the life continuum is the transition from middle age to old age and retirement. Each role change for an individual requires a role change by the individual's significant others. Thus, some individuals may be forced into role changes (because they are significant others) before they are prepared for them. It is important to consider the developmental stage of the individual and his or her significant relationships before intervening.

The second type of transition identified by Meleis (1975) is the situational transition that involves changes in the individual's roles with significant others. These changes may be prompted by the addition or subtraction of persons in the environment resulting, perhaps, from a birth or a death. Such changes have a significant effect on the individual and may require a definition of roles. Because births and deaths frequently occur within the hospital in our society, nurses become involved with clients during these role transitions.

The third type of transition identified by Meleis (1975) occurs when an individual who has been previously healthy becomes ill. This transition into the sick role may require sudden role changes brought about by acute illness, or more gradual role changes reflecting a slower disease process, such as those seen with chronic diseases. Again the nurse may be involved in this type of role transition when an individual seeks medical care or is hospitalized. It is obvious that all three types of role transitions may involve the loss of a role, the acquisition of a role, or a combination of the two.

The result of poor or unsuccessful role transition may be role insufficiency. Role insufficiency results when individuals lack knowledge of how to perform a role. This may involve not knowing the usual feelings and expectations associated with the role. This situation prevents the individual from fulfilling the usual expected behaviors, and this role insufficiency may be perceived by the individual, the significant others, or both. A person may consciously refuse to accept a new role because the associated costs are viewed as outweighing the gains. Voluntary acceptance of a new role is accompanied by expectations of appropriate reinforcements and role clarity (Meleis, 1975).

Behaviors of clients may be used to identify role insufficiency. Meleis (1975) has identified behaviors for developmental, situational, and health-illness transitions. These are categorized into role loss, role acquisition, and combined loss and acquisition. In role loss, grief, mourning, and powerlessness are characteristic of developmental, situational, or health-illness transitions. In role acquisition, anxiety, depression, and withdrawal are observed in developmental and situational transitions. In health-illness transitions of role acquisition, anxiety, depression, and withdrawal are combined with manifestations of role insufficiency. In role changes of concomitant loss and acquisition combinations of all antecedent behaviors and role insufficiency are found in all three types of transitions. Apathy, frustration, unhappiness, aggression, and hostility may also suggest insufficiency in role transition.

COMPONENTS, STRATEGIES, AND THE PROCESS OF ROLE SUPPLEMENTATION

Meleis (1975) views Role Supplementation as composed of components, strategies, and process. The *components* are role clarification and role taking. *Role clarification* is the identification of the specific information and cues required to enact a role. To clarify a role one first identifies the behaviors, sentiments, and goals of a role as they pertain to a situation and involve significant others. When enacting a role the individual needs to understand the role, including the expectations of the significant others.

The second component of Role Supplementation is *role taking*. It is defined as "imaginatively assuming the position or points of view of another person" (Lindesmith and Strauss, 1968, p. 282). This ability to take the role of another individual is an indication of a smooth social interaction and uncomplicated role transition (Meleis, 1975). The concept of role taking originated with Mead (1934). Mead and later Turner (1962) proposed that roles are learned in pairs. Mead's idea of paired roles incorporates the expected behaviors of the significant other. For example, for a person to enact the role of a wife, it is essential to have another individual enacting the role of a husband. The roles of husband and wife are then paired roles that occur simultaneously.

The *strategies* to achieve role clarification and role taking are role modeling, role rehearsal, and reference group interactions (Meleis, 1975). *Role modeling* is learned as a result of observing another person portray the complexities of a role (Bandura, 1963). Mowrer (1960) views this process as imitation that is learned without direct reinforcements and that involves trial and error learning. This imitation or role modeling is the most predominant type of social role learning and results in accurate and relatively smooth transitions in roles. In our highly mobile culture lack of continuous contact with role models may reduce role modeling to a minimum (Meleis, 1975). Nurses may serve as role models for clients learning new roles. By enacting the behaviors of the role, nurses enable their clients to visualize the behaviors of the role. For example, a nurse may serve as a role model for a new mother when interacting with the baby. The nurse through his or her behaviors demonstrates how to stimulate, hold, and feed the newborn.

A second strategy for Role Supplementation is *role rehearsal*, which utilizes the mental enactment of the role and the imagined behaviors of the significant others. Due to the anticipation and planning of future behaviors this strategy becomes a significant prelude to role taking. This fantasy enactment may in reality be very dissimilar to actual role behavior; however, this rehearsal allows the individuals involved to anticipate some actions and sentiments (Meleis, 1975). Role rehearsal allows individuals to interact in the new roles in a learning situation. It enables the individuals involved to examine their roles and discuss the situation prior to taking on the role and its obligations and pressures. The nurse can utilize role rehearsal with individuals in paired roles and help them discuss possible problems, solutions, and behaviors they expect of each other.

The final strategy of Role Supplementation is *reference group interaction*. Many reports on the effectiveness of reference groups in transitional situations have been noted (Meleis, 1975). Examples of such groups included Reach For Recovery (mastectomy clients), I Can Cope (cancer), or Mended Hearts Clubs (open heart surgery). Each of these groups help members adjust to their new roles by discussing common problems and sharing solutions the members have found helpful. Nurses can provide contacts with these groups for their clients when they are appropriate to help facilitate learning new roles.

The *process* to enhance the components of role clarification and role taking and facilitate the strategies of role modeling, role rehearsal, and reference groups is *communication*. Communication, a central concept of Mead (1934), depends on the sharing of significant symbols as the individual anticipates the interpretation others put upon his symbolic gestures. A pattern of meaning is established and lines of intended behaviors are created. It is through open and clear communication of symbols that roles emerge. Nurses can help their clients communicate expectations and interpret symbolic gestures in various roles. By helping individuals identify the meaning these symbols and gestures have for the individuals involved, the nurse assists clients in learning and fulfilling new roles to the best of their abilities.

RESEARCH ON ROLE SUPPLEMENTATION

Since Role Supplementation as a nursing intervention was not identified in nursing literature until 1975 (Meleis, 1975), it is not surprising that little empirical testing of the intervention has been done. Only two articles were found; both were reports of studies by Meleis and associates.

The first study was conducted by Meleis and Swendson (1978) and was designed to test the effect of Role Supplementation as a preventive nursing intervention. The study involved families who were experiencing a transition from a dyadic to a triadic relationship through the birth of a first child. The mothers were 18 to 34 years old and in the fourth gestational month of their pregnancy. The study utilized three groups: an experimental (Role Supplementation) group (n = 12), a control group (n = 36), and a group involved in a special program of individualized care and early hospital discharge (FamCap) (n = 10). Three strategies were used to assist the families in the experimental group to develop a sense of role clarity and mastery associated with the new roles of parenthood: reference group, role modeling, and role rehearsal.

The reference group, made up of husband-wife teams, was led by two nurse clinicians weekly. Group members were given the opportunity to explore ideas and the normal range of feelings and experiences associated with the role of parent. Role modeling was provided by individuals—family or friends, physicians, and nurses—and the couples discussed role modeling in the reference group experiences. Role rehearsal was facilitated by use of a case study in the group. Couples explained how they would handle various situations.

The results of this study found no increase in communication skills, role taking, or congruency in role perceptions. After the intervention, the husbands in the experimental group did have lower anxiety scores post delivery compared with the husbands in the other groups. Wives in the experimental group showed significant differences in their perception and attitudes toward ignoring the infant, protectiveness of the infant, and responsiveness of infant needs (Meleis and Swendson, 1978).

A second report concerning the same study expanded on the effects of the intervention from the participants' viewpoint. Swendson, Meleis, and Jones (1978) used case studies to describe client reactions to the Role Supplementation intervention. The couples believed the intervention made them more aware of changes in life that occur with the birth of a child and offered alternative means of coping with these changes. Role Supplementation helped the husbands understand their new responsibilities and helped couples understand each other's feelings and the needs of the baby. The group discussions helped them realize that many couples shared their anxieties. Couples definitely valued the individual attention from the nurses. Role rehearsal and role modeling were useful in bringing them closer to the reality of the situation. It must be emphasized that this study was based on small sample sizes and that all subjects were aware of their participation in the study, so that the results may have been influenced by the Hawthorne effect.

These studies are only a beginning step in researching the effectiveness of Role Supplementation as a nursing intervention. It is obvious that research of this nature is very costly in terms of time commitments on the part of both the researcher and the participants. Many research tools were utilized to attempt to determine if the intervention resulted in changes in behaviors and attitudes. Home visits were made to obtain needed information post delivery. Members of the experimental group were able to call the nurse at any time with questions during this study. Meleis and Swendson (1978) noted that tools need to be developed that can measure the effectiveness of Role Supplementation as an intervention for developmental, situational, and health-illness transitions.

NURSING DIAGNOSES AND ROLE SUPPLEMENTATION

Which nursing diagnoses could be treated by nurses utilizing Role Supplementation? Gordon (1982a) provides a comprehensive list of nursing diagnoses, giving a definition and the identifying characteristics for each diagnosis. In an attempt to identify which diagnoses could be treated by Role Supplementation, I identified all diagnoses with role difficulties or role transitions as a listed etiology of the diagnosis, since nurses intervene to eliminate the cause and thus eliminate the problem (Gordon, 1982a). Ten diagnoses were identified in this process. In a second attempt to identify diagnoses for Role Supplementation, I examined the defining characteristics of all diagnoses for the behaviors identified by Meleis (1975) as characteristic of role insufficiencies. These behaviors were grief, mourning, powerlessness, anxiety, depression, and withdrawal. Twelve diagnoses were identified from this process. When the two lists were compared, several diagnoses appeared on both:

○ Anticipatory Grieving
○ Alteration in Parenting
○ Body Image Disturbance
○ Dysfunctional Grieving
○ Ineffective Family Coping
○ Ineffective Family Coping: Compromised
○ Ineffective Individual Coping

It would seem that, if both a behavior of role insufficiency and role problems are found in the defining characteristics and are identified as a cause of a diagnosis, Role Supplementation would prove to be an effective nursing intervention. This possibility needs to be tested. Although this procedure identified nursing diagnoses most likely to be treatable by Role Supplementation, the inadequacies of the accepted list of diagnoses preclude jumping to conclusions. Further development of these diagnoses is needed. Not all defining characteristics or etiologies have been identified at this time. This is only a beginning step in an attempt to identify possible diagnoses treatable by Role Supplementation.

RECOMMENDATIONS FOR PRACTICE AND RESEARCH

It seems obvious that research in the areas of role transition, role insufficiency, and role supplementation is greatly needed to identify specific patient behaviors that occur during transitions and inadequate role performance. Validation of the behaviors identified by Meleis (1975) as characteristic of role loss, role acquisition, and a combination of these needs to be done. Nurses need to identify role transitions of a developmental, situational, and health-illness nature with which they deal in practice and collect client behaviors that occur during transitions and role insufficiency.

Meleis (1975) identified three broad areas for the development of testable hypotheses of this nature. These were:

> The clinical definition of the role insufficiency syndrome and its relationship with a variety of role transitions by observing clients during role transitions, describing and collating their behaviors, reactions, and interactions surrounding the transition.
> The development and adaptation of valid tools for the components, strategies, and processes of role supplementation.
> Studies to explore the relationship between role insufficiency and role supplementation. (p. 270)

These areas still need to be explored by nurses. It is essential that nurses apply role theory when working with clients and their significant others.

Inherent in the use of Role Supplementation as an intervention is the need for skills in group process and knowledge of role expectations. More emphasis should be placed in nursing on intervening with clients in groups rather than in one-to-one relationships. This allows the nurse to serve as a role model.

CASE STUDY

This author used Role Supplementation as an intervention, focusing on the component of role clarification and using role rehearsal as the specific strategy. It is this author's viewpoint that one of the strengths of this intervention is the ability to choose the strategies to fit the needs of the client and the significant other. The process of communication was of great importance in this case study. No reference group was needed.

Mr. E., a 68-year-old retired farmer, was admitted to a large university hospital with complaints of anorexia, nausea, and vomiting while in a home-training program for hemodialysis. When he was first diagnosed as having chronic renal failure he had a difficult health-illness transition. He stated that he suddenly became "elderly," was forced to give up his part-time job, and lost his dominant role as husband. In order to preserve his independence and his dreams of traveling upon retirement, he decided to learn home dialysis. It was not until he was admitted with the above-described symptoms that he really assumed the illness role.

Mr. E. was hospitalized for four months, developing hepatitis midway through his hospitalization. He became very dependent and depressed. His wife assumed responsibility for managing their home, and she accompanied him to his hemodialysis treatments and bathed and fed him in the hospital. It was at this point that Mr. E. began expressing dissatisfaction with his behavior. He was depressed, very dependent, and failed to see any improvement in his condition. The nurses were trying to get him ready for discharge, and it was decided that he would not return to home training.

After four months in the sick role, Mr. E. expressed great concern when the doctors began planning for his discharge. His feelings of anxiety about leaving the sick role were increased by the physician's withdrawal of sanction to the sick role. The anxious behaviors exhibited by Mr. E. were as follows:

1. Verbal expressions of not being capable of his own self-care. "I can't feed myself. I can't tolerate sitting long enough to get home. I'd be too weak to get to the house."

2. Verbal expressions of the physicians' not understanding his condition. "If they knew how weak I was, they wouldn't send me home. How can they send me home when they don't know what made me sick?"

Mr. E. demonstrated the behaviors of anxiety, powerlessness, depression, and withdrawal characteristic of role transition. Because of his anxiety, poor role definitions, and problems of inner dynamics of role relationships, the author believed role clarification using role rehearsal would be an effective step. The objective was to identify the behaviors, sentiments, and goals the couple believed were inherent in Mr. E.'s reassuming his previous role. The author did this by working with the couple together and with Mr. E. alone.

The first step was discussing with Mr. E. what abilities were necessary for him to leave the hospital. Mr. E. named three concerns: "I want to be able to eat without vomiting." (It had been three weeks since his last episode.) "I want to be able to walk from the car to the house." "I don't want to be a burden to my wife."

Once the author initiated the topic, the couple was able to discuss Mr. E.'s role. Mrs. E. confirmed his lack of vomiting for three weeks. Mr. E. stated, "Has it been that long?" There was consensus that he should be able to walk from the car to the house. Most important, Mrs. E. expressed her desire to help Mr. E. at home and her ability to handle problems. The conversation progressed as follows:

Mr. E.: "What would you do if I fell on the floor? You can't pick me up."

Mrs. E.: (laughing) "You're right, but I can go to the neighbors for help. You can lie on the floor until I get back, can't you?"

Mr. E.: "Yes, I guess I could."

The ability to discuss what each expected of the other individual was beneficial. Mr. E. realized that his wife did not expect him to return immediately to the previous roles they had shared. Mr. E. agreed to work on increasing his strength by ambulating with the physical therapist.

The second step used by the author was to help Ms. E. increase her husband's feelings of independence since this was considered essential to discharge by the couple. The author suggested that she gradually increase his responsibility for his own meals. At this time she was still feeding him. It was decided to encourage him to decide what foods he would eat first. Progressively Ms. E. was to encourage him to feed himself, with Ms. E. taking over when he became tired. Finally Mr. E. would feed himself unassisted. The author and Ms. E. also discussed gradually including him in decisions required for caring for the home. It was believed that this might help him become reinvolved in decision making.

In using this intervention the author spent one hour with this couple. A relationship had already been established on the basis of three months of weekly visits in the hospital. Three days after the discussion, Mr. E. was walking in the hall three times a day and helping to bathe and feed himself. In six days he was walking in the hall six times a day and feeding and bathing himself without help. At the end of a week Mr. E. was discharged, confident that he and his wife could take care of any problems that might arise. This change of behavior occurred following the implementation of Role Supplementation. In this instance, the behaviors were clarified; in other instances, different strategies of Role Supplementation may be the key to successful intervention.

EDITORS' COMMENTS AND QUESTIONS

Role Supplementation is an intervention in which the nurse can assist the client in transition between roles. The aim is to enhance the transition and prevent role insufficiency. Three strategies are suggested for Role Supplementation. Appropriate nursing diagnoses are identified and a case study is presented. This intervention has had minimal research and suggestions for further study are given.

Questions for Discussion

1. *Discuss the cost and benefits related to this intervention.*

2. *What type of research is needed to document the outcomes related to this intervention?*

3. *Discuss the implications of using a family approach in this intervention.*

References

Bandura, A. The role of imitation in personality development. *Journal of Nursing Education*, 1963, *18*(4), 207–215.

Banton, M. *An introduction to the study of social relations.* New York: Basic Books, 1965.

Burr, W. Role transitions: A reformation of theory. *Journal of Marriage and the Family*, 1972, *34*, 407–416.

Cottrell, L. The adjustment of the individual to his age and sex roles. *American Sociological Review*, 1942, *7*, 617–620.

Dunn, M. S. *A marriage role expectation inventory.* New York: Family Life Publications, 1963.

Gordon, M. *Manual of nursing diagnosis.* New York: McGraw-Hill Book Company, 1982a.

Gordon, M. *Nursing diagnosis: Process and Application.* New York: McGraw-Hill Book Company, 1982b).

Lindesmith, A. R., and Strauss, A. L. *Social psychology* (3rd ed.). New York: Holt, Rinehart and Winston, 1968.

Mead, G. *Mind, self and society.* Chicago: The University of Chicago Press, 1934.

Meleis, A. Role insufficiency and role supplementation. *Nursing Research*, 1975, *24*(4), 264–271.

Meleis, A., and Swendson, L. Role supplementation an empirical test of a nursing intervention. *Nursing Research*, 1978, *27*(1), 11–18.

Mowrer, O. H. *Learning theory and the symbolic process.* New York: John Wiley & Sons, 1960.

Parsons, T. *The social system.* New York: Free Press, 1951.

Schaeffer, E., and Manheimer, H. *Dimensions of prenatal adjustment.* Unpublished paper presented at the Eastern Psychological Association, New York, New York, April 6, 1960.

Swendson, L., Meleis, A., and Jones, D. Role supplementation for new parents—a role mastery plan. *The American Journal of Maternal Child Nursing*, 1978, *3*:(2), 84–91.

Taylor, J. A. A personality scale of manifest anxiety. *Journal Abnormal Social Psychology*, 1953, *48*, 258–290.

Turner, R. H. Role taking: Process vs. conformity. In A. Rose (Ed.), *Human behavior and social processes.* Boston: Houghton-Mifflin, 1962, pp. 20–40.

12

PATIENT TEACHING

BARBARA K. REDMAN
SUE ANN THOMAS

DESCRIPTION OF THE INTERVENTION

Patient Teaching is an interpersonal intervention that uses a stimulus already in the environment or creates a new one to help the patient develop a new thought, skill, attitude, or intention that is permanent enough to be useful in behavior change. Patients are people under the care of a provider or health care institution either intermittently or at a particular time. Much of the theory and practice of Patient Teaching is relevant to teaching others not under care, although the kinds of learning created are sometimes different, as are the approaches for getting into contact with the individuals. *Patient Education* may be thought of as the process of helping someone to learn through planned sequences of teaching and supportive activity. The terms Patient Teaching and Patient Education will be used interchangeably in this chapter.

The goals of Patient Education have historically been quite medicocentric—oriented to the goals of the health care system. Some of these goals have at times put the onus of change on the individual (victim blaming) rather than on society or on health care institutions, where it belonged. Compliance with the prescribed regimen has been a predominant goal of the medical care system, although nursing theory and practice has never been quite so limited in their focus. As institutional care has become more expensive, significant moves have been made toward having patients do medical treatments (such as dialysis) at home. This creates a need for teaching programs. In addition, the predominance of chronic illness requires a considerable emphasis on teaching for management of the illness. Concerns for quality of life have led to new, less compliance-oriented emphases in the teaching for chronic illness management. Nursing's concerns have more clearly focused on the broader concept of self-care—on assisting the patient and family to develop self-care skills and coping abilities for whatever their health situation, acute or chronic, including efforts to develop better health. Of special concern is development of goals based on the patient's and family's perceived needs, which is not just a philosophical point but also necessary for effective learning in many health situations. The education of patients has long been an active element of

160

rehabilitation programs that require major lifestyle changes. These programs traditionally focused on persons with major traumas, such as paraplegia, but the concept of rehabilitation is now being extended to those with major disruptions of heart function, to those with cancer, and to those with other disorders. Patient Education is also a major element in informed consent for treatment and in programs in which clients are being taught how to use the health care system.

Within certain fields, there are patterns of approaches to patient information and behavior. For example, since hypertension has been defined as a disease with an effective treatment, compliance with the medical regimen has been almost the exclusive desired outcome. The care is often given in community or clinic settings or in private practitioners' offices. Patient Education is one element of a construct that might be called the chronic disease treatment model, which also includes systematic monitoring schemes and follow-up. The social learning model (selective reinforcement) is seen as most likely to yield the desired behavior. In the field of cancer, there is some consensus that support beyond that usually included in education is necessary as well as teaching. Some programs emphasize support and some emphasize education, but in both cases the other element is secondary (Johnson and Flaherty, 1980). Comprehensive cancer rehabilitation programs exist, although they have been slow to develop. In a survey of such programs, Patient Education was found to be the most common feature (Harvey, 1982). Finally, changes in treatment modalities or diagnostic approaches create changes in patient education goals and learning conditions, as do decisions to allow known methods to be used by patients. A good example exists in the diabetes education literature, in which recent reports of patient self-monitoring of blood glucose of fast fraction hemoglobin levels have been almost uniformly positive, not only in terms of control but in terms of motivation and reinforcement necessary for learning.

What is conspicuous by its absence in this field is the lack of long-range developmental goals from health learning. Although theories of child development and adult learning are used to match instructional approaches to individuals, in the general Patient Education theory there is no sense of domains of health coping skills that are developed and matured through health experiences. This is unfortunate, since use of such a model is likely to provide much more efficiency in reaching episodic health care behaviors and is likely to create more of a sense of satisfaction in both provider and patient than is the case at present.

Many kinds of information input can constitute the teaching stimulus. Learning frequently occurs from stimuli that were not intended to teach, such as expectations in the environment. For this reason, it is appropriate to think of all contacts with the health care system as teaching stimuli and to make them positive learning experiences. Stimuli may be single messages, printed or spoken, or they may be complex interactions between patient and provider over a long period of time. They may also be experiences that are provider-directed and require learning a large body of knowledge, significant care skills, new interaction patterns with family members, and a strong sense of self-sufficiency. Training for home dialysis is an example of such an experience. It involves massive patterns of stimuli, aimed at multiple goals such as informed consent, adherence to a medical regimen, rehabilitation, coping, and self-care.

The teaching intervention is based at least implicitly on theories of learning. Some very basic features and principles of learning should underlie all teaching practice: the limitations of memory; the effects of anxiety on perception and information processing; the usefulness of getting messages through several senses and of exploiting natural readiness to learn when it is available; the need for active involvement and practice in order to internalize learning and to perfect skills (the amount of time spent actively practicing the task is the critical element). More formal theories of learning may be used. Behavioral learning theory has spawned intervention methods of its own, such as those used in behavior modification, but its principles of reinforcement can be used in all teaching interactions. Cognitive learning theory addresses information processing, problem solving, and the construction of meaning. Theory about the adult learner provides perspectives about how adults organize learning tasks in their lives, how they use previous learning, and how changes in their perspectives create new motivation and consolidation of learning.

The elements of a teaching intervention—goals, teaching methods, including institutional environment, readiness of the learner, evaluation and role within which teaching behaviors are planned and delivered—come together in typical patterns. A common goal for Patient Education is to alter a basic living behavior. Depending on how independent the patient is and on how profound the required behavior change, involvement of the environment may be crucial. Teaching methodologies should be experiential. Teaching must be built into the care-giving process in a cohesive way with the possibility of support for intermittent long-term maintenance of essential behaviors. Evaluation of effectiveness will often leave the nurse in an uncomfortable limbo between demonstration of knowledge, skills and confidence improvement and apparent lack of improvement in physiological parameters of the disease process or adherence to the regimen. This pattern for Patient Education is quite different from that for education in schools, where the goal is to learn intellectual skills and disciplines of knowledge, and the institution is devoted entirely to teaching. Even so, much Patient Education is inadvertently patterned after the school model and thus is much less effective than it could be.

LITERATURE ON PATIENT TEACHING: GENERAL AND RESEARCH

It might be kind to say that the literature on Patient Education is unsystematic! While there is a range of material from anecdotes to textbooks to research reports, with contributions from all of the health disciplines, the lack of a system derives from the fact that there are no comprehensive models into which Patient Education fits. There are, rather, many partial models addressing the learning needs of specific populations, such as those with a particular disease, or a disorder of a particular organ system. The bulk of the Patient Education literature is, then, segregated into these kinds of groupings with almost no cross reference among them: prenatal and postnatal, parenting, diabetes, hypertension, cardiac, pulmonary, cancer, arthritis and rheumatism, and preoperative or preprocedure; there are also smaller amounts of material for enterostomal, dialysis, and burn education, teaching of self-care skills to psychiatric patients, and other situations. There is a huge amount of literature on interventions to increase compliance with medical regimens, much of which incorporates Patient Education. There are related fields, such as genetic counseling and discharge planning, which overlap considerably with educational concerns. In general, the literature on behavior change such as cessation of smoking and control of obesity has found Patient Education not to be as effective as are more purely behavioral interventions.

There are a number of important related bodies of literature on health, of which Patient Education is a part, such as the legal and ethical literature on informed consent, education as an option in health policy, and Patient Education as part of quality assurance. There is a growing literature on organization and delivery of Patient Education, roles of patient educators, successful introduction of Patient Education programs into health care institutions, and financing for these programs.

General bodies of literature in education and human learning have to be applied with care, since they are often oriented to school learning. Each of the activities of teaching has been addressed specifically for patients and adaptations made to health settings (Redman, 1984). Protocols for Patient Education resemble teaching plans, the technology of teaching tools is addressed with special concern about problems of misunderstanding or incomplete learning, and there are many studies of readability of materials for the target groups with which they are being used. Work on instructional design from the field of education has almost never been used, even though millions of dollars are spent on instructional materials. There are special problems with the evaluation literature, not only because methods common in schools may be less appropriate in clinical settings but also because the heart of evaluation is standards of value, and these are confused in the health field, where value has always been measured in terms of mortality and morbidity. How much value should be attached to a better quality of life after a pulmonary rehabilitation program (of which Patient Education is a part) when the disease process is not arrested and the patient cannot return to work? There is a small body of literature specifically on patient learning, primarily in children's conceptions of health and in motivation (health belief model, health locus of control). Anecdotes from practice sometimes display considerable naiveté about learning, with expressions of shock on finding that patients do not remember half of what physicians tell them in an office visit, for example.

Using the literature is often a challenge, since conventional retrieval mechanisms are wholly inadequate. To a large extent, the field is a conglomeration of subliteratures. each defining a teaching model around a particular disease entity, with the learning goal being highly related to the efficacy of the medical treatment known for that disease. If teaching about a particular disease entity is the nurse's focus, for example, a search of the specific literature for the disease is not so difficult. Such a subliterature, however, always suffers from biases and narrow horizons and is not sufficient by itself. There is no standardized language. Sometimes Patient Education is simply defined as information availability, no matter what the learning needs of the patient (Swain and Steckel, 1981). Such a treatment does not adequately represent an educational intervention, since the field is rich in theory on conditions for attitude and behavior change that require considerably more than information availability.

There are several recent review articles that summarize research in Patient Education, some of them using newer forms of synthesis called meta-analysis (Glanz, 1980; Mazzuca, 1982; Mumford, 1982; Posavac, 1980; Reading, 1979). This approach involves the statistical analysis of the summary findings of a group of empirical studies (Glass, 1981) and offers a replicable method by which to draw conclusions about the overall effectiveness of Patient Education as tested in a number of studies. The reviews find Patient Education outcomes (as measured by the studies summarized) on the average to be positive and clearly better than outcomes for patients who had no teaching. What is also clear is that for behaviors considered to be clinically important, purely informational approaches are not the most effective option. In one summary of psychological interventions for surgery and heart attacks (Mumford, Schesinger, and Glass, 1982), approaches intended to offer emotional support and relieve anxiety were more effective than purely informational approaches, although a combination of both approaches seemed clearly superior to either alone. On the average, psychological intervention reduced hospitalization approximately by two days below that of the control group, which makes it a cost-effective intervention. In a summary of controlled experiments of the effectiveness of Patient Education on compliance, physiological progress, and long-range health outcomes, efforts that merely increased patients' knowledge, through an invariant presentation of medical facts or treatment principles intended for all patients with a single chronic medical problem, were rarely successful. More effective were programs that (a) used the patient's own regimen and daily routine as the content of instruction, and (b) attempted to affect the patient's home or work environment in ways that promote effective self-management, such as memory aids, social support, medication monitoring, and telephone follow-up (Mazzuca, 1982).

What is clear from these reviews is that Patient Education must be broadly defined and incorporated into a nursing framework that is focused on problem solving *with* the patient, incorporating his environment, altering his regimen, exploring his feelings and attributions, allowing him freedom to approach the behavior change in his own way, making care accessible both physically and in terms of time, having the provider psychologically accessible, and building follow-up into the interaction. For the provider, at least two process approaches are available to aid in Patient Education. One of these follows the traditional nursing process steps. Another (Green et al., 1980) starts with the desired health status and works backward to identifying the necessary behaviors, categorizing the factors that seem to have direct impact on the behaviors into predisposing, enabling, and reinforcing factors, and intervening on those to remove blocks or reinforce positive forces.

AVAILABLE INTERVENTION TOOLS

There are several kinds of tools available in Patient Education, all of which aid in planning or carrying out the intervention. These tools follow the nursing process steps.

1. The primary tool is the kind of relationship with a provider that was outlined in the previous section.

2. General nursing assessment guides often include some screening questions about health skills, knowledge, and beliefs and serve the purpose of identifying individuals who need Patient Education. If that need is positive, a more detailed educational assessment guide will be used to further pinpoint the areas of learning need.

3. Teaching protocols or standardized nursing care plans provide guidance for preparation and actual delivery of Patient Education. For example, one sample set of protocols included the following items in columnar format: goals and objectives, references for nurse preparation, content to be taught, a list of teaching aids and how to use them, guide questions to ask patients to evaluate learning, and the role of other team members, such as the dietitian. It also included questionnaires and forms for knowledge assessment, physical assessment, physiological well-being survey, and a teaching progress sheet (DeJoseph, 1980).

4. Instructional materials to give to patients or to use with them while teaching are in widespread use. Many printed materials and audiovisual aids are available from commercial sources or voluntary health organizations; many other teaching tools are developed by staff in institutions. Assuring the quality of all materials for specific purposes is a problem. A number of hospitals have televisions systems with regular schedules of programming for patient education. Some have practice settings, such as a facsimile of a small apartment for teaching of transfer, cooking, and other skills for persons with some degree of paralysis. All of these are tools to be used in a patient-provider relationship.

5. Evaluation tools may include audit standards and questionnaires, tests, and observation tools to determine whether the patient has learned. These actually are also intervention tools, since test-taking is usually a learning experience, and because they serve to redirect the teaching process.

A look at the availability of these tools for one area of teaching—diabetes education—will illustrate some concerns about tools, although diabetes is likely to be better developed than are most other areas of Patient Education. Of the respondents (about one third) to a survey in Michigan, 66 per cent indicated they were currently using an assessment form to determine the educational needs of their diabetic patients. Analysis of 203 of these forms found information about the patient's knowledge to be the most common information gathered (present in 75 per cent of the forms), whereas health beliefs and attitudes (such as patient perceptions about the efficacy of the regimen, the perceived seriousness of diabetes, and willingness to comply) were assessed in fewer than 10 per cent of the forms; questions about family interest in learning, a type of indirect measure of the degree of social support available to the patient, were found in 7 per cent of the survey; and 9 per cent attempted to assess adaptation to the disease. Even within the knowledge category there was wide variation, with 82 per cent of the forms assessing knowledge of diet but only 28 per cent knowledge of exercise (Boutaugh, Hull, and Davis, 1982). There are also tools available to measure social coping skills in diabetics (Gross and Johnson, 1981), a Personal Responsibilities Attitude Assessment System used by the Maine Diabetes Control Project (Anderson, Genther, and Alogna, 1982), an educational diagnosis instrument under development (Davis et al., 1981), and a psychometrically sophisticated tool for evaluating diabetes education, also under development (Windsor et al., 1981). There are a wide variety of teaching materials and protocols available for diabetes education.

Without tools and a consistent and coherent structure within which they are to be used (such as a protocol), it is likely that little teaching will be done. A set of tools and protocols communicates to the staff an expectation that teaching will be done. In addition, since staff members are busy and cannot develop tools instantly on their own, they will feel unprepared to teach without these supports. Generally there has been little systematic assessment of staff preparation for Patient Education, and intervention tools are required to assist those who need development. Also of importance are adequate systems for documentation that Patient Teaching has been done and for recording evidence of patient learning. This evidence is most often observation of behaviors and verbal answers to important questions originally explicated in the goals. A program will periodically have to show that it is cost-effective; this can often be done most clearly with the chronic diseases by showing that after teaching, patients have fewer hospitalizations for avoidable complications.

ASSOCIATED NURSING DIAGNOSES AND APPROPRIATE CLIENT GROUPS

Patient Education is relevant for most groups of patients, including many psychiatric patients and those with learning disabilities.

Of the nursing diagnoses approved by participants at the Fourth National Conference (Kim and Moritz, 1982), a number could be helped by Patient Education. One of the most directly relevant is Knowledge Deficit, which can come from lack of exposure, lack of recall, information misinterpretation, lack of interest in learning, or unfamiliarity with information resources. Ineffective Coping by Individuals and Compromised Coping by Families can be due to lack of skill in problem solving or lack of knowledge of how to use present skills and thus be amenable to teaching intervention, as can Family Coping: Potential for Growth and Impaired Home Maintenance Management. There are teaching actions that can be preventive for patients with a diagnosis of Potential for Injury. Teaching may be effective for the subgroup of those diagnosed as Noncompliant who lack knowledge, skills, and motivation, but it may be only a component of the treatment for others with more complex problems; the same may be said for Alterations in Parenting and Sexual Dysfunction. Clients with Self-Care Deficits often require retraining.

RECOMMENDATIONS FOR PRACTICE AND RESEARCH

Although much as been accomplished in defining teaching programs and getting them into operation, much remains to be done to define the intervention strategy with clarity, let alone rigor, and to make certain that good quality practice is being efficiently and consistently delivered.

1. The field should be aware that outcome goals thought achievable to some degree by Patient Education are widely variable in terms of values. Open discussion of this issue should help staff members at institutions who are trying to coordinate and further develop Patient Education programs. Also, there should be a mechanism for identifying new models of desired patient learning which surface periodically, defining them and their usefulness to quality care, and then deliberately implementing them. One that seems to be emerging is a psychoeducational model, in which families of mental patients want not just support but also skill in strategies for coping with their relatives. New models are likely to emerge when treatment patterns are changed or new disease entities or health behaviors are defined.

2. A great deal of work should be done on definitions and measurement of components of Patient Education intervention. This is important in research studies so that treatment variables are replicable and results cumulative. Of further concern is the need to routinely monitor the interventions to see that they are actually being delivered with reasonable fidelity to the definitions of the treatment variable.

3. An unknown amount of the needed Patient Education can be incorporated into ongoing care processes by making conversations purposeful and by having plans for patient learning. Beyond this, other delivery systems, such as classes, will be needed. Most health care institutions are far from comprehensive in their Patient Education services and are likely to be inefficient in those they do deliver. Both weaknesses should be addressed.

4. Very little is known about the quality of most ordinary Patient Education. In many fields, although good models of effective Patient Education are gradually being developed, processes of recognition and diffusion of these superior models are unknown—probably they are haphazard to some degree.

Of equal importance is development of monitoring systems in care of individuals. An example is the study by Bubela (1981) of four patients and their spouses whose treatment for cancer involved constant intra-arterial infusion by catheter for four to six weeks to the site of malignancy . Teaching apparently involved instruction sheets and demonstration of filling the syringe and changing it, discussion of possible side effects and complications, and type of information patients should report. The visiting nurse was to change the dressing. All patients had problems with technical aspects of the care, some quite serious (such as cracked tubing while the patient was asleep, with his awakening in a pool of blood). The visiting nurses were often not the same individuals and may sometimes have to be directed by the patient how to perform the dressing change. All spouses were afraid when they encountered technical problems and worried about pulling the catheter out. It is indeed clear that families needed not only more supervision and a standardized teaching plan (Bubela, 1981)—they also needed to learn under supervision until the tasks were mastered. The fact that this teaching program would be inadequate should have been known when it was planned. Aside from legal liability on the part of the agency, poor quality of Patient Education is poor quality care. Perhaps all such programs should be reviewed and approved before implementation, since personnel in a particular area may not have expertise to predict teaching or learning difficulties.

5. Finally there is evidence that Patient Education is entering a new phase of acceptance and development. A recent editorial appearing in *Cancer Nursing* (Reed-Ash and Gianella, 1982) calls for standardization of the Patient Education process in multiple areas of cancer care, with standardized assessment methods and specific outcome criteria. This kind of consolidation is necessary and can occur through specialty organizations or progressive health care agencies taking responsibility for the consensus-developing activities. What is clear is that nursing must take a leadership role in moving the field this next stage forward, since nursing manpower is the only way Patient Education can be given on a broad basis, and nursing's theoretical base is much more supportive for this kind of care than are those of many other disciplines.

CASE STUDY EXAMPLES

The following case studies illustrate use of a consistent process. The first step is engagement of the patient into a teaching-learning process. The patient must be encouraged to relate the specific factors involved with his or her health care problem; then he or she can begin to identify concerns and goals concerning therapy. Once the patient's needs are identified, the second step begins by determining the nursing diagnosis and negotiation of a plan with active patient involvement. The third step is carrying through the plan with a process of evaluation of effectiveness.

While the nurse's role in Patient Education requires counseling skills, there are differences between counseling and teaching as intervention strategies. Counseling is used when the primary focus of the intervention is on emotions, whereas Teaching is used in situations where a combination of cognitive, affective, and psychomotor skills are to be developed. Generally, in Counseling the therapist encourages the patient to set his or her own goals—the therapist does not have specific goals in mind for the patient. In Patient Teaching the nurse has specific goals for the teaching-learning process, since there are definite areas of content that each patient needs to learn to assume safe self-care. The nurse must negotiate the goals of the Patient Teaching sessions with the patient, but, unlike many counseling situations, the nurse has his or her own specific goals for the session.

The cases also illustrate that in clinical situations, Patient Education methodology includes not only the traditional instructional approaches and aids but also demonstration, counseling, peer group and family discussions, behavior modification, simplifying regimens, community organizing, and other intervention approaches which serve to stimulate learning and help make environments supportive to learning.

Case Study 1

Mrs. F., a 24 year old white female, is seen in the outpatient department by a clinical specialist in nursing. Her chief complaints are tiredness, depression, and weight gain. She weighs 175 pounds and is 5'4" tall. She has been married for the past 6 years. She and her husband have three children, ages 3 years, 1 year, and 2 months. Mrs. F. is currently breast-feeding the 2 month old baby. She and her husband are high school graduates. Her husband is a mechanic.

To assess what factors may be contributing to Mrs. F.'s complaints, the nurse uses open questions about the patient's usual day and her extended family. The nurse finds out that the patient's mother weighs 225 pounds and her father is of normal weight. She has two brothers and one sister, each of whom "are about 40 pounds overweight." Eating large meals plays a strong social function in her extended family. The nurse then asks about the patient's weight gain. She states "she had never been overweight before she had her babies" and "she has put on twenty pounds with each pregnancy just like my mother did." The patient states "I just stay home all day and eat, I finish whatever the children don't eat." The patient then discusses in detail her routine schedule. This reveals that the patient has very little purpose or structure to her day. "Things are the same day after day—I just try to keep up with the children." The patient states she "feels out of control." She says, "For example, the house is a mess" and "the three year old is bad, needs constant attention, and is uncontrollable." The nurse asks about the patient's husband and the patient replies, "He doesn't care, I am supposed to take care of the house and the kids." "All he does is work, days, nights, and weekends." She also states that her immediate family sees her as "childish" and "complaining about every little thing."

The nurse then asks the patient to write down a list of all the foods she had eaten that day. The list shows all convenience foods, no milk products, and very little protein. The patient and nurse then talk about the list of foods. The nurse helps the patient to categorize the foods as carbohydrates, fats, and protein sources. The patient then states that she can see foods on the list that she "shouldn't eat." The nurse then asks if the patient is willing to try to change her eating pattern and therefore lose weight. The patient agrees. Plans are made for the patient to keep a food diary and weigh herself daily. An appointment is made for the next week. The nurse also asks if the husband might be willing to join them at the next appointment.

The first step in any nurse-patient interaction is engagement of the patient. This means encouraging the patient to "tell her story." The patient must trust the nurse enough to tell the nurse the specific facts related to his or her story. A patient who will not discuss probnlems with the nurse generally does not fully comply with the plan of care. The patient must become involved and identify his or her needs.

This patient has three nursing diagnoses: Depression, Ineffective Coping, and Obesity. The next step illustrated in this case is negotiation of a plan of care with active patient involvement. Giving the patient a task to complete in the following week allows the nurse to evaluate the patient's willingness to comply with a negotiated plan. The husband's involvement may or may not be crucial to the successful weight loss or to decreasing Mrs. F.'s depression, but an involved other may help Ms. F. stay motivated to change.

Mrs. F. and her husband attend the next clinic visit. The nurse asks Mr. F. what prompted him to come to the appointment. He states, "Well, she asked me to come. I am upset with her. She has no energy and she is always in a bad mood. I tell her it's all that junk food." The nurse then asks Mr. F. what he would like to see changed and how could he help? Mr. F. replied, "I want to see her happier with herself. I will be glad to help with the kids some and help her to diet by not eating junk myself." The nurse then asks Mrs. F. what she thinks of this. She was frankly surprised. She had viewed Mr. F. as unconcerned; she thought his interest was "super."

The nurse and Mr. and Mrs. F. then review the diet diary and weight record. Ms. F. had lost 3 pounds. She decreased her carbohydrate and junk food intake, but had also frequently skipped meals and had days in which she ate little vegetables or fruit. The nurse suggests some changes in the meal plans to include more fruits and vegetables. The couple indicates their favorite fruits and vegetables, and a plan is made for the next week.

Both Mrs. F. and her husband have active involvement in the plan of therapy. Both have clearly identified what they will do to make this plan work.

In the following weeks Mr. F. continued to support the diet plans. He also agreed to watch the children one night a week. Mrs. F. decided to join a weight loss group on the night he would watch the children. As she got out once a week, Mrs. F. recognized her depression and fatigue were also decreased. She and her husband, at the suggestion of the nurse, began to take a walk after dinner several nights a week. The large family dinners continued to be a source of "high temptation" to overeat for Ms. F. In a discussion with the nurse, Mrs. F. devised her own plan to overcome this problem. She decided to not "diet" on special occasions, but neither would she overeat. She ate small portions of all the food offered, but would refuse "seconds." She succeeded at this attempt. Over the following months Mrs. F.'s plan for weight loss was successful and she found that the changes her dieting had made had helped her in more ways than just the weight loss.

Throughout this case the nurse consistently planned for the evaluation of the effectiveness of therapy. She allowed new problems to be discussed and plans altered to fit different circumstances.

Case Study 2

Mr. J. is a 46 year carpenter. He has been diagnosed as hypertensive for the past 12 years. During this time his medications have been gradually increased. He is currently on Hydrochlorothiazide, 50 mg bid, Propranolol (Inderal), 40 mg bid, and Promazine Hydrochloride (Prazine), 2 mg bid. He is 25 pounds overweight and smokes. He does not participate in any regular exercise program. He is married and has two sons, 14 and 12 years old. His wife is a housewife.

On his routine three month follow-up visit, Mr. J.'s blood pressure is 168/106. The nurse inquires if Mr. J. can think of any reasons why his blood pressure would be so elevated. Mr. J. states he has been on his low salt diet and he has lost 6 pounds. The nurse then asks if he has been taking his medications as prescribed. He replies that he has. She then asks him if he has been having any additional stresses in his life. Mr. J. looks down and replies, "No, I haven't."

The nurse schedules Mr. J. to come back in three days and again have his blood pressure checked. At this point, the nurse is concerned. She does not understand why Mr. J.'s blood pressure would be so high. She also worries that Mr. J. is not able to discuss with her his concern.

On the next visit his blood pressure is 140/85. The nurse asks Mr. J. if he can account for the difference. With a small smile on his face, Mr. J. says, "No." The nurse then asks Mr. J. to tell her about the last three days. This is an effort on the nurse's part to allow Mr. J. to relate some factors that may be influencing his blood pressure. Mr. J. does not open up and "tell his story." He gives a brief, curt description of going to work, watching television, and other routine events. After failing to engage Mr. J., the nurse then asks Mr. J. how he intends to keep his blood pressure down at this level. He replies that he does "not intend to keep his blood pressure down." The nurse asks what would keep him from wanting to maintain a lower blood pressure. Mr. J. quietly states that he is a man and will not have his "manhood" taken from him. The nurse then encourages Mr. J. to describe the difficulties he has been experiencing. Mr. J. describes a lack of sexual arousal and decreased ability to perform sexually with his wife. He also states that since he stopped his medication one month ago, these "problems" had disappeared.

The nurse then asks Mr. J. to tell her what medication he was on when he had last been to clinic. He replies, "None." The nurse then asks Mr. J. to discuss with her what hypertension is and the consequences of continued elevated pressures.

Mr. J. has finally allowed the nurse to know the difficulties he is experiencing. He has engaged in a therapeutic relationship with her.

During the discussion it is evident to the nurse that Mr. J. knows little about his hypertension and its complications. She tells him in simple terms the prognosis of untreated hypertension. He seems to be concerned. He states, "A man must provide for his family and I can't do that if I have a heart attack or stroke. But I'm really caught in between, I can't live like it was on the medicines and I won't live without them."

The nurse decides on the following nursing diagnoses: Knowledge Deficit about hypertension and Sexual Dysfunction related to hypertension drugs. Mr. J. is willing to negotiate a plan of therapy with the nurse, but needs more information on the possible courses of action.

The nurse then tells Mr. J. that medications can be changed to reduce the side effects he is experiencing. She also tells him there are a few things he could do for himself to improve his health. They discuss weight loss, regular exercise, and stopping smoking.

Over the next several months Mr. J. and the nurse meet frequently to discuss the new medication regimen and his efforts at weight loss, exercise, and cessation of smoking. His wife attends these sessions and is an active participant in planning meals and encouraging Mr. J. to continue his graduated exercise program. They also have an opportunity to discuss their concerns about sexuality. Mr. J. loses weight and maintains a well-planned exercise program; in addition his problems with impotency decrease. He reports that since he and his wife have begun to talk more about their sexuality, he has become more relaxed. His blood pressure has decreased and his medications have also been decreased.

Frequent visits with the nurse provide support for Mr. J. and his wife. They actively discuss both personal and medical problems with her. The nurse is able to evaluate the effectiveness of their plan by monitoring Mr. J.'s blood pressure and personal response to the therapy.

Case Study 3

Joan is a 17 year old unmarried pregnant woman. She is in her 20th week. She is in her senior year of high school and is continuing her studies despite her pregnancy. Her blood pressure has been elevated in the last two visits: 145–150/100–104. She has gained 40 pounds. She has been put on a diuretic.

The nurse working with Joan finds it difficult to engage her. Joan answers all questions with a "yes" or "no." The nurse has tried to encourage Joan to tell her about herself, but Joan has refused.

Joan's mother accompanies Joan to most visits. She asks some questions about Joan's pregnancy, but seems hostile to Joan and rarely talks to her.

The nurse recognizes the importance for Joan to relate openly, but thinks that perhaps the one-to-one relationship with the nurse is threatening to Joan.

The nurse asks Joan if she would like to meet with some other pregnant teenagers for a twice a month group session. Joan reluctantly agrees to attend.

The nurse thinks that the sharing in a group session may allow Joan to "open up" about her own problem. The nurse also assumes that Joan needs to learn a great deal about pregnancy, delivery, and care of the newborn. It is more cost-effective to do this type of teaching in a group setting. The nurse will continue to see Joan every two weeks, but on the alternate weeks Joan will attend the nurse-supervised group meetings.

In the first meeting, the six teenagers seemed reluctant to talk, but during the prolonged break for juice and low calorie snacks the girls seemed to warm up to the group. The agenda of the group was negotiated with the girls. Each girl named the issues she wanted to discuss. The nurse then grouped the issues into topical areas. The sessions allowed for much group discussion and questions.

As Joan's participation in the group sessions increased, so did her comfort in her visits with the nurse. Her weight gain over the next six weeks was four pounds. She began asking many questions about nutrition and hypertension. She went on a low sodium diet and her blood pressure decreased to 130/90. The diuretic was discontinued.

The group provided a stimulus for Joan to discuss her concerns with her peers. She became more in control of her own health planning with group support. The group members formed a close-knit group and decided to continue to meet to help each other through the early days of motherhood.

The nurse provided the structure, information, and guidance to ensure good group process. The teenagers needed each other to decrease their isolation and encourage sharing of concerns. Joan's mother also benefited from the group sessions. She had been feeling overly responsible and angry about Joan's pregnancy. As Joan became more independent, her mother felt less burdened by Joan's pregnancy. Joan and her mother began discussing child care alternatives and Joan's mother was delighted to find out Joan had found a day care center to take care of the baby.

This situation illustrates the complex interrelationship of health care problems. There are many social, family, emotional, and health issues in this case study. The nurse is responsible for helping to set health care goals with the patient and her family. To do this, he or she also must help the family to seek other resources, develop coping skills, and facilitate communication between family members.

EDITORS' COMMENTS AND QUESTIONS

The goal of Patient Teaching has changed from enhancing compliance with the medical regimen to assisting the client to assume responsibility for self-care. Redman and Thomas emphasize that Patient Teaching is more than information giving. It is a means of helping the client develop a combination of cognitive, affective, and psychomotor skills. Although there is a large literature on Patient Teaching, it tends to be organized around specific disease entitites. There is no information on Patient Teaching related to the diagnosis of Knowledge Deficit, and there are few guidelines on how to assess readiness for learning.

Questions for Discussion
1. *Distinguish between Patient Teaching and Counseling.*
2. *Which is more effective, structured or unstructured Patient Teaching?*
3. *How can various tools for Patient Teaching be standardized?*
4. *How can the outcome of Patient Teaching be documented?*
5. *Does every client need Patient Teaching?*
6. *How can Knowledge Deficit be assessed?*

References
Anderson, R. M., Genther, R. W., and Alogna, M. Diabetes patient education from philosophy to delivery. *Diabetes Educator*, 1982, 9(1), 33–36.

Boutaugh, M. L., Hull, A. L., and Davis, W. K. An examination of diabetes educational assessment forms. *Diabetes Educator*, 1982, 7(4), 29–34.

Bubela, N. Technical and psychological problems and concerns arising from the outpatient treatment of cancer with direct intraarterial infusion. *Cancer Nursing*, 1981, 4, 305–309.

Davis, W. K., Hull, A. L., and Boutaugh, M. Factors affecting the educational diagnoses of diabetic patients. *Diabetes Care*, 1981, 4, 275–278.

DeJoseph, J. F. Writing and evaluating educational protocols. In Squyres, W. P. (Ed.), *Patient education; an inquiry into the state of the art*. New York: Springer-Verlag, 1980.

Glanz, K. Compliance with dietary regimen: Its magnitude, measurement and determinants. *Preventive Medicine*, 1980, 9, 787–804.

Glass, G. R., McGaw, B., and Smith, M. L. *Meta-analyses in social research*. Beverly Hills, Calif.: Sage Publications, 1981.

Green, L. W., Kreuter, M. W., Deeds, S. G., and Partridge, K. B. *Health education planning; a diagnostic approach*. Palo Alto, Calif.: Mayfield Publications, 1980.

Gross, A. M., and Johnson, W. G. The Diabetes Assertiveness Test: A measure of social coping skills in pre-adolescent diabetes. *Diabetes Educator*, 1981, 7(2), 26–27.

Harvey, R. F., Jellinek, H. M., and Habeck, R. V. Cancer rehabilitation: An analysis of 36 program approaches. *Journal of the American Medical Association*, 1982, 2127–2131.

Johnson, J., and Flaherty, M. The nurse and cancer patient education. *Seminars in Oncology*, 1980, 7(1), 63–70.

Kim, M. J., and Moritz, D. A. (Eds). *Classification of nursing diagnoses.* New York: McGraw-Hill Book Company, 1982.

Mazzuca, S. A. Does patient education in chronic disease have therapeutic value? *Journal of Chronic Diseases, 1982, 35,* 521–529.

Mumford, E., Schlesinger, H. J., and Glass, G. V. The effects of psychological intervention in recovery from surgery and heart attacks; an analysis of the literature. *American Journal of Public Health, 1982, 72,* 141–151.

Posavac, E. J. Evaluation of patient education programs: A meta analysis. *Evaluation and the Health Professions, 1980, 3*(1), 47–62.

Reading, A. Short term effects of psychological preparation for surgery. *Social Science and Medicine, 1979, 13A,* 641–654.

Redman, B. K. *The process of patient education* (5th ed.). St. Louis: C. V. Mosby, 1984.

Reed-Ash, C., and Gianella, A. Patient education. *Cancer Nursing, 1982, 5,* 261.

Swain, M. A., and Steckel, S. B. Influencing adherence among hypertensives. *Research in Nursing and Health, 1981, 4,* 213–222.

Windsor, R. A., Roseman, J., Gartseff, G., and Kirk, K. A. Qualitative issues in developing educational diagnostic instruments and assessment procedures for diabetic patients. *Diabetes Care, 1981, 4,* 468–475.

13

VALUES CLARIFICATION.

JAMES Z. WILBERDING

Values Clarification is an intervention developed by educators. It is designed to assist people to learn the process of "valuing" and thereby be clearer about their own values. Because values are one basis for decision making, Values Clarification is relevant in nursing as clients assume more responsibility for decisions about their care. Since the nurse's goal is to assist and support the client, the nurse should understand the values clarification process. In some instances, the nurse may choose to initiate the process as an intervention.

VALUES AS DISTINCT FROM ATTITUDES, BELIEFS, AND OPINIONS

Before exploring Values Clarification as a process it is helpful to distinguish *values* from certain other affective concepts, particularly attitudes, beliefs, and opinions. Attitudes are dispositions toward a particular thing. They have cognitive, affective, and behavioral components and some level of permanence (Gordon, 1975; Steele and Harmon, 1979). According to Gordon, "attitudes have specified referents, while values are more generalized" (1975, p. 9). Steele and Harmon define beliefs as "a special class of attitudes in which the cognitive component is based more on faith than on fact. They represent a personal confidence in the validity of some idea, person, or object" (1979, p. 3). Gordon's definition is broader than Steele and Harmon's, as it includes more bases for a belief than just faith. He writes:

> Beliefs are propositions to which individuals assent at varying degrees of certitude ranging from conjecture to conviction. Beliefs are verifiable in that at least theoretically they can be shown to be true or false. A person's belief may be (1) validated, where direct or indirect evidence already has been examined, (2) unvalidated but taken on faith, or (3) unvalidated but questioned. Beliefs may be held at various levels of confidence depending

*I would like to include an expression of appreciation to the psychiatric nursing staff at the Iowa City V. A. Medical Center for their comments on the value sheet in Table 13–1.

173

upon the conclusiveness of the evidence to the individual or the degree of faith manifested in it. Beliefs are taken to refer to past or present phenomena. (Gordon, 1975, p. 7)

Opinions, according to Gordon, "represent judgements regarding a course of action in terms of implicitly or explicitly stated consequences" (1975, p. 7). Opinions, then, might be considered more in the intellectual realm than in the affective, but people usually have feelings about their opinions. On the other hand, according to Steele and Harmon, "A *value* is an affective disposition towards a person, object, or idea" (1979, p. 1). Experience is a major source of values. Thus, different people have different values and these are changeable, according to Raths, Harmon, and Simon (1966). Gordon disagrees to some extent, for he writes that values "tend to persist over time and are resistant to change" (1975, p. 10). Gordon defines values as "constructs representing generalized behaviors or states of affairs that are considered by the individual to be important" (1975, p. 2). Thus, Gordon brings in behaviors as a component of values, whereas Steele and Harmon left them at the level of affect. Gordon (1975) also recognizes that values involve choice—the preferring of one thing to another. This discussion supports the assertion of Raths and colleagues (1966) that there is no consensus on the definition of *value*. They state rather broadly that "a value represents something important in human existence" (Raths et al., 1966, p. 9) and that values are "those elements that show how a person has decided to use his life" (p. 6). Raths and associates give criteria for a value that are more definitive and will be considered later in the chapter.

The variety of definitions does not diminish the importance of values. An important function of values, according to Simon, Howe, and Kirschenbaum (1972), is to serve as a basis for our decisions and choices. According to these authors, health is an area of potential value conflict. Health, of course, is a major concern of the nurse and thus the nurse is appropriately concerned with value conflicts about health. At least one nursing theory states that "the humanistic nursing effort is directed toward increasing the possibilities of making responsible choices" (Paterson and Zderad, 1976, p. 17). If choice involves value decisions, the nurse will be interested in his or her client's valuing ability. In the realm of health care decisions, Curtin puts the case for concern for values more strongly:

> Insofar as patients' values are ignored, or replaced with others' values, patients cease to exist as unique human beings. Depersonalization may be partial or complete, but those individuals will die as the persons they were. If the depersonalization is complete, those individuals will not be able to create new values and goals in their life and they will lose a sense of meaning or purpose in their existence. (Curtin, 1979, p. 7)

Thus, if we are committed as nurses to the well-being of the whole person, we will be interested in supporting their unique wholeness as individuals with appropriate intervention in the area of values. At the same time we will avoid the imposition of our own values.

THE PROCESS OF VALUING

In 1966 Raths and associates catalogued factors that impinged on children's values. These included great changes in social institutions, broken families, lessened contact with parents, exposure to violence and strange behavior in the media without an opportunity to discuss these with the family, lessened contact with and importance of religion, greater mobility, and more choices.

They postulated that children do not learn well because of lack of clarity about the purpose of life. These children were likely to be apathetic, flighty, uncertain, inconsistent, and possibly drifters, overconformers, overdissenters, role players, and underachievers (Raths et al., 1966). A common problem of children so affected is confusion in values, according to Raths and colleagues (1966).

There are three traditional ways of helping children acquire values (Kirschenbaum, 1977; Simon et al., 1972). Moralizing is one of these and basically consists of telling the child what is right or wrong. Modeling, which seeks to set an example for others to follow, is another traditional way (Kirschenbaum, 1977). The problem with these approaches is that there are many different sources of moralizing and modeling, such as parents, religions, entertainment, and peers. This only adds to the confusion (Kirschenbaum, 1977; Simon et al., 1972); nevertheless moralizing and modeling have been traditional parental prerogatives. A third approach is the laissez faire attitude, which consists of letting children do what they want in the belief that things will turn out all right. It is quite likely that this will lead the child to confusion (Simon et al., 1972). A different but nontraditional approach is Values Clarification as propounded by Raths and others (Kirschenbaum, 1977; Raths et al., 1966, 1978; Simon et al., 1972). The process described by Raths and colleagues will be discussed from this point as applying to both children and adults, although the focus of their writings was on children.

Raths and co-workers (1966) call Values Clarification a theory. The theory applies critical thinking techniques to matters that are in the affective domain (Raths et al., 1966). Values Clarification is a method whereby persons are encouraged to undertake the process of valuing and there is emphasis on the human "capacity for intelligent, self-directed behavior" (Raths et al., 1966, p. 46). The point seems to be that valuing is more than an affective process, that it requires intellectual activity in the form of critical thought to be brought to completion.

There are seven essential steps in the valuing process as described by Raths and associates:

1. Choosing freely.
2. Choosing from among alternatives.
3. Choosing after thoughtful consideration of the consequences of each alternative.
4. Prizing and cherishing.
5. Affirming.
6. Acting upon choices.
7. Repeating. (Raths et al., 1966, pp. 28–29)

For clarification it should be pointed out that steps 4 and 5 involve feeling happy about the choice made in the first three steps and being willing to publicly affirm this choice. Step 7, repeating, means that we act repeatedly on our choice in life. The seven steps may be summarized as choosing, prizing, and acting (Raths et al., 1966, p. 30).

According to the theory, these steps function as criteria for what is and what is not a value. A true value meets all seven of the criteria. The steps are listed here in the order in which they are usually placed in the literature. They may not necessarily occur in this order. For example, someone may perform an act repeatedly, such as visiting with an elderly neighbor. It may be that only later, after some reflection, does he discover that he prizes this experience and that this contact with an aging person represents a value for him. There are "expressions which approach values, but which do not meet all of the criteria" (Raths et al., p. 30). These are value indicators. Examples of these are goals, aspirations, interests, feelings, and worries (Raths et al., 1966, pp. 30–33). These value indicators may become values as the valuing process is applied to them (Raths et al., 1966, p. 33).

According to Raths and colleagues (1978), there are three sources of content for clarification. These include value indicators, personal issues, and social issues. In nursing, all three of these sources may need to be considered in the community health situation. The nurse in acute care is more likely to be confronted with a client's personal issue, such as choosing surgery or radiation for cancer treatment.

In initiating Values Clarification, the helper and client focus on a life issue, the helper communicates acceptance of the client, and the helper invites the client to progress through the seven steps of valuing (Raths et al., 1978, p. 48). It should be added that a basic component of Values Clarification is for the helper to maintain a nonjudgmental stance (Raths et al., 1978). The client's decisions are accepted. Coupled with this is the need for individual autonomy, i.e., the client chooses freely without coercion from the helper.

Kirschenbaum criticizes the seven criteria proposed by Raths and associates, primarily on the grounds that they are not operational. In addressing the criteria of prizing and cherishing, he asks, "*How* proud must someone be of a belief before it may be considered a 'value'?" (Kirschenbaum, 1977, p. 9). He is also careful to point out that Values Clarification does not mean simply clarity about one's own values without consideration of others' values. The personal and social consequences of an individual's position are important in the clarification process (Kirschenbaum, 1977). Kirschenbaum's criticisms and ethical commentary are an important element in the literature on this topic. Prior to Kirschenbaum's affirming that the consequences of values are important, the major ethical emphasis of values clarification literature was on the individual's right to choose values autonomously.

The better defined ethical position of Kirschenbaum is evident in his definition of the valuing process: "a process by which we increase the likelihood that our living in general or a decision in particular will, first, have positive value for us, and, second, be constructive in the social context" (Kirschenbaum, 1977, pp. 9–10). Values Clarification aims to teach this. According to Kirschenbaum, "values clarification can be defined as an approach that utilizes questions and activities designed to teach the valuing process and that helps people skillfully to apply the valuing processes to value-rich areas in their lives" (1977, p. 12). Kirschenbaum (1977) views the valuing process as consisting of five dimensions: (1) thinking, (2) feeling, (3) choosing, (4) communicating, and (5) acting. Kirschenbaum formulated three hypotheses based on the theory, which relate to children. Unfortunately, the nursing profession has not yet tested formal hypotheses from the theory, although it is evident from the literature that nurses are predicting outcomes for persons who undergo Values Clarification. For example: "The end result is a person with more awareness, empathy, and insight than a person who has not had this experience" (Steele and Harmon, 1979, p. 9). We await the formalization and testing of this prediction.

NURSING APPLICATION

The most serious development of a rationale for Values Clarification as a nursing intervention is by Gadow (1979, 1980 a, b, 1981). She believes that self-care is a philosophical basis of nursing. By self-care, Gadow means a type of care that respects the client's autonomy. Gadow views autonomy as a fundamental human right. Self-determination is an expression of this right, and self-determination calls for decisions to be made that express the patient's values (Gadow, 1980a). Thus, throughout her writings, Gadow proposes that the nurse act as an advocate for this type of care by assisting the patient in clarifying his or her values. Gadow does not offer an elaborate methodology for this clarification but does propose discussions between nurse and client as one mode of intervention (Gadow, 1981). There is no mention of the methods used by Raths and colleagues in Gadow's work; she has conceptualized Values Clarification independently on the basis of her dual background as nurse and philosopher.

Other nurses who write on Values Clarification have drawn from the work of Raths and associates (Berger et al., 1975; Coletta, 1978; Rheinscheld, 1980; Rosner, 1975; Steele and Harmon, 1979; Uustal, 1977, 1978, 1980). Thus, we have the rather odd situation of nurses' basing an intervention on a theoretical framework from another discipline when one of their own, colleagues, Gadow, has independently developed a nursing-based framework for it. The appeal of the Raths and co-workers' theory may lie in the fact that there are numerous published collections of tools for Values Clarification based on this theory.

Uustal's writing focuses on using Values Clarification as a tool for personal growth and ethical reflection by nurses. She touches on Values Clarification as useful in patient teaching. She believes that Values Clarification could be a way of finding out what the patient wants to learn so that this could be taught first (Uustal, 1978). Her understanding of the theory set forth by Raths and associates becomes questionable when she writes, "How does the nurse stimulate a person to value high level wellness?" (Uustal, 1978, p. 206). Neither Raths and colleagues nor Gadow views Values Clarification as stimulating an individual to adopt any value. Rather the person is supposed to engage in *valuing*. Period. Choice of values is up to the client. The nurse who would use Values Clarification as an intervention would have to seriously reflect on whether he or she could accept a client's values if they differed greatly from hers or those of other professionals. The ultimate question is whether the nurse can accept the client as an autonomous agent.

RESEARCH ON VALUES CLARIFICATION

There is a great need for research on Values Clarification as a nursing intervention. Rheinscheld (1980) has published an article in which she hypothesizes that the patient who is noncompliant with his prescription for reduced activity after a myocardial infarction might become more compliant following Values Clarification. She believes that once his values become clearer, he will see the dissonance between his values and behavior and, if he values health, will change his behavior. The assumption here is that the patient will value health more than the forbidden activities. In many cases, such an assumption is unwarranted. Rheinscheld (1980) goes on to recount a case report of such a patient and describes a method for allowing him to prioritize his values. Unfortunately, she does not report whether the particular patient's behavior changed. Thus, Rheinscheld offers a testable hypothesis but no case data to support it, much less experimental evidence.

Rosner reports on "action research" (1975, p. 410) on Values Clarification done by school nurses. According to Rosner, "While this type of research lacks the rigid control of laboratory research, it is of value to educators since it provides an orderly, disciplined base for change" (1975, p. 410). Action research is also described as "a type of research in which one of the purposes is to change the behavior of the researchers themselves, and in which they themselves are the consumers of the research" (Rosner, 1975, p. 410). The study involved five nurses in a school district using Values Clarification with students in various areas such as drug education, teenage pregnancy counseling, and Red Cross work. Rosner reports that one of the nurses believed the Values Clarification project enhanced students' sense of self-worth about service to others and all nurses had positive feelings about the experience. However, student response to the techniques was neither analyzed descriptively nor measured. Thus, the study yields no hard evidence of the effect of Values Clarification on clients.

Berger and associates (1975) conducted an exploratory study of Values Clarification as an aid in assisting chronic heart patients to examine their lifestyles, set priorities, and make changes necessitated by their disease conditions. Value-clarifying strategies were used on a one-to-one basis with a convenience sample of 20 cardiac patients. Some of these exercises were adapted from the book *Values Clarification* (Simon et al., 1972). After a baseline assessment of history and lifestyle, each patient participated in eight clarifying strategies, four in the hospital and four at home after discharge. The strategies were designed to help patients set goals regarding their lifestyles. Patients were then asked to rate themselves in their progress toward the goals set by themselves and were interviewed about their reactions to the Values Clarification approach. It was found that after reviewing their lifestyles, 15 of the 20 patients were able to set behavioral objectives for themselves to deal with area of conflict. In their self-evaluation, 13 of the 20 patients said they had acted on their goals. The investigators believed that conducting strategies in the home was helpful because it was a quieter and more "real" environment and afforded family involvement. Use of strategies on a one-to-one basis was believed to permit a safe way of discussing topics that would be difficult to handle in a group. Chi square analysis demonstrated "a close relationship between age and the patient's willingness to engage in decision making as it related to changes in life style ($p < .05$)" (Berger et al., 1975, p. 198). All patients in the age range of 51 to 60 years in the study acted on self-set goals, but this was not true of other age groups. According to their findings, Values Clarification may help cardiac patients cope with their illness.

The available nursing research on Values Clarification has been described. The bulk of research on the intervention is found in education. Raths and colleagues (1966, 1978) published reports of research on the subject. An example of these studies is one by Klevan (Raths et al., 1978), who looked at college students' responses to Values Clarification in an education course. There were two unmatched control groups. Effect of the treatment was measured according to "(1) changes in consistency of attitudes, (2) expressions of purposefulness, and (3) expressions of friendliness among class members" (Raths et al., 1978). The treatments consisted of value-clarifying discussions with the type of issues in education applying critical thinking. Students in the experimental group were found to have developed more consistent attitudes and personal purposes. Friendliness was unchanged. The results cannot be attributed to the experimental treatment alone owing to uncontrolled variables (Raths et al., 1978).

Governali and Sechrist (1980) criticize the weak research done on Values Clarification. In their study, they hypothesized that college students would change their ranking on Rokeach's Value Survey after one experience with a value-clarifying technique. The subjects were divided into a directive group in which the instructor focused discussion on six "focus" values after subjects read a value-oriented story, a nondirective group in which open discussion of the story ensued but without calling attention to "focus" values, a group in which subjects read the story and answered questions about it in writing without discussion, and a nontreatment control group. Prior to the Values Clarification experience, the subjects ranked 18 values on Rokeach's Value Survey. They also did this after the Values Clarification experience. Nonparametric statistical analysis was done. Little shifting in value rankings was found after the treatment. From this we may conclude that Values Clarification has little effect on value ranking. But we must remember that the subjects were exposed only to a single Values Clarification period using one type of exercise. Perhaps a longer treatment period would yield different results. It might also be asked how the hypothesis of the study came about. Raths and associates (1966) view Values Clarification not as a way to change value rankings but as a way to teach valuing.

Other educational studies have shown Values Clarification to have some effect. Salzano (1975) evaluated the effects of Values Clarification on self-image using the Tennessee Self-Concept Scale. Although he found no significant difference between his control (no Values Clarification) and experimental (received Values Clarification) groups, he believed that Values Clarification had some impact on the experimental subjects because the total positive subscores of the Tennessee Scale showed dramatic increases or decreases from one individual to another. Graham (1976) found that persons who had undergone Values Clarification made more value-based choices than persons who had not been exposed to Values Clarification.

The effectiveness of Values Clarification as a nursing intervention, then, is not yet evident in nursing research. Educational research leads us to believe that the technique has some effect, but better studies are needed. We cannot be certain that effects demonstrated in educational settings will translate to the nursing setting.

USING VALUES CLARIFICATION

There is a wealth of intervention tools described in the Values Clarification literature (Raths et al., 1966, 1978; Simon and Clark, 1975; Simon et al., 1972). Two techniques that are applicable in the nursing situation, the clarifying response and the value sheet, will be discussed here. A number of the other techniques described in the literature are for classroom use. They might have some applicability for the nurse working in a school or community group situation but probably not for the nurse working in acute care. The clarifying response is useful for work with individuals, and the value sheet is useful for group endeavors.

The clarifying response is a technique devised by Raths and colleagues whereby questions are asked of clients with the aim of getting them to reflect on their situations and what is important to them. The interaction is usually brief because the objective is to get the client to think on his or her own, and this can only be done quietly and often when the client is alone (Raths et al., 1978). Brevity also prevents the client from feeling "cross-examined" (Raths et al., 1978, p. 57). Thus, the nurse does not expect the client to solve immediately whatever problem he or she is dealing with at the end of a clarifying dialogue. Rather, the nurse expects that the client will be more able to think through the situation. The technique is described in the following example.

A nurse finds a post myocardial infarction patient with the oxygen turned off, smoking a cigarette while eating potato chips brought into the hospital by a friend. The patient has been advised to stop smoking and maintain a low sodium, low fat diet.

Client:	Don't lecture me. I know I'm not supposed to do this.
Nurse:	Is this what you want to do?
Client:	I've been dying to all the while I've been here.
Nurse:	How do you feel about your diet?
Client:	I hate it. . . . You know I love to cook . . . rich things with creamy sauces. I love giving dinner parties and I love good food.
Nurse:	What other things are important to you?
Client:	My children and grandchildren. My oldest granddaughter stays with me while attending college to save money.
Nurse:	You hate your diet and smoking restrictions but love your social life and family. Given your condition can you have all your favorite foods, smoke, and expect a lot of time with your friends and family? Think about it.

This exchange is brief but it attempts to get the client to assess what she prizes and what the consequences of her behavior will be. The nurse's last remark encourages the client to think about possible consequences of her behavior. The nurse avoids judgment and coercion and merely encourages consideration of the issues, maintaining an accepting attitude toward the patient (Raths et al., 1978).

The value sheet would be used in a more structured situation, such as a parenting class for families with preschool children. At the top of the value sheet the clients find a statement that the nurse believes will have value implications for them. The statement is followed by a series of questions that lead the clients through the value-clarifying process with regard to the issue raised by the statement. Each client writes out his or her answers to the questions. These may be used as discussion material later (Raths et al., 1978). Table 13–1 provides an example of a values sheet for use in a parenting class.

Table 13–1. VALUE SHEET ON CHILD DISCIPLINE

Situation:
Four year old Marty recently saw chicks hatch from eggs at a museum. He was delighted and fascinated and asked endless questions about the process. A water leak in the basement preoccupies Marty's parents and he slips into the kichen, climbs onto a chair, opens the refrigerator door and retrieves a full carton of eggs. Marty has been forbidden by his parents in the past to open the refrigerator. In closing the door, Marty losses his balance and falls from he chair. He is unhurt but crying with fright, the eggs lying broken around him.

Questions:
1. Name as many forms of child discipline as you can think of.
2. In a two-parent family, is it sometimes preferable for one parent to deal with disciplinary matters rather than the other? Why?
3. In what ways can parents deal with their anger at a child? How would you? How would you like to?
4. How do you feel about your disciplinary methods? Do you feel good about the way you manage discipline? Explain.
5. Imagine yourself to be Marty's parent. Does the above situation call for disciplinary measures? Why? Which of the techniques you mentioned in question 1 would you use in the situation? Why?

The question on this value sheet take in all three aspects of the valuing process: choosing, prizing, and acting. Specifically, Questions 1 through 3 explore alternative choices, Question 4 examines prizing, and Question 5 covers acting.

Whatever technique the nurse uses, he or she must maintain an accepting attitude toward the client. The client's individuality should be kept in mind, and in particular the clarifying response should be tailored to the client's needs (Raths et al., 1978). The nurse should also be permissive. If the client chooses not to participate, that choice is respected (Raths et al., 1978). Many other clarifying techniques are described elsewhere, and the reader is encouraged to consult other works (Pender, 1982; Raths et al., 1966, 1978; Simon et al., 1972; Steel and Harmon, 1979).

APPROPRIATE CLIENTS

Before choosing a nursing intervention it is necessary to determine the nursing diagnosis. Inadequate Decision Making is a nursing diagnosis to which Values Clarification is suited as an intervention.

Most nursing literature views decision making in the light of how *nurses* make decisions (Bailey and Claus, 1975; Gill, 1979; Grier, 1976, 1977; Grier and Schnitzler, 1979; McDonald and Harms, 1966; Sculco, 1978; Taylor, 1979). It is possible to summarize a definition of decision making based on the nursing literature and impose it on the client. Following this approach we could conclude that the antecedent conditions of decision making are the existence of a discrepancy between what is and what could or ought to be in the life of a person (Bailey and Claus, 1975) and the existence of alternative actions for dealing with that discrepancy (Grier, 1976, 1977; McDonald and Harms, 1966). The behaviors of decision making consist of acknowledging preferences for alternatives available (Grier, 1976), assigning probabilities to outcomes of alternative actions (Grier, 1976; McDonald and Harms, 1966), and awareness of and ranking of the value of the possible outcomes of the alternative actions (Grier,1976; Shontz, 1974). Taking risks may also be involved in some decisions (Grier and Schnitzlar, 1979).

Descriptive studies of *clients* involved in decision making are much needed. The foregoing summary of decision making should be considered tentative until it is validated by research. It is evident that awareness of and ranking of values are part of decision making. Therefore, we may hypothesize that Values Clarification would facilitate a client's decision making. Inadequate Decision Making would result from lack of clarity about values.

Clients sometimes have important treatment decisions to make, such as a cancer patient who must choose between radiation and surgery. The nurse in a community setting may encounter a pregnant client who must decide whether or not to marry the man who fathered her child and whether to keep the child. All such clients would need to be assessed in terms of the antecedent conditions and behaviors of decision making before the nurse initiated Values Clarification. Their permission to participate in Values Clarification should also be sought. Values Clarification should not be used with persons with serious emotional problems (Raths et al., 1966).

Spiritual Distress and Spiritual Despair (Kim and Moritz, 1982) are other nursing diagnoses for which the nurse may choose Values Clarification as an intervention. Spiritual Distress is partially characterized by a "challenged belief and value system" (Kim and Moritz, 1982, p. 333) and Spiritual Despair is partially characterized by a loss of belief in one's value system (Kim and Moritz, 1982, p. 334).

RECOMMENDATIONS FOR PRACTICE AND RESEARCH

It is important to recognize that using Values Clarification in its nonjudgmental, permissive form assumes that the client is an autonomous agent responsible for his or her own care. Can the nurse accept, nonjudgmentally and permissively, a decision by a patient that leads to illness rather than health? Even if the nurse could do this on a personal level, could he or she do it on a professional level? The nurse may privately believe that a person has the right to harm himself if he so wishes, but as a professional he or she is held accountable under professional ethics.

The code of ethics of the International Council of Nurses states the fourfold responsibility of the nurse: "To promote health, to prevent illness, to restore health and to alleviate suffering" (Beauchamp and Childress, 1979, p. 296). If a nurse has a client who after undergoing Values Clarification chooses to treat his cancer with herbs because he prizes the unproved alternative over chemotherapy, she must ask herself if the intervention has led to restoration of health or alleviation of suffering.

Even if the nurse could justify the above outcome to herself he or she would also have to face colleagues, superiors, and the public. Legally a person has no right to harm himself or others. But if the nurse uses Values Clarification with a client who decides that he prizes death over the permanent disfigurement caused by a burn, can he or she continue to maintain a permissive, nonjudgmental stance?

The ethical and legal questions that have been posed *must* be answered by the individual nurse before he or she begins using Values Clarification. The totally permissive approach is probably inappropriate and even illegal in some circumstances. Therefore, each situation in which Values Clarification might be used must be evaluated carefully.

There is a great need for research on Values Clarification as a nursing intervention. No experimental studies have been conducted by nurses in this area. It must be admitted that values are difficult to study because they are subjective. Thus, measurable behaviors must be found that will provide parameters by which to judge the effectiveness of Values Clarification in experimental studies.

Case Study

D.L. was a 23 year old mechanic from a small midwestern town. In December he developed a persistent headache and shortness of breath. A chiropractor advised him to eat a regular diet of three balanced meals per day rather than the one meal per day which he had been accustomed to eat. The headache was unrelieved. D.L. began to experience fatigue and malaise and went to see a medical doctor. After blood counts and a bone marrow biopsy were done, D.L. was admitted to a teaching hospital in early January. There, blood counts and a bone marrow biopsy were repeated and D.L. was told that he had acute lymphocytic leukemia.

D.L. was begun on a course of chemotherapy consisting of a combination of Vincristine, Doxorubicin (Adriamycin), L-Asparaginase, and Prednisone.

The medical team offered D.L. the possibility of having a bone marrow transplant for his leukemia when he obtained a remission. Chemotherapy effected a remission and so a bone marrow transplant was possible. It was up to D.L. to decide whether to have it.

The existence of a discrepancy and alternative courses of action are antecedent conditions for decision making. Both were present in this case. The discrepancy was that D.L. was now very ill, whereas he had been healthy prior to December. His alternatives consisted of continuing with chemotherapy for three to four years until a cure was achieved, having the transplant during the present remission, or having the transplant after obtaining a second remission. He was told the probabilities of survival for each of the alternatives. He had a 60 per cent chance of survival with the transplant, and a 10 per cent chance of getting leukemia again after the transplant. An important consideration in the matter was that with his type of leukemia, he had a 73 per cent chance of surviving 48 months and longer with chemotherapy alone.

Because D.L. was confronted with a difficult decision and was uncertain, I decided to use Values Clarification with him. I believed his uncertainty may have led to Inadequate Decision Making. Using clarifying responses, I listened for D.L.'s value-oriented statements with regard to the bone marrow transplant, such as "I think I'll wait until next winter to have it so I'll have another summer to enjoy." I would then reflect the value part back to D.L. with a statement like "You want to enjoy another summer" to promote further consideration and thinking on this. I also asked, "What do you think you want to do about the bone marrow?" This was done in brief dialogues over several visits. Direct questions drew D.L. out more than did reflective questions.

D.L. eventually decided against having the bone marrow transplant. From our discussion it was evident that his decision was based on the probabilities of survival associated with his alternatives. Survival is a value, and the probability of survival is what D.L. based his decision on. The difficulty here is evaluating to what degree our value-clarifying interactions affected his decision making. It is certain that they caused him to think about what he wanted. Since D.L. was a religious person from the Christian tradition, it is probable that at least intellectually death may not have seemed a great threat. Thus, there was a choice involved. After making his choice, D.L.'s affect indicated a feeling of peace with regard to his decision. He seemed comfortable, and comfort is a basic nursing goal. Follow-up interviews with patients like D.L. might be useful in determining the amount of help which Values Clarification provides in decision making. Such interviews would allow for exploration of the decision-making process. In D.L.'s case, time and distance made such interviews impossible.

EDITORS' COMMENTS AND QUESTIONS

Many clients must make difficult legal and ethical decisions concerning their health care. Self-understanding of the personal value system is often necessary before choices about personal lifestyle can be made. Wilberding describes a nonjudgmental intervention, Values Clarification, which can assist a client in making these important decisions.

Questions for Discussion

1. What do you do when your personal values conflict with your client's values? For example, many nurses refuse to work with clients having abortions.

2. What do you do when the client's and family's values are in conflict? For example, the need to donate an organ for transplant.

3. What do you do when the client makes choices that promote illness rather than health? For example, when the client attempts suicide.

4. Where do you stand on the quality of life debate? How do you feel about euthanasia?

References

Bailey, J. T., and Claus, K. E. *Decision making in nursing*. St. Louis: C. V. Mosby, 1975.

Beauchamp, T. L., and Childress, J. F. *Principles of biomedical ethics*. New York: Oxford University Press, 1979.

Berger, B., Hopp, J. W., and Raettig, V. Values clarification and the cardiac patient. *Health Education Monographs*, 1975, *3*, 191–199.

Coletta, S. S. Values clarification in nursing: Why? *American Journal of Nursing*, 1978, 78, 2057.

Curtin, L. L. The nurse as advocate: A philosophical foundation for nursing. *Advances in Nursing Science*, 1979, April, 1–10.

Gadow, S. Advocacy nursing and new meanings of aging. *Nursing Clinics of North America*, 1979, *14*, 81–91.

Gadow, S. Toward a new philosophy of nursing. *Nursing Law and Ethics*, October 1980a, 1–2, 6.

Gadow, S. Existential advocacy: Philosophical foundation of nursing. In S. F. Spicker and S. Gadow (Eds.), *Nursing: Images and ideals*. New York: Springer-Verlag, Company, 1980b.

Gadow, S. Advocacy: an ethical model for assisting patients with treatment decisions. In C. B. Wong and J. P. Swazey (Eds.), *Dilemmas of dying: Policies and procedures for decisions not to treat*. Boston: G. K. Hall Medical Publishers, 1981.

Gill, S. Leadership guidelines for decision-making. *Imprint*, 1979, September, 29–31, 44.

Gordon, L. V. *The measurement of inter-personal values*. Chicago: Science Research Associates, 1975.

Governali, J. F., and Sechrist, W. C. Clarifying values in a health education setting: An experimental analysis. *Journal of School Health*, 1980, *50*, 151–154.

Graham, M. D. The process of teaching decision-making through values clarification and its effects on students' future choices as measured by changes in the self-concept (doctoral dissertation, Saint Louis University, 1976). *Dissertation Abstracts International*, 1976, *37*, 1885–A (University Microfilms No. 76–22, 540).

Greenberg, J. S. Behavior modification and values clarification and their research implications, *Journal of School Health*, 1975, *45*, 91–95.

Grier, M. R. Decision making about patient care. *Nursing Research*, 1976, *25*, 105–110.

Grier, M. R. Choosing living arrangements for the elderly. *International Journal of Nursing Studies*, 1977, *14*, 69–76.

Grier, M. R., and Schnitzler, C. P. Nurses' propensity to risk. *Nursing Research*, 1979, *28*, 186–191.

Kim, M. J., and Moritz, D. A. (Eds.). *Classification of nursing diagnoses*. New York: McGraw-Hill Book Company, 1982.

Kirschenbaum, H. *Advanced value clarification*. LaJolla, Calif.: University Associates, 1977.

Kohnke, M. F. *Advocacy: Risk and reality*. St. Louis: C. V. Mosby, 1982.

McDonald, F. J., and Harms, T. A theoretical model for an experimental curriculum. *Nursing Outlook*, 1966, August, 48–51.

Moore, M. L. Effects of value clarification on dogmatism, critical thinking, and self-actualization (doctoral dissertation, Arizona State University, 1976). *Dissertation Abstracts International*, 1976, *37*, 907-A (University Microfilms No. 76–18, 586).

Osman, J. D. A rationale for using value clarification in health education. *Journal of School Health*, 1973, *43*, 621–623.

Osman, J. D. The use of selected value-clarifying strategies in health education. *Journal of School Health*, 1974, *44*, 21–25.

Paterson, J. G., and Zderad, L. T. *Humanistic nursing*. New York: John Wiley & Sons, 1976.

Pender, N. J. *Health promotion in nursing practice*. Norwalk, Conn.: Appleton-Century-Crofts, 1982.

Raths, L. E., Harmin, M., and Simon, S. B. *Values and teaching: Working with values in the classroom*. Columbus, Ohio: Charles E. Merrill Books, 1966.

Raths, L. E., Harmin, M., and Simon, S. B. *Values and teaching: Working with values in the classroom* (2nd ed.). Columbus, Ohio: Charles E. Merrill Publishing Company, 1978.

Rheinscheld, M. J. Values clarification and the post—myocardial infarction patient. *Aviation. Space, and Environmental Medicine*, 1980, *51*, 521–523.

Rosner, A. C. Values clarification and the school nurse. *Journal of School Health*, 1975, *45*, 410–413.

Salzano, M. A. The effects of a values clarification program on the self-image of capable continuation high school students (doctoral dissertation, United States International University, 1975, *36*, 1418-B (University Microfilms No. 75–20, 258).

Sculco, C. D. Development of a taxonomy for the nursing process. *Journal of Nursing Education*, 1978, June, 40–48.

Shontz, F. C. Forces influencing the decision to seek medical care. *Rehabilitation Psychology*, 1974, *21*, 86–94.

Simon, S. B., and Clark, J. *Beginning values clarification*. San Diego: Pennant Press, 1975.

Simon, S. B., Howe, L. W., and Kirschenbaum, H. *Values clarification: A handbook of practical strategies for teachers and students*. New York: Hart Publishing Company, 1972.

Steele, S. M., and Harmon, V. M. *Values clarification in nursing*. New York: Appleton-Century-Crofts, 1979.

Taylor, A. G. Decision making in nursing. *Imprint*, 1979, September, 32–35.

Uustal, D. The use of values clarification in nursing practice. *Journal of Continuing Education in Nursing*, 1977, May–June, 8–13.

Uustal, D. Values clarification in nursing: Application to practice. *American Journal of Nursing*, 1978, *78*, 2058–2063.

Uustal, D. Exploring values in nursing. *AORN Journal*, 1980, *31*, 183–193.

14

SUPPORT GROUPS

CAROLYN K. DREESSEN KINNEY
REBECCA MANNETTER
MARTHA CARPENTER

Use of groups as a means of providing support for identified segments of the general population has a relatively long history. Self-help organizations such as Alcoholics Anonymous (AA), which began in the 1930s, reflect a group approach well established as a viable method of effecting change in the behaviors and attitudes of their members. The structure of an AA group provides an intensive support system not only in the regularly scheduled meetings but on an individual basis, whenever a member is in need of support (Lieberman et al., 1979).

Theoretical examination of support groups, particularly those of a self-help nature, has been a recent development. Research relative to the efficacy of small groups has most often focused on those groups that could be controlled and studied in a laboratory or clinical setting. Professionals are now becoming more interested in exploring the use of small groups to reach many client populations. In addition, the study of informal social networks and their role in both the mitigation of stress and handling of life's dilemmas has also become more widespread. Such study has increased our understanding of how professionals can enhance adaptive capabilities of the people they serve.

A support group as a mode of intervention represents a merging of two theoretical perspectives: social support and small groups. Social support is defined as the feeling of being sustained through need gratification (Weiss, 1974) as well as the gaining of knowledge that allows individuals to recognize that others care for and love them and that they belong to a "network of mutual obligations" (Cobb, 1976, p. 300). A small group can be defined as a planned gathering of individuals in a face-to-face encounter, which meets with some regularity over time and is designed to accomplish some common compatible goal (Lago and Hoffman, 1977–1978). Very simply, a support group is one that provides some measure of social support for its members through the use of the group environment.

Attempts to classify and characterize the different types of support groups are numerous, and a wide variety of descriptive labels have been used, such as self-help groups, mutual aid groups, integrity groups, and information-educational groups. In general, support groups take some common theme related to a handicapping condition or stressful life experience. Each support group tends to develop its own purpose, depending upon the makeup of the group and the structure imposed on it by the group members or initiators. For the purposes of this chapter, a framework will be presented which can be used by the professional nurse to determine the type of support group most appropriate for a given client. This framework is based on the social support needs of the client and will provide direction for the formulation of independent nursing diagnoses.

LITERATURE REVIEW

Social Support

Social support has been discussed in the social and behavioral sciences as a construct that assists an individual in coping with stressful events and maintaining health. Several investigators have shown relationships between psychosocial events and illness or poor recovery from illness (Cassell, 1974, 1976; Cobb, 1976; Hogue, 1977; Kaplan, Cassell, and Gore, 1977). It also has been found that some individuals who are exposed to stressful life events and who subsequently do not become ill "may be protected by coping resources, social assets, or social integration" (Hogue, 1977, p. 66).

Assessment of social support as adequate or inadequate has been described as a way to decide whether intervention is needed. If social support is readily available to an individual in time of need and the individual utilizes the support, intervention is not necessary. Intervention is indicated, however, when the availability of social support or the utilization of social support by an individual is assessed as inadequate. Assessing social support has been proposed by Murawski, Penman, and Schmitt (1978) to include the following (pp. 370–371):

1. An inventory of persons or institutions believed to constitute interpersonal support system including some measure of the nature, strength and availability of such support in health and in time of illness.
2. An assessment of background characteristics which define the individual's social obligations (roles) within the primary support group.
3. An assessment of the beliefs about the sources of support available to meet role obligations during a time of illness.
4. A measure of a pattern of social affiliation.
5. A measure of need for social affiliation.

Brandt and Weinert (1981) have developed the Personal Resource Questionnaire (PRQ) as a measure of the variety of social support sources. Part one of the questionnaire provides "descriptive information about the person's resources, the satisfaction with these resources, and whether or not there is a confidant" (Brandt and Weinert, 1981, p. 277). The second part of the PRQ provides a measure of perceived social support. At present the tool is intended for research, with plans by the authors to further develop the PRQ to be used in clinical assessment concerning the kind and amount of social support needed to buffer life stressors.

Weiss (1974) has categorized social support into six needs, which correspond to six relationship provisions. Each provision is normally a part of different relationships, but in combination these form a supportive network. These six needs are *attachment*, being secure and comfortable and having a sense of place in an intimate relationship; *social integration*, being able to share common concerns and experience a network of relationships in which the individual has the opportunity for companionship, participation in social events, and exchange of services; *opportunity for nurturance*, being responsible for the well-being of another, wherein the person providing the nurturance has a sense of commitment and being depended on; *reassurance of worth*, being competent in a social role and respected or admired and valued in a colleague relationship; *sense of reliable alliance*, being counted on for continued assistance whether or not there is mutual affection or reciprocation; and *obtaining of guidance*, being able to have access to a trustworthy and authoritative person who can furnish support and assistance in formulating of a plan of action during stressful times.

Each of these social support needs can be met to some extent in a support group, depending on the original intent of the group and the progress and growth of the members as the group evolves. Support groups can be organized or recommended by the nurse on the basis of the client's perceived support need or the needs that are assessed and diagnosed by the nurse. It must be recognized that a support group may have one area of need as the major focus, but other needs of members may be met through the group process throughout the life of the group. For example, a support group designed to function as a means of providing information related to coping with a disease condition common to all its members would fall under the category of meeting the need for obtaining guidance. However, this educational group may also meet the members' needs for social integration through social interactions required for group maintenance, such as transportation to meetings and determination of meeting times and places. The primary focus of the group structure would be on providing guidance with the sharing and companionship aspect developing on an incidental basis.

Conversely, a support group could be initiated solely to meet the social integration needs of its members, which is the case in many self-help groups. Then, through the course of the group meetings, the members might determine they are in need of information from a knowledgeable expert and decide to devote some group sessions to a more structured educational format.

A support group for a small gathering of professionals, such as hospital staff nurses, is an example of a group primarily designed to meet the need for reassurance of worth. However, in the process of the group's discussions, the younger and less experienced nurses could learn new skills from the more knowledgeable members, thus meeting his or her need for guidance from an authoritative person. Examples of these and other types of support groups and their relationships to social support needs are discussed later in this chapter.

Group Dynamics

The study of small group dynamics has provided an increasing understanding of why a group is an effective way of providing people with social support and meeting their relational needs. A group environment has unique therapeutic elements that are not as readily available in other relationships. Yalom (1975) has identified 11 curative factors that are evident in group processes. Six of these factors are described by Loomis (1979) as being relevant to support groups.

Imparting of information—teaching or sharing information and knowledge—has been an implicit if not explicit objective of support groups. Boisvert (1976) states that one of the major objectives for a group of coronary patients following surgery was to provide health information. Information seeking regarding a disease process has been a mechanism used by medical patients to improve their coping through discussion groups and information sharing groups (Pavlou, Hartings, and Davis, 1978).

Universality is the sharing of common experiences and recognition that others have similar concerns and problems. The use of discussions in group meetings for patients following coronary surgery allowed participants to share common experiences, thus facilitating the successful rehabilitation and transition from the hospital to the home (Boisvert, 1976). Such discussion groups have also provided a means of improving coping skills of individuals with chronic illnesses, specifically multiple sclerosis (Pavlou et al., 1978). Groups can be used as a way of promoting adaptive coping through affiliation with others who share the same illness or who have loved ones with similar medical conditions.

Group cohesiveness, the sense of belonging and acceptance, is a "necessary condition for the therapeutic functioning and outcomes of most, if not all, health care groups" (Loomis, 1979, p. 35). Sharing, learning, identification, and instillation of hope are more likely to occur when the group is cohesive. Support groups will be less able to meet their specific objectives if participants do not feel a sense of commitment and attraction to the group.

Instillation of hope, or the feeling of optimism, occurs in support groups when individuals see others have successfully dealt with their problems. Spiegel and Yalom (1978) specifically identify anxiety, anger, and isolation as problems that have successfully been solved by women with metastatic breast cancer through the hope provided in group settings. Once common problems have been dealt with effectively by some group members, others in the group become hopeful that they too can solve these or similar problems.

Altrusim, or helping others in an unselfish manner, occurs in support groups when individuals realize they have something to offer other group members, as Spiegel and Yalom (1978) found for individuals with metastatic breast cancer.

Interpersonal learning, interacting effectively with others, is inherent in many of the previously discussed curative factors. As new coping skills, problem solving techniques, viewpoints, and attitudes are experienced and incorporated into an individual's behavior, interpersonal learning occurs (Loomis, 1979). Such group objectives as learning stress management (Webster et al., 1982), improving coping skills (Pavlou et al., 1978; Whitman et al., 1979), facilitating rehabilitation (Kerstein, 1980), providing health teaching (Boisvert, 1976), and fostering grief work (Spiegel and Yalom, 1978) enable interpersonal learning to take place.

NURSING DIAGNOSES

Nursing has long recognized that identification of patient needs can provide a method of organizing nursing care. Maslow's hierarchy of needs (1970) has been used extensively as a way of determining which needs, based upon the perception and condition of the individual, are addressed most effectively by the nurse. More recently, Orem (1980) has identified the individual's capacity for self-care as the appropriate focus of nursing interventions. When the self-care capacity does not meet health care demands, a deficit is said to occur. In this context, needs related to social support can be said to reflect deficits in the individual's capacity to meet the demands of daily living. A support group as described here becomes the vehicle used by the nurse to assist individuals in meeting their needs for social support.

Nursing diagnoses can be determined using a framework that aligns the social support needs as identified by Weiss (1974) with the potential benefits of support groups as identified by Yalom (1975) and Loomis (1979) (Table 14–1). Diagnoses recognized by the National Group for Classification of Nursing Diagnoses and which have a direct association with social support needs and group benefits will be addressed specifically. Many other nursing diagnoses may be identified that are not mentioned here. This discussion merely provides examples of diagnoses that readily come to mind.

The Need for Obtaining Guidance

The diagnosis of Knowledge Deficit is clearly related to the need for obtaining guidance. By imparting information, support groups clarify and expand material that is new to the client, as in the case of an unfamiliar medical diagnosis and the resultant impact on the individual and family.

Knowledge may serve to supplement what is already known or offer alternatives to mythlike or inaccurate beliefs held by the client. Realistic problem solving and the formulation of a feasible line of action are based on obtaining accurate information (Gussow and Tracy, 1976; Powell, 1975). Through the imparting of information, the professional supports the belief that respect for the client's own best choice is a basic health care principle. Shared power through the exchange of information is vital to the concept of self-care (Gussow and Tracy, 1976; Orem, 1980).

The Need for Reassurance of Worth

Lack of self-esteem and self-worth are concomitants of a Disturbance in Self-Concept. The mutual aid afforded by support group interactions creates an arena for the display and recognition of altruistic behavior (Loomis, 1979). The client gives of his or her own experience. Self-worth is defined and

Table 14–1. RELATIONSHIP OF SOCIAL SUPPORT NEED AND GROUP BENEFITS TO NURSING DIAGNOSES

Social Support Need	Nursing Diagnoses	Group Benefits
Obtaining guidance	Knowledge Deficit	Imparting information
Reassurance of worth	Disturbance in Self-Concept	Altruism Interpersonal learning
Reliable alliance	Social Isolation Noncompliance Potential for Violence Potential for Injury	Cohesion Interpersonal learning Universality
Opportunities for nurturance	Spiritual Distress Powerlessness	Instillation of hope Altruism Cohesion
Attachment	Fear Anxiety Grieving	Universality Cohesion
Social integration	Diversional Activity Deficit Parenting and Family Process Alteration	Interpersonal learning Cohesion

esteem develops as individuals recognize and are recognized as being able to give (Lago and Hoffman, 1977–1978). The sharing of what one is counters the idea that one is nothing. It is in this area that the group may give a type of support not often found in the client's family (Dimond and Jones, 1983). Family membership presupposes roles in a hierarchical structure, but the group affords mutual interaction with equals. Familial dependency and its secondary gains may be examined in the group, where self-reliance is valued. Group members learn from each other how to handle family relationships and can begin to imitate the coping skills demonstrated and reported in group sessions.

The Need for a Sense of Reliable Alliance

The diagnosis of Social Isolation identifies a lack of dependable and supportive relationships. The benefit of group cohesion implies the formation of reliable and trusted alliances (Loomis, 1979). Relationships build as group members identify more closely with each other and their common purpose.

The reciprocity inherent in a viable alliance, which is associated with the desire to belong and interact, encourages adherence to the rules (Cole, O'Connor, and Bennett, 1979). The support of rational behavior may also prove beneficial in cases of Noncompliance, Potential for Violence, and Potential for Injury. Cohesive group ties may represent an alternative to long-term relationships that have been lost (Dimond and Jones, 1983). Affirmation by the group of the client's real and potential capacities serves to refocus the client's behaviors (Cassel, 1976; Cole et al., 1979; Powell, 1975). Belonging presents reponsibilities outside the self and may lead to the formation of reliable relationships, which then enable the individual to discard self-recriminating and destructive behavior.

The Need for Opportunities for Nurturance

Through the instillation of hope, support group participants nurture each other. Inherent in the human condition is a sense of the future and expectation that it will be better than the present, which may appear unbearable. Spiritual Distress and Powerlessness reflect hopelessness regarding the future. Alone, the client has no choice but to endure without joy or even choose to end it all. Group sharing and cohesion present to the client alternative courses of action. Mutual sharing allows the client to draw on the strength of others. The spiritual strength of others nurtures those adjusting to new demands on spirituality. Clients nurture each other's hopes for the future and are encouraged to a more optimistic view (Spiegel and Yalom, 1978).

The Need for Attachment

Although each individual is unique in his or her own being, there are many experiences that are shared in common. Fear, Anxiety, and Grieving are universal emotions. For many, experiences leading to these responses are a very real part of life even if they have not reached problematic levels. Individuals identified as having these diagnoses may tend to feel that no one can understand. The discovery through a group that others are concerned and even share such feelings is reported as having a therapeutic effect (Powell, 1975; Spiegel and Yalom, 1978). Simply knowing that one is not alone with this emotional pain serves to encourage adjustment and recovery.

The Need for Social Integration

Appropriate and productive interaction is one result of interpersonal learning. Alternative ways of thinking, acting, and problem solving are possible outcomes of experience sharing. Diagnoses identifying problems in coping are most closely related to the need for social integration. Coping is defined by Cobb (1976) as the "manipulation of the environment in the service of self" (p. 311). Sharing of experiences within the group expands the client's options for productive manipulation of the environment. The client is bolstered by evidence that others have coped (Cole et al., 1979; Gussow and Tracy, 1976).

Sharing experiences increases knowledge about activities available, thus benefiting those with Diversional Activity Deficit (Lago and Hoffman, 1977–1978). This sharing may also preclude the client's failing as others share their less productive experiences. In such a way, failure may also be seen as a learning experience rather than total devastation. The client learns to use new knowledge as it is shared with group members.

Parenting and Family Process Alterations are diagnoses in which interpersonal learning in support groups has direct benefit. Group members serve as role models and supportive fellows through stages of adjustment (Powell, 1975). Individual behaviors are reflected in group interactions. Clients are supported in the difficult task of looking at themselves, as well as their life events, from a more distant and perhaps more objective viewpoint (Ross, Collen, and Soghikian, 1977; Pavlou et al., 1978). Social integration is enhanced as personal social space is defined in relationship with others in the environment.

RECOMMENDATIONS FOR PRACTICE

Before setting up or referring a client to a support group, many factors must be considered. Who the leaders are, what approach is utilized, and what group process model is followed should be explored. The structure of the group needs to be determined as well, including the duration, frequency, and timing of group meetings. The location of the meetings is an additional consideration, especially when there are mobility or transportation problems for some participants.

Client Selection. A primary consideration when suggesting support group intervention is the client's perception of the need(s) to be met (Norbeck, 1981). This perception may be revealed through a discussion of the structure and interactions of the client's present support system. An intact system is to be fostered and protected. Such intervening variables as the client's present stage of development, present resources, ability to use those resources, and present and past means of need gratification should be considered if the support group is to be a viable and productive intervention (Hogue, 1977; Norbeck, 1981).

The PRQ mentioned earlier is a structured method of obtaining information about the client's resources and perceived social support. Another, less formalized method of determining a client's resource potential and social support needs is to follow the line of inquiry recommended by Erickson, Tomlin, and Swain (1983). The client's network of social support can be determined by such questions as "Where do you get your support?" "With whom do you talk things over?" "How do you keep going?" "Is there anyone who provides you with reinforcement and helps you solve problems?" "Do you have family members or friends nearby and available?"

It is also important to obtain information related to how the client perceives the social support obtained from this network. Families may "at first sight seem very reinforcing but when the client's perspective is asked are revealed to be energy draining rather than energizing" (Erickson et al., 1983, p. 125). The nurse can help clients assess whether their dependency needs are being met by asking questions such as "Do you feel you are being supported by your family or friends or are you the one doing the supporting?" Deciding the appropriateness of a support group can be a collaborative effort between the client and nurse once the client's support needs have been mutually examined and determined.

Timing. Support groups appear to be most beneficial during transitional stages (Dimond and Jones, 1983). Transitional stages are periods of adjustment to a new lifestyle replacing one that was interrupted by crisis or loss. One-to-one relationships are most productive during acute crises or in deficit situations. When the crisis has passed or when the deficit is recognized as permanent, the adjustment process begins. It is during this period that support groups are most appropriate. Proper timing is an important aspect in assessment of the fit between the needs of the client and the benefits of the group.

Group Leadership. The leadership style can range from a nondirective to a more structured, directive approach. A nondirective technique appears to be the approach support group leaders employ when the structure of the supportive group meeting is for sharing of experiences and feelings (social integration). A more directed and structured approach may be used by support group leaders when the group has a predetermined format or schedule designed for education purposes (obtaining guidance).

Boisvert (1976) stated that in leading groups for patients following coronary surgery, a modified nondirective technique was used, with emphasis on the following approaches: (1) support and clarification, (2) information and correction of erroneous notions or perceptions, (3) problem solving for current difficulties experienced by the patient, and (4) reinforcement of feeling expression associated with heart disease and the rehabilitation (p. 26).

Spiegel and Yalom (1978) relate that the role of the leader is to identify topic themes that occur in the group discussion. Keeping the group from becoming a nonproductive social gathering as well as clarifying group themes was seen as an important therapeutic tool in working with cancer patients (Whitman et al., 1979).

When the leader is functioning more as a group facilitator, the goal is to foster the emergence of a process enabling group members to be more effective in seeking help from and giving help to one another. The desire for the group to become an alternate care-providing system encourages each member to "maintain a higher standard of self-care" (Cole et al., 1979, p. 332). Eight principles have been identified that may be utilized to facilitate the group process of new support groups:

1. Monitor and direct active involvement of group members.
2. Encourage the expression and sharing of experiential knowledge.
3. Encourage the expression of mutual aid.
4. Encourage appropriate referrals to professionals for information.
5. Emphasize personal responsibility and control.
6. Maintain positive pressure for behavior change.
7. Emphasize the importance of active coping.
8. Minimize leader input (Cole et al., 1979).

Leaders of support groups may be varied in their preparation. The leader or facilitator may be a professional, a paraprofessional, or a lay person. One or more individuals may initiate and lead support groups. When two or more individuals lead a group, it is sometimes beneficial to have a man and a woman lead together. Leadership of groups can also rotate when different sessions of the group have different leaders.

Group Process. Awareness of the group process is also an important responsibility of the leader or facilitator. By creating a relaxed, accepting atmosphere a support group can provide the group members with opportunities to clarify group themes, share personal feelings and experiences, and interact with other group members.

Two models of group process were identified in the literature relevant to the development of support groups. Yalom's group stages (1975) were used to identify the group process occurring in discussion groups for multiple sclerosis individuals (Pavlou et al., 1978). The first stage is the orientation phase, wherein individuals are looking for approval and acceptance within the group. Next, the members are preoccupied with finding who is dominant in the group, who has control in the group, and who has power within the group. The third stage of the formative group is the occurrence of group cohesiveness. After the formative stages have been completed the working phase of the group occurs, with the final stages of termination occurring after the work phase is completed.

Stages of group development identified by Garland, Jones, and Kolodney (1973) were used when discussing the activities of support groups for nurses (Webster et al., 1982). Again, five stages of group development were identified. The first stage is preaffiliation, wherein individuals decide whether they will participate or belong to the group. The second stage is identified as the power and control stage, in which the autonomy of each member is developed. Again, as in Yalom's second stage, conflicts for control occur at this stage. Intimacy is the third stage, and this is the stage at which interpersonal sharing, concern, and dependency occur within the group. The fourth stage, differentiation, is similar to Yalom's third and fourth stages as the group becomes cohesive and mutual support occurs. Separation is the final stage and is the process where the group comes to an end. The progression of a group through the identified stages has an effect on how well the group benefits are operating. Further discussion of group stages and process can be found in Chapter 16 of this book.

Structure of the Group. The structure of support groups varies depending upon the desires of facilitators and group members. No concrete guidelines for the structure or formation of support groups are found in the literature. Most authors agree that homogeneity of group members regarding their specific illness or situation is mandatory for support groups. Examples of some populations that have benefited from support groups include alcoholics (AA), dying patients (Spiegel and Yalom, 1978), drug-dependent individuals (Synanon), patients with cancer (Whitman et al., 1979), vascular-disease amputees (Kerstein, 1980), patients following coronary surgery (Boisvert, 1976), individuals with multiple sclerosis (Pavlou et al., 1978), and nurses on an intensive care burn unit (Webster et al., 1982).

The specific characteristics of individuals who participate in support groups have not been determined. Aiken (1982) reported a pilot study designed to examine whether individuals with cancer who utilized psychological support groups were from nuclear or extended family structures. She hypothesized that the greater proportion of individuals would be from nuclear families. Her pilot study did not significantly uphold her hypothesis, but did indicate the need to determine the characteristics of individuals who participate in support groups.

Membership of support groups may consist of individuals with common problems, family members, friends, or interested visitors. Support group membership may be limited or open, depending upon the desires of the members and the leaders or facilitators and the purpose of the group.

Participants of the groups may be required to sign a contract at the beginning of their involvement in the group. This contract usually is a way of formally showing commitment to the support group. The literature reveals that few support groups require contracts unless the structure of the group is well defined and there is need for the experience to be directive in nature.

RECOMMENDATIONS FOR RESEARCH

The literature about support groups primarily includes thoughts, feelings, and experiences that collectively underscore the therapeutic value of the group approach. Scientifically designed studies collecting empirical data to support the relationship between needs and group benefits are needed. Future studies might focus on the development of tools to measure success or failure of support group intervention. Empirical measures are specifically needed in the following areas:

1. Psychological mechanisms through which social support operates (Cobb, 1976).

2. Specific needs met through social support: grieving (Spiegel and Yalom, 1978), chronic illness (Dimond and Jones, 1983), mental distress (Loomis, 1979), worried but well persons (Ross et al., 1977).

3. Individuals most likely to use and benefit from support groups (Aiken, 1982).

4. Specific leadership types most effective in support groups (Yalom, 1975).

5. Relationship of internal versus external group focus to therapeutic value (Lusky and Ingman, 1979).

Longitudinal studies concerned with the effects of support groups over time are needed to evaluate their derived benefits. Studies involving support groups are most difficult to design owing to the extremely sensitive and diverse nature of each individual's concerns as well as the highly complex structure of social support.

The use of support groups continues to challenge professional investigation. Although they are not a panacea, support groups present fertile ground for research. Much has yet to be discovered about the curative and preventive mechanisms of group interaction (Cobb, 1976). It is hoped that the framework presented here will be used as a guide for development and implementation of support groups as well as a basis for research examinations of the efficacy of support groups as a nursing intervention.

CASE STUDY

A support group established for individuals with multiple sclerosis (MS) is an example of how a small group can be used to meet the members' needs for social support. The group was initiated as a collaborative effort between three nurses and a woman with MS. This woman, J.V., expressed an interest to one of the nurses in starting such a group. After further discussion with her it was assessed that she was experiencing social support needs related to reassurance of worth, social integration, and obtaining guidance. These three needs provided the impetus for starting the MS support group. It was believed that if J.V. experienced these needs, then it was likely other people with MS did also. The specific nursing diagnoses related to these needs were Disturbance in Self Concept, Diversional Activity Deficit, and Knowledge Deficit.

It was decided to survey the community of people known to have MS in order to assess if interest warranted starting a support group. A questionnaire was developed with J.V.'s help asking the potential group members to identify concerns they would want to explore in a group setting and their level of interest in such a group.

Following return of the questionnaires an organizational meeting was held, with J.V. functioning as the leader. This role bolstered her self-concept and allowed her to begin meeting her need for reassurance of worth. Other group members were encouraged to share in the decisions regarding meeting topics, identification of guest experts who could talk with the group about specific concerns, and dissemination of publicity about the upcoming meetings. The nurses functioned as group facilitators rather than experts in an effort to maximize involvement of the group members. All tasks related to the functioning of the group were handled by group members, thus helping them to begin meeting their social support needs of reassurance of worth and sense of reliable alliance.

Subsequent group meetings were initially quite structured, with guest experts presenting material related to the chosen topic for that meeting. The group members seemed to be most comfortable with this approach, at first, which indicated that their need for obtaining guidance was great. Chosen meeting topics were yoga and exercise, pain management, stress management, depression, and self-esteem. Gradually the group sessions became more unstructured, with an increasing amount of personal sharing occurring, thus allowing the members to begin addressing their need for social integration. By the time the self-esteem topic was addressed members were becoming much more comfortable in the group environment and they were beginning to discuss their thoughts and feelings more freely.

An examination of the group sessions revealed that group members were utilizing information presented at the group meetings. Some members who attended the group on yoga were organizing a yoga class for other individuals with MS in the community. Also one member, who had been experiencing a burning discomfort, reported she was obtaining relief by using a TENS (transcutaneous electrical nerve stimulator) unit acquired through consultation with the physical therapist who presented pain management at an earlier meeting.

When it became necessary for the nurses to discontinue attending the group meetings the members were asked to evaluate the group experience. They were given a questionnaire which they were to complete anonymously and send to one of the nurses. The questionnaire covered such issues as whether the group had been beneficial to them, what concerns they had which still needed exploring, how this group compared to any previous experiences with such groups, and whether they wanted the group to continue.

Responses to the evaluation questionnaire revealed an unanimous vote for continuation of the group. Also, the group members indicated they wanted to continue with the positive, supportive experience that developed in the group, not just come to meetings directed at having an "expert" present material. This indicated that the need for social integration was becoming a more predominant need shared by the group members.

The group did continue under J.V.'s leadership, with other members increasingly assuming more responsibility for the functioning of the group. Based upon the questionnaire responses, it is likely that all six of the social support needs were met to some extent in some, if not all, of the group members. The group became self-sustaining, thus providing the group members with the opportunity to enhance their self-care capacity and to provide and receive social support in an independent manner with others who shared their disability.

EDITORS' COMMENTS AND QUESTIONS

In this chapter, the authors merge two theoretical perspectives, group process and social support, to provide a framework for the intervention. A model demonstrates how nursing diagnoses result from a social support need and how group benefits can assist in treating the diagnoses. The work of these authors provides a framework for future researchers to study the benefits of support groups.

Questions for Discussion

1. Do nurses need special training to lead a support group?

2. When should a client be referred to a support group? How do you assess both the client and the group before making this decision?

3. What kind of commitment are you making when you organize a support group?

4. What type of research is needed to document the outcome of support groups?

References

Aiken, S. Family structure and utilization of cancer support groups. *Oncology Nursing Forum,* 1982, 9(1), 22–26.

Boisvert, C. Convalescence following coronary surgery: A group experience. *Canadian Nurse,* 1976, November, 26–27.

Brandt, P. A., and Weinert, C. The PRQ—a social support measure. *Nursing Research,* 1981, 30, 277–280.

Caplan, G. *Support systems and community mental health.* New York: Behavioral Publications, 1974.

Cassel, J. An epidemiological perspective of psychosocial factors in disease etiology. *American Journal of Public Health,* 1974, 64, 1040–1043.

Cassel, J. The contribution of the social environment to lost resistance. *American Journal of Epidemiology,* 1976, 104, 107–123.

Cobb, S. Social support as a moderator of life stress. *Psychosomatic Medicine,* 1976, 38, 300–314.

Cole, S., O'Connor, S., and Bennett, L. Self-help groups for clinic patients with chronic illness. *Primary Care* 1979, 6(2), 325–340.

Coleman, L. J. Orem's self-care concept of nursing. In J. Riehl and Roy, C. (Eds.), *Conceptual models for nursing practice.* New York: Appleton-Century-Crofts, 1980.

Dimond, M. Social support and adaptation to chronic illness: The case of maintenance hemodialysis. *Research in Nursing and Health,* 1979, 2, 101–108.

Dimond, M., and Jones, S.. *Chronic illness across the life span.* Norwalk, Conn.: Appleton-Century-Crofts, 1983.

Erickson, H., Tomlin, E., and Swain, M. *Modeling and role-modeling: A theory and paradigm for nursing.* Englewood Cliffs, N.J.: Prentice-Hall, 1983.

Garland, J., Jones, H., and Kolodney, R. A model for stages of development in social work groups. In J. Bernstein (Ed.), *Explorations in group work: Essays in theory and practice.* Boston: Charles Rivers Books, Inc., 1976.

Gussow, Z., and Tracy, G. The role of self-help club in adaptation to chronic illness and disability. *Social Science and Medicine* 1976, 10, 407–414.

Hogue, C. C. Support systems for health promotion. In J. E. Hall and Weaver, B. R. (Eds.), *Distributive nursing practice: A systems approach to community health.* Philadelphia: J. B. Lippincott, 1977.

Kaplan, B., Cassel, J., and Gore, D. Social support and health. *Medical Care,* 1977, 15 (Supplements), 47–58.

Kerstein, M. D. Group rehabilitation for the vascular-disease amputee. *Journal of the American Geriatrics Society*, 1980, *28*, 40–41.

Lago, D., and Hoffman, S. Structured group interaction: An intervention strategy for the continued development of elderly populations. *International journal of Aging and Human Development*, 1977–1978, *8*, 311–324.

Lieberman, M., Borman, L., and associates. *Self-help groups for coping with crisis*. San Francisco: Jossey-Bass Publications, 1979.

Loomis, M. E. *Group process for nurses*. St. Louis: C. V. Mosby, 1979.

Lusky, R., and Ingman, S. The pros, cons and pitfalls of self-help rehabilitation programs. *Social Science and Medicine*, 1979, 13A, 113–121.

Maslow, A. H. *Motivation and personality* (2nd ed.). New York: Harper and Row, 1970.

Murawski, B. J., Penman, D., and Schmitt, M. Social support in health and illness: The concept and its measurement. *Cancer Nursing*, 1978, October, 365–371.

Norbeck, J. S. Social support: A model for clinical research and application. *Advances in Nursing Science*, 1981, July, 43–59.

Orem, D. E. *Nursing: Concepts of practice* (2nd ed.). New York: McGraw-Hill Book Company, 1980.

Pavlou, M., Hartings, M., and Davis, F. A. Discussion groups for medical patients: A vehicle for improved coping. *Psychotherapy and Psychosomatics*, 1978, *30*, 105–115.

Powell, T. J. The use of self-help groups as supportive reference communities. *American Journal of Orthopsychiatry*, 1975, *45*, 756–764.

Ross, H. S., Collen, F. B., and Soghikian, K. Pilot study of discussion groups for "worried well" patients in an ambulatory care setting. *Health Education Monographs*, 1977, *5*, 51–61.

Spiegel, D., and Yalom, I. D. A support group for dying patients. *International Journal of Group Psychotherapy*, 1978, *28*, 233–245.

Webster, S., Kelly, L. A., Johst, B., Weber, R., and Wickes, L. The support group: A method of stress management. *Nursing Management*, 1982, *13*, 26–30.

Weiss, R. The provision of social relationships. In X. Rabin (Ed.), *Doing unto others*, Englewood Cliffs, N. J.: Prentice-Hall, 1974, pp. 17–26.

Weiss, R. Transition states and other stressful situations: Their nature and programs for their management. In G. Caplan and Killiea, M. (Eds.), *Support systems and mutual help: Multidisciplinary explorations*. New York: Grune & Stratton, 1976, pp. 213–232.

Whitman, H. H., Gustafson, J. P., and Coleman, F. W. Group approaches for cancer patients: Leaders and members. *American Journal of Nursing*, 1979, *79*, 910–916.

Yalom, I. D. *The theory and practice of groups psychotherapy* (2nd ed.). New York: Basic Books, 1975.

15

EXERCISE PROGRAM

JANET DAVIDSON ALLAN

The need to change the sedentary habits of the adult American population is well recognized. Physical inactivity has been linked to premature cardiovascular disease, obesity, orthopedic problems, and emotional distress. Although the President's Council on Physical Fitness and Sports Medicine Newsletter (1979) reported a twofold increase in exercise participation since the 1974 report, at present only 35 per cent of adult Americans exercise regularly. Several other studies confirm this estimate (Harris et al., 1978; *Healthy People*, 1979). The elderly are particularly vulnerable to the effects of inactivity. Many individuals are not aware of the benefits of regular activity or the principles involved in exercise training. As a result, many people who do try to become fit often incur injuries and become discouraged, which causes them to discontinue training activities.

Evidence for the role of regular exercise in the primary and secondary prevention of cardiovascular disease, our leading cause of death and disability, is growing (Froelicher, 1978). Most health maintenance recommendations advocate the modification of lifestyles to include regular, moderate aerobic exercise. Nurses, as part of their involvement in health promotion, need knowledge of exercise training in order to make appropriate assessments and develop management plans with the healthy exercising adult.

The purposes of this chapter are (1) to review the fundamental elements of physical fitness and the beneficial effects of regular exercise; (2) to provide a model for assessment of the adult client; and (3) to delineate strategies for the development of aerobic exercise programs.

WHAT IS EXERCISE?

Human physical performance capacity has three major determinants: capacity for energy output (aerobic and anaerobic mechanisms), neuromuscular functions (strength, technique, and coordination), and psychological factors (motivation and strategies) (Åstrand and Rodahl, 1970). Simply, physical exercise is defined as action or activity involving physical and mental exertion. Sustaining such exertion physically involves muscular strength, muscular endurance, flexibility, and cardiopulmonary (aerobic) endurance (Åstrand and Rodahl, 1970; Getchell, 1976). Psychological factors play an important role in both the initiation and continuance of an exercise program.

Muscle strength is the ability of a muscle group to produce a force against resistance (Getchell, 1976). Exercises involving muscle strength are often called isometric (or static) activities; common samples are lifting, holding, or carrying objects of all kinds. This type of exercise has little effect on cardiac conditioning (Haissely, 1974; Lind, 1970). *Flexibility* refers to the range of movement of a joint or joints (Getchell, 1976). Exercises involving flexibility are called calisthenics; examples include arm swinging, neck rotation, or torso and hip bending (flexion and extension). These types of exercises are useful during warm-up periods prior to cardiac endurance activities. *Muscle endurance* is the ability of a muscle group to perform a repeated action for an extended period of time (Getchell, 1976). Activities calling for muscle endurance include repeated pushups, situps, or jumping in place. Exercises that promote *cardiopulmonary endurance* or fitness are called aerobic exercises. They are rhythmic, repetitive exercises that create a demand for increasingly larger amounts of oxygen by using large muscle groups. Examples include swimming, jogging, biking, running, and race walking. Implicit in the definition of aerobic exercises are the concepts of repetition and training. Thus, cardiac endurance is the ability of the body to participate in vigorous exercise for an extended period of time (Åstrand and Rodahl, 1970).

Although this chapter will focus upon cardiopulmonary fitness, the use of muscle endurance and flexibility exercises will also be discussed. Many individuals, for a variety of reasons, will not be able to participate in aerobic activities but would benefit from a general exercise program.

THE BENEFITS OF EXERCISE

Many studies (Blackburn, 1977; Brand et al., 1976; Fox et al., 1972; Morris et al., 1953; Paffenbarger, 1978; Paffenbarger et al., 1970, 1977) over the past 30 years have explored the relationship between physical activity or sedentary lifestyle and coronary heart disease (CHD). Inactivity, along with smoking, hypertension, family history, high serum lipid levels, stress, diabetes, and obesity, is often included among the multiple factors contributing to CHD in industrialized countries. Although smoking, hypertension, and hypercholesterolemia are the three cardinal risk factors for CHD, there is increasing evidence that physical inactivity should be considered the fourth (Froelicher, 1977). In fact, there is growing evidence that regular physical activity can prevent CHD (Brand et al., 1976; Froelicher, 1977; Paffenbarger, 1978; Paffenbarger et al., 1977).

Support for this hypothesis has come from two human sources: population studies and clinical studies. Population studies have revealed that persons with more physically demanding occupations or leisure activities have lower rates of CHD (Brand et al., 1976; Morris et al., 1953; Paffenbarger, 1978; Paffenbarger et al., 1970, 1977; Pollock et al., 1971). Clinical studies have demonstrated that the cardiovascular functional capacity of patients with CHD can be dramatically improved by physical training (Bonanno and Lies, 1974; Froelicher, 1977; Wenger, 1978). This brief review will focus upon population studies.

The first report of a statistically significant relationship between physical activity and CHD was the famous London Transport System study of Morris and associates (1953). This study found that bus conductors, who were more physically active because of climbing stairs on the double decker buses, had a lower incidence and a more benign form of CHD than did the sedentary bus drivers. A similar relationship was found in comparing postal clerks and postal delivery men (Morris et al., 1953). Other similar studies also demonstrated a trend of less severe CHD and decreased mortality rates in more physically active individuals (Bonanno and Lies, 1974; Fox et al., 1972a; Froelicher, 1978).

Later studies led to further exploration of the relationship between quantity of exertion and the amount of preventive value. Skinner and associates (1966) found that the difference in daily calorie expenditure associated with a significant decrease in CHD prevalence was only 400 to 500 calories.* Paffenbarger and co-workers (1970), in their study of San Francisco longshoremen, found a 25 per cent reduction in CHD death rates over a control group, with a 925 kilocalorie per day increase in caloric expenditure. Paffenbarger and colleagues (1977) and Brand and associates (1976), in more recent studies of longshoremen, and Paffenbarger (1978), in a study of college men, found the risk of CHD to be inversely related to activity level at work. Physical activity may be at quite low levels of intensity and still afford a beneficial effect. These studies emphasize the beneficial effect of long-term physical activity habits at all levels of energy expenditure.

Other studies examine more broadly the association of health and activity. The Alameda County Study (Belloc and Breslow, 1972; Wiley and Comacho, 1980) reported several lifestyle parameters to be positively associated with health. Belloc and Breslow initially reported on this longitudinal study, which entailed a survey conducted in 1965 on 4000 adults aged 20 to 70 years. They found seven lifestyle variables or health practices to be associated with a general index of health. These practices included no smoking, moderate drinking, seven to eight hours of sleep per night, regular meals, particularly breakfast, not eating between meals, moderate weight, and weekly physical activity (Belloc and Breslow, 1972). Physical activity, such as gardening or long walks, even at minimal levels was associated with positive health status. Wiley and Comacho, reporting on the same population eight years later (1980), found five health practices to be predictive of future positive health status. These included not smoking, seven to eight hours of sleep per night, moderate drinking, regular physical activity, and moderate weight.

As mentioned previously, the elderly are particularly vulnerable to the effects of inactivity. *Healthy People* (1979), the report of the Surgeon General on health promotion, states that fewer than 25 per cent of noninstitutionalized adults 65 years of age and older participate in regular exercise. Accidents (particularly falls, which account for 60 per cent) are the sixth leading cause of death among the elderly and, in part, can be attributed to a sedentary lifestyle that is not just "the aging process" (de Vries, 1979; *Healthy People*, 1979). The study by Harris and co-workers (1978) reports that only 30 per cent of adults 50 years old and older exercise regularly.

In summary, although this is a difficult area to research because of the confounding variables and the poor characterization of physical activity, studies do seem to suggest that moderate habitual activity can significantly reduce the incidence and severity of CHD and generally improve health status in all age groups. How does habitual exercise affect the body and specifically reduce CHD morbidity and mortality?

---

*Carrying 80 pounds for 1 hour will utilize 600 calories (Fox et al., 1972a, p. 27)

SPECIFIC BENEFITS OF AEROBIC EXERCISE

Regular, long-term aerobic exercise results in a number of physiological alterations that are probably beneficial (Table 15–1). Studies have suggested that elevated plasma levels of high density lipoproteins (HDL) may be associated with a lowered risk of CHD (Gordon et al., 1977; Miller and Miller, 1975) and that vigorous exercise may result in elevated HDL levels (Ratliff et al., 1978). Other biochemical changes include increased fibrinolytic activity (Williams et al., 1980) and decreased platelet aggregation, leading to rapid clot dissolution. Clot formation is considered one factor in causing myocardial infarction. A decrease in catecholamines may account for both decrease in blood pressure and decrease in the perception of stress.

Hypertension increases the risk of CHD twofold (Blackburn, 1977). Decrease in blood pressure is one of the major positive hemodynamic effects of exercise (Froelicher, 1978). Moderate exercise seems to produce decreases in diastolic blood pressure in normal individuals (Mann et al., 1969; Pollock et al., 1971) and in hypertensive men (Boyer and Kasch, 1970). Pollock and associates found, in a study of middle-aged unconditioned men, that training in vigorous walking had a significant effect on diastolic blood pressure and body composition. Many of the hemodynamic changes seen with chronic aerobic exercise result from an increase in stroke volume and lower heart rate. These hemodynamic changes, which occur in older individuals also (Froelicher, 1978), will be described more fully in a later section.

Exercise is recognized to have several other, less direct beneficial effects. For example, a training program may result in a decrease in cigarette smoking. Studies have suggested that exercise may reduce stress and improve the sense of psychological well-being. Eliot and associates (1976), in their review of the mechanisms by which aerobic exercise enhances cardiovascular function, advocate exercise as a therapeutic intervention for the relief of stress. Others report improved self-image and decreased depression (Fox et al., 1972a; Heinzelmann and Bagley, 1970). In one of the few nursing studies on exercise, Goldberg and Fitzpatrick (1980) report increased morale among institutionalized elderly individuals after the initiation of a movement therapy program.

Table 15–1. EFFECTS OF REGULAR AEROBIC EXERCISE THAT ARE BENEFICIAL TO HEALTH

Hemodynamic
- Lower resting heart rate
- Lower heart rate at each level of exercise
- Lower cardiac output at each level of exercise
- Lower blood pressure
- Increase in stroke volume
- Increase in collateral cardiac circulation
- Increase in maximal oxygen consumption
- Faster return to normal heart rate after exercise

Biochemical
- Decrease in catecholamines
- Increase in fibrinolysis
- Decrease in platelet aggregation
- Increase in alpha-lipoproteins
- Increase in mitochondrial function in muscle

Morphologic
- Increase in muscle fiber size
- Increase in coronary vascularity
- Increase in muscle mechanical efficiency

These studies suggest that exercise training can be useful in the promotion of psychological as well as physical well-being.

The primary benefit of exercise training is related to improving cardiovascular efficiency. The major physiological responses to aerobic exercise result in lowered heart rate, increases in stroke volume, and increases in oxygen extraction by large muscles (Froelicher, 1978). In this body energy system, the capacity of muscles to take up oxygen is considered the limiting factor. Studies suggest that with training there is an increase in mitochondrial and enzymatic activity in both cardiac and peripheral muscles that results in greater oxygen extraction (Blomqvist, 1978). The net result of these adaptive changes is that after endurance training an individual is able to perform more physical work at lower heart rates.

CARDIAC FITNESS: QUANTIFICATION OF AEROBIC EXERCISE

How much aerobic exercise is necessary to result in cardiovascular fitness? The amount of exercise necessary to accomplish cardiovascular fitness is related to the concept of maximum oxygen uptake (MVO_2)—the maximum amount of oxygen that can be utilized by the body. Maximum oxygen uptake measures the maximal amount of physical work that an individual can perform, using large muscles, in a given period of time. It is the most direct measure of exercise capacity. There is a maximal point for each individual. The amount of activity required to provide beneficial effects on the cardiovascular system occurs at between 60 and 80 per cent of the maximum aerobic capacity (Blomqvist, 1978). There is little added benefit to exercise beyond this 80 per cent level. The major difference between sedentary and active individuals is the percentage of maximum cardiac capacity used for a given amount of work.

Determination of the MVO_2, which is age related, is necessary in order to prescribe the appropriate amount of exercise. For each individual there is an intensity (amount) of exercise that is enough to condition the muscles and the cardiovascular system. This is the concept of "target zone."

MVO_2 in clinical practice is not measured directly. However, there is a linear relationship between MVO_2 and heart rate. In normal individuals, the points of maximal oxygen uptake and maximal obtainable heart rate are positively correlated. Sixty to 80 per cent MVO_2 correlates with 70 to 85 per cent of the maximal obtainable heart rate.

The maximal obtainable heart rate can be determined from specific exercise tests, such as the treadmill, bicycle ergometer, or age-predicted heart rate charts (Merriman, 1978). Exercise testing provides information about the cardiovascular system that is unobtainable in a routine health assessment. The bicycle ergometer and treadmill, the most commonly used in the United States, record heart rate, blood pressure, electrocardiographic, and symptomatic responses as an individual exercises to an exhaustion endpoint (Bruce, 1974). Both the person's exercise capacity and functional limitations are measured. The heart rate obtained can be used to determine the target zone (70 to 85 per cent of maximal heart rate), which is used to gauge the intensity of an exercise program.

In populations without coronary disease or major coronary risk factors, age-predicted heart rate charts (Table 15–2) can be used to determine maximum heart rate. Such charts can be used to calculate an individual's target zone (70 to 85 per cent heart rate) and show the normal decline in maximal heart rate

Table 15–2. MAXIMUM HEART RATE AND TARGET ZONE BY AGE

	Maximum Heart Rate Beats/Minute									
	208	200	194	188	182	176	171	165	159	153
85% level	177	170	165	160	155	150	145	140	135	130
70% level	146	140	136	132	128	124	119	115	111	107
Age	20	25	30	35	40	45	50	55	60	65

Adapted from Zohman (1974) and Hellerstein (1969).

with age. Men and women of the same age can reach similar maximal heart rates. The target zone or heart rate is the key to any safe aerobic exercise program.

Table 15–2 shows the maximum attainable heart rate and the target zone for ages 20 to 65 years. For example, an individual 45 years old is predicted to be able to achieve a maximum heart rate of 176 at maximal exercise capacity. His or her target zone to be achieved during an exercise program would be a heart rate of 124 to 150. If an age-predicted chart is not available, the maximum heart rate can be calculated by subtracting the person's age in years from 220. For example, the predicted maximum heart rate for a 45 year old would equal $220 - 45 = 175$. To find the target zone, find 85 and 70 per cent of 175.

ASSESSMENT

An exercise intervention fitness plan must include a heart rate level so that the individual can monitor his or her own activity within an effective and safe zone. One controversial area in exercise prescription is whether to base the heart rate level on electrocardiographic exercise testing or an age-predicted chart. Disagreement relates to the reliability of the treadmill test as a diagnostic tool, the appropriate male population to be screened, and its applicability to women (Morris and McHenry, 1978). The decision to base the exercise heart rate prescription on either of these two options should be made following a focused health assessment.

Most adults, whether seeking help for an exercise program or for another concern, will have been leading sedentary lives and can be considered unconditioned. As documented in the study by Harris and colleagues (1978), individuals who exercised the least were over 30 years old, women, non-white, living in rural or inner city areas, and earning less than $15,000 per year. Most adults also have varying risk factors for cardiovascular disease or other functional impairments. Clear guidelines are needed to identify those patients who require extensive evaluation, including exercise testing or physician supervision, and those patients who might safely utilize the age-predicted heart rate and for whom the nurse can help plan an exercise program. These guidelines will be useful whether the nurse has primary responsibility for a client's care or is working in collaboration with another health professional.

Assessment of the individual for exercise prescription should include a focused health history and physical examination, and selected laboratory parameters. The purposes of this assessment are the following:

1. To determine the presence of risk factors for or presence of CHD.

2. To identify the existence of other health problems or functional difficulties that might modify or preclude exercise prescription.

Table 15–3. HEALTH HISTORY FOR EXERCISE PRESCRIPTION

I. *Present Health Status* (includes aspects of past health and family history):
   A. *Presence of Coronary Artery Disease* (actual or suspected)
      1. Do you have angina pectoris (or do you ever get a pressure or pain or tightness in your chest if excited, exercising, eating, or walking against a cold wind)?
      2. Do you have or have you had palpitations or rapid heart beats or irregular heart beats?
      3. Have you ever had a heart attack (myocardial infarction, coronary occlusion, or coronary thrombosis)?
      4. Have you ever had rheumatic fever?
      5. Have you had a cardiogram taken while exercising that was not normal?
      6. Do you take or have you taken any of the following: nitroglycerin (small pill that you put under your tongue for chest pain), digitalis, or quinidine for your heart?
   B. *Risk Factors for Coronary Heart Disease*
      1. Do you have hypertension or high blood pressure? What is the treatment plan (diet, drugs, exercise, relaxation, herbal remedies)?
      2. Do you have elevated cholesterol (high fat in the blood)? Are you on a special diet or taking medication?
      3. Do you smoke now? How much? Did you ever smoke? When did you quit?
      4. Has anyone in your family had a heart attack or heart trouble or high cholesterol before the age of 50?
      5. Do you have diabetes mellitus or high blood sugar? What is the treatment plan (diet, oral agents, insulin)?
   C. *Other Potentially Limiting Conditions*
      1. Do you have any chronic illnesses?
      2. Ask about: asthma, emphysema, hyperthyroidism, anemia, any arthritis, back, joint, visual, or auditory problems (current or past) that limit activity, renal disease, chronic infectious processes (chronic hepatitis), and obesity (greater than 30 per cent of ideal weight).

II. *Past Health History*
   Ask about any other major hospitalizations and surgeries; medications (prescribed and over-the-counter), major allergies, immunization status, and last skin test for tuberculosis.

III. *Personal Social History*
   A. Explore individual's health beliefs about health in general and exercise specifically. Include data on the following: general concern about health; priorities and positive health activities; past experience with health care system and providers; perceptions about susceptibility for heart disease and the potential severity of heart disease.
   B. Explore reasons for wishing to start an exercise program and expectations. Include data on the following: past exercise experiences; knowledge abut exercise; beliefs in the benefits of exercise; exercise interests; daily schedule (work and home); personal (financial) and community resources and client support systems (family and friends' concerns and knowledge about exercise).

3. To collect psychosocial and environmental data that would individualize the exercise plan (American College of Sports Medicine, 1975).

Table 15–3 outlines a health history to be used to evaluate an individual prior to exercise prescription. It incorporates a focused assessment for the presence of risk factors for coronary heart disease, actual CHD, and other health problems that might modify or preclude exercise. For the elderly, major hearing or vision losses are particularly important to evaluate. The psychosocial history provides important data about the individual's current health beliefs, lifestyle, and past experiences that will provide clues about motivation for exercising. Harris and co-workers (1978) reported that the majority of individuals took up exercise to stay healthy, feel better, or lose weight. Only 17 per cent were advised to exercise by a health professional. The psychosocial history will be discussed further later in this chapter.

The physical examination should parallel the history by focusing primarily upon the cardiac, respiratory, and musculoskeletal systems. Laboratory studies should include determination of lipid levels, urinalysis, complete blood count (for heavily menstruating women and the elderly), and any other studies that are indicated by the history and physical examination.

This assessment enables the nurse to identify those individuals who can safely use the age-predicted heart rate and those individuals who require further evaluation, perhaps even a physician-supervised exercise program. Fair, Allan-Rosenaur, and Thurston (1979) developed a useful patient categorization scheme: *Category I* comprises those with no risk factors or disease and *Category II* is made up of persons with risk factors or disease.

Category I: No Risk Factors or Disease. The nurse and patient can utilize the age-predicted heart rate to plan an exercise program for the individual under 45 years old. Men over 45 should be referred for stress testing; if it is negative, exercise prescription can proceed utilizing the heart rate from the test (Morris and McHenry, 1978). There is little evidence that asymptomatic women should be screened by exercise testing. The patient with a positive stress test should be referred to a physician for further evaluation.

Category II: Risk Factors and/or Disease. Two questions should be answered: (1) Does this patient need stress testing? (2) Can this patient safely perform an exercise test (Fair et al., 1979)?

For those individuals under 45 years old the nurse should seek consultation to determine whether the risk factors or other health problems are slight enough to allow the use of age-predicted heart rate or severe enough to warrant exercise testing or physician consultation. A 30 year old man who smokes and has moderate hypertension should be referred to a physician before being exercise tested. A 37 year old woman with moderately elevated lipid levels who smokes five cigarettes per day and has chronic mild low back pain presents a common clinical situation for which the literature offers no clear guidelines. The health professional is left to apply clinical judgment and seek peer consultation in making decisions about these marginal situations.

All individuals over 45 years old should undergo exercise stress testing. Consultation with a physician is advisable prior to referring any individual in Category II for testing (Blocker, 1976; Merriman, 1978). Absolute contraindications to exercise testing or participation in a conditioning program include recent myocardial infarction; recent pulmonary embolism; congestive heart failure; heart block (second and third degree); aortic aneurysm; acute myocarditis; severe valvular disease (aortic stenosis); and uncontrolled arrhythmia (Blocker, 1976; Cooper, 1970; Wilmore, 1976).

Within the previously mentioned broad parameters, there are clients with specific nursing diagnoses for whom the intervention of an Exercise Program is useful. The most general diagnosis that can be applied to the vast majority of clients is Health Maintenance Alteration due to a sedentary lifestyle. More specifically, exercise is a useful intervention in clients with the following diagnoses (Kim and Moritz, 1982): Sleep Pattern Disturbance secondary to stress; Self-Concept Disturbance secondary to changes in body image; Body Elimination Disturbances (constipation) secondary to decreased activity; Grieving for actual or perceived loss; Cardiac Output Alterations secondary to increased peripheral resistance or volume; Nutritional Alterations secondary to more or potential for more than body requirements; and Mobility Impairment secondary to pain, musculoskeletal neurological impairment, or anxiety and depression. There are several potential diagnosis for which exercise could be utilized as an appropriate intervention: Potential for Injury (particularly in the elderly); Potential for Decreased Cardiac Output and Tissue Perfusion; Potential for Increased Clot Formation; and Potential for Decreased High Density Lipoproteins.

INTERVENTION

Recognizing the need for increased physical activity and translating this awareness into action or behavioral change are unrelated events. A successful exercise intervention includes the designing of an Exercise Program that has three major goals: (1) increasing the individual's awareness of the need for physical activity; (2) teaching individuals how to safely achieve cardiovascular fitness; and (3) assisting individuals to maintain this lifestyle change.

Increasing Individual Awareness

Although there is a vast literature on health behavior, little is really known about what motivates individuals to make changes in their lifestyles. Research that has focused on attitude change has identified many of the complexities involved in beliefs and preferences (Roberts, 1975). We learn that an individual adheres to a program of physical activity for a variety of reasons: potential health benefits, sense of well-being, encouragement from spouse, or social camaraderie. However, we are still left with trying to understand under what conditions a person will change a course of action (lifestyle behavior) in response to an expert opinion, persuasive campaign, a peer-network pressure, or internal clues.

Other research has focused upon decision-making models (Farquhar, 1975, 1978; Kasl and Cobb, 1966; Rosenstock, 1966), which attempt to reveal the conditions under which people make a decision to pursue a new course of action or adhere to a decision they have already enacted. The well-known Health Belief Model (HBM) is a theory based on decision-making concepts of valence or attractiveness of a goal to an individual and subjective probability or personal estimate of attaining the goal (Kasl and Cobb, 1966). The theory provides one theoretical framework for predicting the likelihood of an individual's deciding upon and undertaking a recommended preventive health action. Preventive health behavior is any behavior undertaken for the purpose of promoting wellness, preventing disease, or detecting disease in an asymptomatic stage. The theory argues that whether or not an individual will undertake a health action depends on specific personal perceptions as well as interpersonal and situational factors.

The relevant perceptions that are postulated to determine a health decision include (1) importance of general health and health-related activities; (2) sense of susceptibility; (3) potential seriousness of a symptom or problem; and (4) the proposed action's ability to reduce severity or susceptibility (Becker and Maiman, 1975; Kasl and Cobb, 1966). Interpersonal factors that influence decision making include (1) concern of personal network, particularly family, and expectations of friends; (2) general family patterns of health behavior; and (3) information from media or health professionals (Kasl and Cobb, 1966; Pender, 1975). An individual's relationship with a specific health provider, which includes an evaluation of his or her competence and ability to understand the patient's concern, is very important (Hulka et al., 1976). Situational factors that encompass broader aspects of influence include societal and group norms and cultural practices related to health.

The HBM also stipulates that a cue to action or a challenge must occur to trigger the appropriate behavior by making the individual consciously aware of his or her feelings about a health threat. Such cues can be internal, such as the perception of a symptom, or external, such as a message through popular media (television special), or an interpersonal interaction (recommendation to exercise from a health provider) (Becker and Maiman, 1979). In other words, how does an individual identify inactivity as a social or health problem? Recent studies of this model have demonstrated stronger correlations between health beliefs and concurrent adherence to a health behavior. This suggests that positive health beliefs become stronger with actualization and continuation of a particular health plan. Nursing research is needed in the area of health beliefs about, and adherence to, health promotion activities.

In developing an exercise prescription with a client, the nurse must have knowledge of the factors that influence health behavior. The particular factors outlined in the HBM can be integrated into the health history and intervention plan. As research indicates, beliefs change as the individual has positive experiences with the health intervention. The nurse needs to reassess the client's beliefs periodically during the monitoring phase of the intervention.

As stated previously, a challenge must occur to make an individual aware that a sedentary lifestyle constitutes a threat to health. The power of health assessment and health diagnosis in increasing individual awareness of the risks of a sedentary lifestyle should not be underestimated. There is notoriously little emphasis on health promotion in our medical care system. The nurse who focuses upon health issues with clients often receives a very positive response. In that regard, the provision of health information, specifically about physical fitness, cannot be overemphasized. Harris and colleagues (1978) reported that while only 17 per cent of patients received exercise information from a health professional, over 60 per cent expected the provider to give such information. Several visits may need to be spent providing such information before a patient is ready to plan an exercise program.

Other techniques besides the actual health diagnosis and physical examination that the nurse can utilize to increase individual awareness or readiness for change are suggested by Farquhar (1975, 1978). Using decision-making theory and aspects of the HBM, he lists three steps for self-directed change: (1) enhance cognitive structure and motivation, (2) teach specific methods of achieving a particular change, and (3) teach specific methods of maintaining change over time (Farquhar, 1978).

Techniques for enhancing cognitive structure and motivation in relation to exercise include providing information about the risks of a sedentary lifestyle and the ways of reducing such risks. Another useful technique is client self-assessment. Ask the individual to list his or her current beliefs about exercise, current activity patterns (weekdays, weekends, holidays), and barriers to making changes. The client can do this task orally or keep a written log and bring it to a subsequent visit. Farquhar (1978) also suggests a technique of "self-monologues" to identify belief barriers. These consist of paired positive and negative statements. An example of positive self-talk is, "Walking up three flights of stairs to the office will be good for me"; negative self-talk would be, "I don't have time to exercise."

The aforementioned steps are essential prior to developing an exercise plan with a client. Clients will be at different stages of readiness for proceeding to the second step, the actual exercise prescription. Often health professionals move directly from identification of the patient as sedentary to exercise prescription and wonder why the patient often does not adhere to the program or even return for future visits.

Achieving Fitness: Specific Exercise Prescription

The goal of the exercise prescription is to design with the client a training program that will safely achieve or maintain a conditioned cardiovascular system (Fair et al., 1979). The prescription has eight major aspects: (1) type of activity; (2) intensity; (3) frequency; (4) duration of the exercise; (5) warm-up and cool-down exercises; (6) education about conditions warranting cessation or modification of the program; (7) method for monitoring intensity (Fair et al., 1979); and (8) an individualized program, which also constitutes the third step of the nursing intervention.

Type of Activity

A repetitive endurance type of exercise or one that uses large muscle groups is recommended. Examples of such exercises are rope skipping, cycling (rolling or stationary bicycle), swimming, brisk walking, jogging, running, stair climbing, skiing, and dancing. Physically disabled clients may utilize walking, modified stationary bicycles, or wheelchair propulsion (Wilmore, 1976). Walking and running are particularly suited to older clients because they avoid the isometric tension in upper limbs created by cycling (de Vries, 1979), a tension that increases blood pressure.

Frequency, Intensity, and Duration

Frequency refers to how many days per week the exercise should be performed. The majority of sports researchers recommend that exercising five times per week produces significantly better results than exercising three times per week (Merriman, 1978). However, several studies (Fox et al., 1972; Merriman, 1978; Pollack et al., 1971) have shown that fitness can be attained and maintained on a frequency of three times per week. There should be an interval of no more than one to two days between each exercise period.

Intensity is critical to improvement in cardiovascular fitness. It requires exercising at a heart rate within each individual's age-specified target zone, 70 to 85 per cent of maximal attainable heart rate (Table 15–2). Progression to a fitness level is very crucial in exercise prescription and relies heavily on monitoring of heart rates during activity. Teaching this skill will be discussed later in this chapter.

Duration refers both to the specific length of time the individual should exercise and to the amount of time required for conditioning. The majority of researchers conclude that each exercise session should be 20 to 30 minutes in duration (Merriman, 1978; Wilmore, 1976). Pollock and associates (1977) found that 87 male subjects had an 8.7 per cent increase in MVO_2 with training 15 minutes three times per week and a 17.8 per cent increase with 30 minutes of exercise three times per week. It usually requires 20 to 30 weeks of regular activity for adults to reach optimal training level.

In summary, the prescription should include a specific endurance activity, performed three times per week, for 20 to 30 minutes within the individual's target zone. Less conditioned individuals should start at the lower range of their target zones, 70 to 75 per cent of maximal heart rate. de Vries (1979) suggests that elderly persons exercise in the 60 to 75 per cent heart rate by taking 60 per cent of the maximal heart rate for the 60 or 65 year old individual.

Warm-Up and Cool-Down Phases

These two periods are an integral part of all exercise programs even though they do not provide a conditioning effect. The warm-up phase prepares the body for sustained activity by increasing blood flow and stretching postural muscles. It is a period of adaptation that prevents a sudden increase in work load on the heart, the circulatory system, and the muscles and joints. The warm-up sequence should be designed to gradually increase the intensity of exercise, include rhythmic exercises that stretch muscles, and put joints through their full range of motion (Myers, 1975).

For 5 to 10 minutes, as your heart rate slowly reaches its target zone, follow this sequence:

1. Initiate rhythmic movements starting with joint range of motion, such as performing a forward and backward crawl (circumduction, extension, and flexion of shoulder gridle); walk with hands clasped behind head, while twisting side to side (circulation, rotation of trunk); or do knee bends (Cooper, 1972; Myers, 1975).

2. Do stretching exercises, such as touching toes (hip, thigh, and back extensors), raising hands over head and bending from side to side (lateral trunk muscles), progressing to alternate knee hugs (back muscles), straight leg raises (knee and hip muscles), assuming sprinter's position with heel pointed (hamstrings), and walking rapidly in a circle (Cooper, 1972; Myers, 1975).

The cooling-down period is equally important after the period of endurance exercise, to prevent syncope that can result from a sudden decrease in the supply of blood to large muscle groups. For 5 to 10 minutes the individual should (1) continue to use large muscle groups—for example, jogging but at a slower pace, (2) slow down to a few minutes of walking, and (3) employ range of motion, stretching, and static muscle contraction and relaxation activities (Cooper, 1972).

Conditions Warranting Cessation of or Alteration in the Exercise Program

Major Problems. The nurse needs to provide clear instructions to the client to stop exercising and seek health advice if any of the conditions listed in Table 15–4 occur. Investigation of the cause of these symptoms must be made before a client resumes exercising. Every prescription should include a written list of these symptoms (Fair et al., 1979), which often occur because clients do not progress slowly in their training program.

Other Considerations: Minor Illness, Climate, Eating, and Exercise. Patients need to consider discontinuation of their training program during episodes of minor illness. Deconditioning occurs very rapidly; studies report an initial loss beginning in three days and a 50 per cent loss of the original improvement in three months (Merriman, 1978). The implication of these data is that the intensity of the exercise prescription needs to be decreased when the client resumes an exercise program.

Table 15–4. SYMPTOMS THAT WARRANT CESSATION OF EXERCISE

Pain in chest, arm, neck, or jaw
Irregular heart rate
Dizziness, lightheadedness
Persistent shortness of breath after exercise
Unexplained weight loss
Nausea or vomiting during or after exercise
Prolonged fatigue or lethargy
Uncoordinated gait or weakness
Muscle or joint pain or joint swelling

From Cooper, K. Guidelines in the management of the exercising patient. *Journal of the American Medical Association*, 1970, *211*, 1663–1667. Reprinted by permission.

Climate is another factor in altering exercise programs. The ideal exercise weather is 40°F to 85°F with humidity less than 60 per cent and wind velocity less than 15 mph (Cooper, 1972). Exercise in hotter climates should be scheduled for cooler periods of the day. Salt and water replacement is recommended for individuals who sweat profusely. If high temperatures and humidity are persistent yearly features in a particular region, exercising can be done indoors. Cold weather is less dangerous, but the individual must extend his or her cool-down period to avoid excessive chilling.

It seems advisable to avoid vigorous exercise after a large meal. However, there is little evidence either for or against exercising on an empty stomach or after a light snack. The important point is to develop a regular routine that is tailored to the individual's normal pattern. Vigorous exercise does tend to suppress appetite, so it may be scheduled to assist in weight reduction.

Monitoring Intensity and Individualizing the Program

Besides providing instruction about intensity, frequency, duration, and modifying circumstances, every client must be taught how to monitor the intensity of his or her exercise program. As already noted, intensity is based upon exercising at a heart rate equal to 70 to 85 per cent of the individual's maximal heart rate (target zone). The nurse must instruct the client to monitor intensity by counting the pulse rate. Using a 10 second heart rate representative of his or her target zone, the client needs to count the pulse rate at the wrist or neck immediately upon stopping exercise. He or she must find the pulse quickly, count for 10 seconds, multiply times 6, and compare this number with the target zone range. If the pulse rate exceeds the target zone, the client needs to reduce the intensity of the exercise. If the pulse rate is lower than the target zone, the client needs to increase the intensity of the exercise. Intensity can be altered by manipulating two parameters: vigor and time.

Monitoring intensity also includes the concept of progressing to a fitness level. It is useful to think of an exercise program as consisting of two phases: a training phase to develop the individual to a desired level of fitness, and a maintenance phase in which the individual tries to maintain optimal fitness. The client frequently moves too quickly into a fitness program during the training phase, exceeding his or her target rate, and often incurring injury and becoming discouraged.

In the training phase, the client with specific guidelines uses the 10 second pulse rate to develop an exercise pattern that includes a below target zone 10 minute warm-up period, a 30 minute aerobic exercise period within the target zone, and a 10 minute cool-down period in which the heart rate moves slowly out of the target zone. Initially, clients must monitor their pulse frequently so that they will not exceed their target zone. Providing specific written instructions to clients regarding progression is very useful. Fair and associates (1979) developed a useful written instruction sheet (see Tables 15–5 and 15–6). As illustrated in these tables, it is important for the nurse to provide detailed instructions concerning the client's 10 second heart rate, exercise schedule, warm-up and cool-down activities, and specific activities that lead to a sound progression into the conditioning exercise.

There are some general guidelines for progression into a fitness program. Most authors (Blocker, 1976; Cooper, 1972; de Vries, 1979; Myers, 1975) recommend that all deconditioned individuals begin with a walking program. Such a program provides the client with an opportunity not only to work out an exercise schedule but also to practice monitoring intensity.

Table 15–5. EXERCISE PLAN

Name: John Smith   Age: 30

10 Second Exercise Heart Rate Prescription   Conditioning Exercise (circle)

a. Target Zone	136–165 bpm/25 beats/10 sec	Walking	Jogging
b. Stress ECG	N/A	Swimming	Biking
		Other	

Frequency: Weeks 1–8: 4 × Week (Minimum); 3 Day Maximum Interval; Week 9 on: 3 × Week

Mon.	Tues.	Wed.	Thurs.	Fri.	Sat.	Sun.
6:30–7:30 am		6:30–7:30 am		6:30–7:30 am		10–11 am

EXERCISE ROUTINE

Warm-Up
5–10 min: forward/backward crawl; toe touching, side bending; straight leg raises and sprinter's position.

Conditioning
Weeks 1–3: alternate jogging, walking 1 minute, then jogging and walking 2 minutes to cover one mile in 18 min. If exercise heart rate is exceeded, increase walking for 2 minutes, jogging 1 minute. Week 4 on: systematically increase pace to cover 1.5 miles in 22 min.

Cool-Down
5–10 min: continue using large muscle groups, slower jogging 3 min; slow walking for 5 min. Then, 5 min period of alternating stretching and range of motion exercises.

STOP EXERCISE

Seek medical advice if any of these symptoms occur:
—Chest, arm, or joint pain
—Increased shortness of breath
—Irregular heart beat
—Lightheadedness, fainting
—Nausea and vomiting with exercise
—Unexplained weight changes
—Muscle or joint problems
—Prolonged fatigue
—Unexplained changes in exercise tolerance

Adapted from Fair, J., Allan-Rosenaur, J., and Thurston, E. Exercise management. *Nurse Practitioner*, 1979, May-June, pp. 13–18. Reprinted by permission.

Tables 15–7 and 15–8 provide two examples of a walking program for two different age groups. For the 50 year old and older age group, the individual walks a mile in 18 to 20 minutes (3 mph rate). In these initial stages, the client should walk a quarter of a mile, count the pulse, and adjust the pace of walking accordingly. Walking is a particularly good exercise for the elderly; an individual who is not able to progress to jogging can receive major benefits from a walking program. For some individuals who are unable to be outside, a walking program can be carried out in a gym or recreation center. Younger individuals and some conditioned elderly persons may want to proceed to a jogging program once they are able to walk a mile in 13 minutes without exceeding their target zone.

Table 15–9 illustrates a progressive jogging program. The client should gradually increase the jogging time guided by the target zone. A person who can jog 1.25 miles in 12 minutes is considered to have reached a conditioned level that will maintain fitness (Hellerstein et al., 1969).

212   LIFESTYLE ALTERATION

Table 15–6. EXERCISE PLAN

Name: Mabel Smithers   Age: 60

10 Second Exercise Heart Rate Prescription   Conditioning Exercise (circle)

    a. Target Zone*   96–111 bpm/16 beats/10 sec   Walking   Jogging
    b. Stress ECG   negative   Swimming   Biking
                                                         Other _____

Frequency: Weeks 1–6: 4 × Week (Minimum); 2 Day Maximum Interval; Week 7 on: 3 × Week

Mon.	Tues.	Wed.	Thurs.	Fri.	Sat.	Sun.
10 am - 11 am		10 am - 11 am		10 am - 11 am		4 pm - 5 pm

EXERCISE ROUTINE

Warm-Up
5–10 min: range of motion (arms over head forward/backward crawl), stretching (touch toes knee bent, bend side to side), and walking in a circle.

Conditioning
Weeks 1–3: walk 1 mile/20 min. Weeks 4–6: walk 1.5 miles/24, 22, 21 min. Weeks 7–10: walk 2 miles in 32 min. If exercise heart rate not reached, increase pace of walking. If exercise heart rate exceeded, slow pace.

Cool-Down
5–10 min: continue to use large muscles—slower walking for 5 min. Then 5 min period of alternating muscle stretching exercise (raise hands over head).

STOP EXERCISE

    Seek medical advice if any of these symptoms occur:
    —Chest, arm, or joint pain
    —Increased shortness of breath   —Unexplained weight changes
    —Irregular heart beat   —Muscle or joint problems
    —Lightheadedness, fainting   —Prolonged fatigue
    —Nausea and vomiting with exercise   —Unexplained changes in exercise tolerance

*60–70% level of maximal heart rate.
Adapted from Fair, J., Allan-Rosenaur, J., and Thurston, E. Exercise management. *Nurse Practitioner*, 1979, May-June, pp. 13–18. Reprinted by permission.

Table 15–7. PROGRESSIVE WALKING PROGRAM (AGE 50 YEARS AND OVER)

Week	Frequency/Week	Distance (miles)	Time/Pace
1–2	4–5	1.0	18–20 min/slow
3	4–5	1.0	15–17 min/moderate
4	4–5	1.5	24 min/moderate
5	4–5	1.5	22½ min/moderate
6	4–5	1.5	21½ min/moderate
7	4–5	2.0	32 min/moderate
12	3	3.0	44 min/moderate-fast
16	3	4.0	55 min/moderate-fast

Adapted from Blocker (1976) and Cooper (1972).

Table 15–8. PROGRESSIVE WALKING PROGRAM (AGE 30 YEARS AND UNDER)

Week	Frequency/Week	Distance (miles)	Time/Pace (min)
1–2	4–5	1.0	15.0
3	4–5	1.0	13.0
4	4–5	1.0	21½
5	4–5	1.5	21.0
6	4–5	1.5	20½
7	4–5	2.0	28.0
12	3–4	3.0	40.0

Adapted from Blocker (1976) and Cooper (1972).

Other conditioning exercises such as swimming (Table 15–10), biking (indoor and outdoor), and rope jumping should be planned in a similar manner. Swimming is an excellent exercise for individuals of all ages. It has the advantage of being useful for clients who have musculoskeletal or neurological disabilities that make walking or jogging too difficult. Hot showers should be included in the warm-up period for swimmers, in order to decrease musculoskeletal difficulties (Blocker, 1976).

Research indicates that adults reach an optimal training level sometime after 20 to 30 weeks of regular physical activity. At approximately six months, maximal aerobic power gains tend to plateau. The degree of improvement is related to the initial state of deconditioning. Before delineating ways in which the nurse can help the client maintain a fitness program, clothing and the prevention of common injuries will be briefly discussed.

Prevention of Common Injuries

According to *Running Times* (1978), a large portion of all aches, pains, and injuries suffered by runners, joggers, and walkers are related to a lack of shock absorption or a lack of motion control. The body absorbs shock as the impact of the poorly padded foot on a hard surface transmits force through the heel and leg. On the other hand, lack of motion control results from excessive flattening out of the foot as it moves through the gait cycle. The most common running injuries caused by these two factors, in order of frequency, are knee pain, muscle tightness, shin splints, ankle pain, low back pain, arch pain, tendinitis, hip and calf pain, and toenail problems (*Running Times*, 1979). These injuries also relate to the factors that include the type of running surface and patterns of running (*Running Times*, 1978, 1979). The *Running Times* (1979) survey also reported that runners with the lowest percentage of injuries ran slowly, ran frequently (six times per week), had low mileages (less than 30 miles/week), and ran on relatively soft surfaces such as grass, dirt, and

Table 15–9. PROGRESSIVE JOGGING PROGRAM (AGES 30 TO 50 YEARS)

Week	Frequency/Week	Distance	Jog	Walk	Time (min)
1–3	4–5	1 mile	1 min	1 min (130 yd)	18
			2 min	2 min (260 yd)	
			1 min	1 min	
			2 min	2 min	
			1 min	2 min	
4–8	4–5	1.5 miles	Systematically increase weeks 1–3 schedule		22
12–16	3	2 miles	Systematically increase weeks 4–10 schedule		19

Adapted from Harris et al. (1967) and Cooper (1972).

Table 15–10. SWIMMING PROGRAM (AGES 30 TO 50 YEARS)

Week	Frequency/Week	Number and Length of Swims	Time (min)
1–2	4–5	4 25-yd swims (100 yds)	2.3
3	4–5	3 50-yd swims (150 yd)	3
4–5	4–5	4 50-yd swims (200 yd)	4
6–8	4–5	3 100-yd swims (300 yd)	6.15–6½
9–12	4–5	4 100-yd swims (400 yd)	8½–9
13–15	3	450–550 yd	10–10½
16–19	3	550–650 yd	12–12½
20–30	3	650–800 yd	12–16½
Thereafter	3	800–1000 yd	18–20

Adapted from Blocker (1976) and Cooper (1972).

asphalt. The reader desiring more information should seek other sources for specific details about running injuries (Friedman and Knight, 1978).

Running, jogging, and walking are done in a heel-to-toe gait, which also places pressure on the gastrocnemius and soleus muscles of the calf and stretches the Achilles tendon. Running shoes need to provide maximum cushioning to prevent overstretching of muscles and tendons and to provide strong support to control excess motion and guide the foot as it moves. Shoes should be lightweight; have a good arch support, a 1 inch heel, and a cushioned sole; and fit well enough to prevent the foot from slipping within the shoe. Shoes are the most important clothing investment for a runner, jogger, or walker for the prevention of injuries. Other clothing should be selected according to the activity and the climatic conditions.

Individualized Program: Maintaining the Exercise Program

Successful maintenance of a change in behavior or lifestyle is vital but notoriously difficult (Farquhar, 1978; Haynes et al., 1979). Although this aspect of exercise as a nursing intervention is discussed last, it is probably the most important. The process of individualizing or tailoring a prescription for the individual is the major strategy used not only for initiation of change but also for maintenance. This process of tailoring, which underpins the entire exercise intervention, is the cornerstone to successful initiation of and adherence to a particular plan, and begins when the nurse first encounters the client. As discussed previously, a variety of techniques can be utilized to individualize the intervention: focused nursing assessment; client self-assessment; client self-monologues; and a specific weekly exercise program. Data related to daily patterns, preferences, past experience, health beliefs, personal resources, and social supports are utilized not only to increase client readiness but also to tailor the actual exercise or plan.

Making a plan with the client should involve an agreement about objectives or goals of care and mutual expectations. Goals of care, of course, are important because they provide clear direction for the nurse and client, guide the selection of specific intervention techniques, and provide a means for evaluation and recognition of change. One technique that is particularly helpful in developing a plan of action with the client is the contract (Fink, 1979; Herje, 1980; Steckel, 1980). Contracting as an intervention is specifically described in Chapter 6. An example of a contract for the intervention of exercise appears in Table 15–11.

Table 15–11. CONTRACT FOR EXERCISE

Goal: Establish regular walking program
Intermediate Behavior (Week 1):
  1. Keep written diary of all activities for one week.
  2. List pros and cons of exercise.
  3. List resources in neighborhood and work.
  4. List social support from work colleagues and family.

Contract:
I, *Mr. Wiley*, will bring diary of list of exercise activities, pros
and cons, resources, and social supports from work and home to
the next visit. The nurse will evaluate my current activities and
help me plan a beginning walking program.

Signed: Ms. Franks, RN
Signed: Mr. Wiley
Date: 6/3/83
Reward: I will buy a new shirt.

Contracting is an ideal strategy for providing clients with an individualized experience in behavior change and concurrent means of developing positive health beliefs about that change. The use of other patient education techniques, the development of a positive therapeutic relationship, and regular follow-up visits may enhance the client's successful execution of the exercise plan (Haynes et al., 1979; Hulka, 1976).

CASE STUDY

C. W. is a 40 year old married high school teacher who comes to the clinic concerned about being overweight and having a family history of heart disease. He feels that he is unhealthy and needs to change his lifestyle.

Present History

Mr. W., who is 6 feet tall, has weighed 200 lb since age 30 years and has unsuccessfully attempted to lose weight numerous times using self-initiated "fad" diets. He eats two meals per day, lunch (at school) and dinner (at home), and has a diet consisting of high cholesterol and high salt foods: bread or pasta products and few fruits and vegetables. He has never had blood cholesterol measured. Mr. W.'s father, who is living, had a myocardial infarction (MI) at age 45 years. Mr. W. believes that he is at risk for an MI since he is fat and sedentary like his father. The rest of the family history is negative for diabetes, heart disease, hypertension, or hypercholesterolemia. Mr. W. denies chest pain, high blood pressure, palpitations, or any history of rheumatic fever. He has never had an electrocardiogram. He has no history of other chronic illness or current concerns. Mr. W. does not smoke, drinks 2 ounces of whiskey per day, and does not exercise regularly.

Past Health

History reveals no major surgeries or hospitalizations. Mr. W. takes no prescribed medication, has no allergies, and was last skin-tested for tuberculosis and immunized in the service (1968).

Personal Social History

Mr. W. has been married for 15 years, has two children, 12 and 10 years, and describes his relationship with his wife, who also teaches, as very good. Mrs. W. in fact urged the client to have a checkup and get help with his concerns. Mr. W. has taught science at the same school for 10 years and generally enjoys his job. He is financially secure. Until recently, Mr. W. felt that he was young, had no illnesses, and did not need to be concerned about his health. At a recent college reunion he was shocked both by the early death of a few friends and by the youthfulness of others. As he stated, "I suddenly felt old, ugly, and worried that I'd have an MI like my dad and not be able to fully participate in life's activities." His past experiences with the health care system have been minimal but positive. With regard to exercise, Mr. W. wishes to learn how to jog, because it will "improve my heart," but is afraid it will be too hard to maintain: "I'm lazy." He has not exercised since college and has never run. He would like to exercise at lunch but does not know how to go about this. He thinks that his family will be supportive of this plan.

Objective
General Findings. 6 feet, 198 lb.; blood pressure, 130/84; pulse, 84; respirations, 18. Overweight black male in no distress.

Thorax/Lungs. No lung abnormalities. Equal expansion, and diaphragmatic excursion 3 cm bilaterally. Resonant to percussion and clear to auscultation.

Cardiovascular. Normal sinus rhythm. $S_1 > S_2$. No murmurs or extra sounds. No bruits. Pulses 2+ and equal.

Musculoskeletal. No spinal deformities. Full range of motion in all joints. Good muscle mass.

Laboratory. ECG and urinalysis normal. Cholesterol, 240 mg/dl.

Nursing Diagnoses
1. Health Maintenance Alteration, secondary to sedentary lifestyle.
2. Nutrition Alteration, more than body requirements.
3. Potential for:
    a. decreased cardiac output.
    b. decreased tissue perfusion.
    c. decreased high density lipoprotein.
    d. increased clot formation.
    e. self-concept disturbance—body image.

Plan
Exercise Program. Mr. W. will begin a progressive walking program (see Tables 15–7 and 15–8) for 2 to 4 weeks; when he is able to walk a mile comfortably in 13 minutes, he can begin the jogging program (see Table 15–9). Initially, to enhance cognitive structure and motivation and to obtain more specific data, a contract was established with Mr. W. (see Table 15–11). In progressive visits, the nurse will move to assist Mr. W. with specific aspects of initiating and maintaining an Exercise Program, teaching him how to monitor his pulse, helping him develop a specific exercise plan (see Table 15–5 and 15–6), and selecting the appropriate time, climate, and clothing.

Nutrition. Concurrently the nurse will work with Mr. W. to develop a plan for improvement of his nutritional intake and weight loss.

SUMMARY
The need to change the sedentary habits of adult Americans is well recognized. With the increasing emphasis on exercise as an important health-promoting behavior, it is important that nurses have knowledge of exercise training in order to appropriately assess and develop management plans with the healthy exercising adult. This chapter provided a review of the fundamental elements of physical fitness and the beneficial effects of regular exercise; a model for assessment of the adult client; and specific strategies for the development of a fitness program with the client. The mechanics of the exercise prescription are straightforward, but the tailoring of an individualized program that provides the guidance and support necessary for the initiation and maintenance of lifestyle change is more difficult.

Although there is a growing body of knowledge that nursing can utilize in developing exercise intervention plans, more research needs to be done. We know very little about those factors that prompt individuals to make a decision to pursue a new course of action or to maintain this new behavior. Nurses have an important role, not only as researchers, but also as skilled clinicians, in taking leadership in the whole neglected area of promotion of health in the adult population.

EDITORS' COMMENTS AND QUESTIONS

This chapter presents the nurse with valuable suggestions on how to assess a client's status before beginning an Exercise Program. It also describes the eight components of an exercise prescription and provides a format for writing the exercise prescription. Allan gives suggestions on motivational activities and goal-setting activities that are crucial in maintaining long-term adherence to an Exercise Program.

Questions for Discussion

1. *What type of assessment needs to be completed before starting a sedentary client on an Exercise Program?*

2. *Compare the benefits of aerobic versus nonaerobic exercise.*

3. *Can nurses promote a health practice such as exercise when they themselves are poor role models for health practices?*

4. *How does the nurse's role in an Exercise Program differ from the role of the exercise physiologist?*

5. *How can the nurse facilitate maintenance of an Exercise Program?*

References

American College of Sports Medicine. *Guidelines for graded exercise testing and exercise prescription.* Philadelphia: Lea & Febiger, 1975.

Åstrand, P. O., and Rodahl, K. *Textbook of work physiology.* Philadelphia: F. A. Davis, 1970.

Becker, M. H., and Maiman, L. A. Sociobehavioral determinants of compliance with health and medical care recommendations. *Medical Care,* 1975, *13,* 10–24.

Becker, M., et al. Patient perceptions and compliance: Recent studies of the health belief model. In R. B. Haynes, D. W. Taylor, D. Sackett (Eds.), *Compliance in health care.* Baltimore: Johns Hopkins University Press, 1979, pp. 78–109.

Belloc, N., and Breslow, L. Relationship of physical health status and health practices. *Preventive Medicine,* 1972, *1,* 409–421.

Blackburn, H. Coronary disease prevention: Controversy and professional attitudes. *Advances in Cardiology,* 1977, *20,* 10–26.

Blocker, W. Physical activities. *Postgraduate Medicine,* 1976, *60,* 56–61.

Blomqvist, C. G. Exercise physiology: Clinical aspects. In N. Wenger (Ed.), *Exercise and the heart.* Philadelphia: F. A. Davis, 1978, pp. 1–12.

Bonanno, J., and Lies, J. Effects of physical training on coronary risk factors. *American Journal of Cardiology,* 1974, *33,* 760–764.

Boyer, J. L., and Kasch, F. W. Exercise therapy in hypertensive men. *Journal of the American Medical Association,* 1970, *211,* 1668–1671.

Brand, R., et al. Job activity and fatal heart attacks studied by logistic risk analysis. *Circulation,* 1976, *54* (Suppl. II), 511.

Bruce, R. Method of exercise testing. *American Journal of Cardiology,* 1974, *33,* 715–720.

Cooper, K. Guidelines in the management of the exercising patient. *Journal of the American Medical Association,* 1970, *211,* 1663–1667.

Cooper, K. *The new aerobics.* New York: Bantam Books, 1972.

de Vries, H. Tips on prescribing exercise regimens for your older patient. *Geriatrics,* 1979, *4,* 75–81.

Eliot, R. S., Forker, A. D., and Robertson, R. J. Aerobic exercise as a therapeutic modality in the relief of stress. *Advances in Cardiology,* 1976, *18,* 231–242.

Fair, J., Allan-Rosenaur, J., and Thurston, E. Exercise management. *Nurse Practitioner*, 1979, May–June, 13–18.

Farquhar, J. Research in attitude change and motivation of health practices. In A. Enelow and J. Henderson (Eds.), *Applying behavioral science to cardiovascular risk*. Chicago: American Heart Association, 1975, pp. 58–62.

Farquhar, J. *The American way of life need not be hazardous to your health*. New York: W. W. Norton, 1978.

Fink, D. Tailoring the consensual regimen. In R. B. Haynes, D. W. Taylor, and D. Sackett (Eds.), *Compliance in health care*. Baltimore: Johns Hopkins University Press, 1979, pp. 110–118.

Fox, S. M., Naughton, J. P., and Gorman, P. A. Physical activity and cardiovascular health. I. Potential for prevention of coronary heart disease and possible mechanisms. *Modern Concepts of Cardiovascular Disease*, 1972a, 41, 17–20.

Fox, S. M., Naughton, J. P., and Gorman, P. A. Physical activity and cardiovascular health. III. The exercise prescription: Frequency and type of activity. *Modern Concepts of Cardiovascular Disease*, 1972b, 41, 25–30.

Friedman, B., and Knight, K. Running for life, health, and pleasure. *American Journal of Nursing*, 1978, 4, 602–607.

Froelicher, V. Does exercise conditioning delay progression of myocardial ischemia in coronary heart disease? *Cardiovascular Clinics*, 1977, 8, 11–16.

Froelicher, V. Exercise and the prevention of coronary atherosclerotic heart disease. In N. Wenger (Ed.), *Exercise and the heart*. Philadelphia: F. A. Davis, 1978, pp. 13–23.

Getchell, B. *Physical fitness: A way of life*. New York: John Wiley & Sons, 1976.

Goldberg, W., and Fitzpatrick, J. Movement therapy with the aged. *Nursing Research*, 1980, 29, 339–346.

Gordon, T., et al. High density lipoprotein as a protective factor against coronary heart disease: The Framingham Study. *American Journal of Medicine*, 1977, 62, 707–14.

Haissley, J. Comparative response to isometric (static) and dynamic exercise tests in coronary disease. *American Journal of Cardiology*, 1974, 33, 791–796.

Harris, L., et al. *Health maintenance*. Mutual Pacific Life Insurance Co., 1978.

Harris, W. E., et al. Jogging: An adult exercise program. *Journal of the American Medical Association*, 1967, 201, 759–761.

Haynes, R. B., Taylor, D. W., and Sockett, D. (Eds.). *Compliance in health care*. Baltimore; Williams & Wilkins, 1979.

Healthy people. The Surgeon General's report on health promotion and disease prevention background papers, DPHEW/PHH. Washington, D.C.: U.S. Government Printing Office, 1979.

Heinzelmann, F., and Bagley, R. W. Response to physical activity programs and their effect on health behavior. *Public Health Reports*, 1970, 85, 905–911.

Hellerstein, H. K., Levitas, I. M., Fox, S. M., et al. Walk, jog, run or play in shape. *Hospital Physician*, 1969, 51, 77–85.

Herje, P. Hows and whys of patient contracting. *Nurse Educator*, 1980, January–February, 30–34.

Hulka, B., et al. Communication, compliance and concordance between physicians and patients with prescribed medications. *American Journal of Public Health*, 1976, 66, 847–853.

Kasl, S. V., and Cobb, S. Health behavior, illness behavior, and sick role behavior. Part 1. *Archives of Environmental Health*, 1966, 12, 246–266.

Kim, M. J., and Moritz, D. (Eds.). *Classification of nursing diagnoses*. New York: McGraw-Hill Book Company, 1982.

Lind, A. Editorial: Cardiovascular responses to static exercise (isometrics, anyone?). *Circulation*, 1970, 40, 173–176.

Mann, G., et al. Exercise to prevent coronary heart disease. *American Journal of Medicine*, 1969, 46, 12–27.

Merriman, J. E. Exercise prescription for apparently healthy individuals and for cardiac patients. In K. Wenger (Ed.), *Exercise and the heart*. Philadelphia: F. A. Davis, 1978, pp. 81–92.

Miller, G. J., and Miller, N. E. Plasma high-density lipoprotein concentration and development of ischaemic heart disease. *Lancet*, 1975, 1, 16–19.

Morris, J., Heady, J., Raffle, P., Roberts, C., and Parks, J. Coronary heart disease and physical activity of work. *Lancet*, 1953, 2, 1053–1057, 1111–1120.

Morris, S., and McHenry, P. Role of exercise stress testing in healthy subjects and patients with coronary heart disease. *American Journal of Cardiology*, 1978, 42, 659–666.

Myers, C. *The official YMCA physical fitness book*. New York: Popular Library, 1975.

Paffenbarger, R. Physical activity as an index of heart attack risk in college alumni. *American Journal of Epidemiology*, 1978, 108, 161–175.

Paffenbarger, R., et al. Work activity of longshoremen as related to death from coronary heart disease and stroke. *New England Journal of Medicine*, 1970, 282, 1109–1114.

Paffenbarger, R., et al. Work-energy level, personal characteristics, and fatal heart attack: A birth cohort effect. *American Journal of Epidemiology*, 1977, 105, 200–213.

Pender, N. A conceptual model for preventive health behavior. *Nursing Outlook*, 1975, 23, 385–390.

Pollock, M. L., et al. Effects of walking on body composition and cardiovascular function in middle aged men. *Journal of Applied Physiology*, 1971, 30, 126–130.

Pollock, M. L., et al. Effects of frequency and duration of training on attrition and incidence of injury. *Medicine and Science in Sports*, 1977, *9*, 31–38.

President's Council on Physical Fitness and Sports Medicine Newsletter. Washington, D.C.: U.S. Government Printing Office, 1979.

Ratliff, R., Elliot, K., and Rubenstein, C. Plasma lipid and lipoprotein changes with chronic training. *Medicine and Science Sports*, 1978, *10*, 55 (abstract).

Roberts, D. Attitude change research and motivation of individuals. In A. Enelow and J. Henderson (Eds.), *Applying behavioral science to cardiovascular risk.* Chicago: American Heart Association, 1975, pp. 42–57.

Rosenstock, I. M. Why people use health services. *Millbank Memorial Fund Quarterly*, 1966, *44*, 94–127.

Running Times. 1978, *10*, 12–20.

Running Times. 1979, *3*, 25–26.

Skinner, J., et al. Social status, physical activity, and coronary proneness. *Journal of Chronic Disease*, 1966, *19*, 773–783.

Steckel, S. Contracting with patient selected reinforcers. *American Journal of Nursing*, 1980, *9*, 1596–1599.

Wenger, N. *Exercise and the heart.* Philadelphia: F. A. Davis, 1978.

Wiley, J. A., and Comacho, T. C. Lifestyle and future health: Evidence from Alameda. *Preventive Medicine*, 1980, *9*, 1–21.

Williams, R., et al. Physical conditioning augments the fibrinolytic response to venous occlusion in healthy adults. *New England Journal of Medicine*, 1980, *302*, 987–991.

Wilmore, J. Exercise prescription: Role of the psychiatrist and allied health professional. *Archives of Physical Medicine and Rehabilitation*, 1976, *57*, 315–319.

Zohman, L. *Beyond diet . . . exercise your way to fitness and heart health.* Mazola Corn Oil, CPC International, 1974.

16

GROUP PSYCHOTHERAPY

VERONICA WIELAND
SANDRA CUMMINGS

DESCRIPTION OF INTERVENTION

Group Psychotherapy has been defined as a method of psychotherapy in which the emotional reactions of members of the group are understood as being reflections of their interpersonal conflicts (Smith, 1970). In this modality of treatment it is the clients' relationship abilities, their interpersonal conflicts, and their problematical communicative patterns that become the focus and concern of the leader. These issues are both cognitively and affectively explored in a group whose purpose is to provide the clients with the opportunity not only to verbalize their concerns and problems but also to experience them in the "here and now" of the group. A psychotherapy group replicates the interpersonal world of the clients. Significance is given to the relevance of their interpersonal history as a major determinant in why they behave as they do (Yalom, 1975).

The nursing intervention of Group Psychotherapy is illustrated in this chapter through the application of the five stages of group development. Groups go through actual observable stages, and these stages can be classified into *Me Centeredness; the Awful Me; the Very Good Me; the Union of the Awful and Very Good Me;* and *Me Letting Go.* These titles are descriptive of the overall behavioral themes in the development of the group. These stages are fluid and in a constant state of change; they go forward and backward. The nurse may see a group in the Very Good Me stage one week, and the next week the group may be in the Me Centeredness stage. A number of factors influence this fluidity, such as member termination, introduction of new members into the group, the credibility of the therapist, the resistance to change, and unclear norms and expectations (Misel, 1975).

The conceptualization of these titles resulted from the authors' extensive work with inpatient and outpatient psychotherapy groups. Frequently these groups were supervised by experts in Group Psychotherapy. These groups consistently were videotaped or audiotaped. The authors also utilized a process recorder, who wrote verbatim the communications occurring in the group. By reviewing these data the authors were able to determine the stages of group development and to develop the intervention.

Although the descriptive language varies according to author, there is considerable consistency regarding the basic stages of group development (Yalom, 1975). Tuckman (1965) describes four developmental sequences in small groups; Martin and Hill (1957) describe six phases. Whitaker and Liebeman (1964) talk about the brief, formative stage and the extended, established phase of Group Therapy. An analysis of the orientation phase of Group Therapy is discussed by Sweeney and Drage (1968). The termination process of groups and its relationship to the separation-individuation process is described by Kauff (1977). The developmental stages of 18 sessions of Group Therapy are described by Heckel, Holmes, and Salzberg (1967).

There is little in the literature, however, dealing with how the leader applies the knowledge of Group Psychotherapy developmental stages. Misel (1975) discusses five stages of group development and emphasizes the importance of the leader's role in each of these stages. If the leader is credible, he or she can move the group into the working stage. The quicker the group moves into the working stage, the better the leader is as a therapist. Smith (1970) describes three stages of group development and discusses the nurse's role in each stage.

Lacoursiere (1980) focuses on the significance of the leader's being able to understand the similarity between the stages of group and individual development. If the nurse understands this sameness, he or she will be able to help clients (1) develop a level of insight about their interpersonal behaviors; (2) identify each stage of group development with their individual developmental stages; and (3) maintain a separate identity while joining with others.

Yalom (1975) stresses the importance of the group leader's knowing the developmental stages of the group. This knowledge enables the group leader to guide with a sense of direction, to assist the group in forming therapeutic norms, to prevent the group from establishing norms that hinder therapy, to diagnose group blockage, and to intervene in such a way as to allow the group to proceed. In order for nurses to intervene with their knowledge of the five stages of group development, they need the tools of *process illumination* and *here and now activation* (Yalom, 1975).

The term "process illumination" refers to relationship implications of interpersonal transactions. It is concerned not only with the verbal content, but also with the how and why, especially if it illuminates some aspects of the client's relationship with others and those with whom he or she is interacting. The leader considers the meta-communication aspect of the message or the communication about the communication (Cathart and Samouar, 1979). For example, when a client in a group begins to talk about missing an old childhood friend, it may be important to consider *how* and *why* he is discussing the topic. Is his affect congruent with the content? To whom is he addressing the comment? How are his responses being received by other clients? Is he talking about a member of the group who is absent? Is he talking about someone he has felt has been supportive and caring? It becomes the leader's responsibility to raise questions and make comments that encourage exploration so the significant meaning of the message is understood.

"Here and now activation" is another important tool used by the leader to facilitate the group movement through the stages of development. The members then begin to create their own interpersonal world within the present group experience. The leader needs to think in terms of here and now (Moreno, 1964). When he or she does so long enough, the group is reflexively steered into the here and now. Whenever an issue is raised in the group, it becomes important to think, "How can I relate this content to the group's life in the here and now?" The leader moves the focus from outside to inside, from the abstract to the specific, from the generic to the personal (Yalom, 1975).

For example, if a client describes a hostile confrontation with a friend, the leader may inquire, "If you were to be angry like that with anyone in the group, with whom would it be?" Also, the leader must help members discuss their feelings about the group itself as well as toward individual members (Yalom, 1975). It often is therapeutic to ask how members are viewing the group's movement—do they feel the group is moving too quickly or too slowly, for example?

In addition to group developmental knowledge, the nurse needs to have an understanding of individual psychodynamics, stages of the human life cycle, and psychotherapy (Smith, 1970). This foundation helps the nurse determine the genesis of the clients' interpersonal problems and their resistances and blockages to achieving change.

Priority is given to the nurse's knowledge and application of the stages of group development. This intervention helps him or her to continue to focus on group process rather than on individual problems. The tools of process illumination and here and now activation help achieve the goals of this intervention. Table 16–1 is a summation of this intervention and includes the goals, the tools, and the outcome.

SELECTION OF CLIENTS

The most important criterion for inclusion in Group Psychotherapy is the client's level of motivation. Motivation is required not only when relief of symptoms and discomfort is desired, but also when the situation requires a willingness to change by working hard to find other ways of dealing with problems (Mann, 1973).

Table 16–1. GROUP PSYCHOTHERAPY: KNOWLEDGE AND APPLICATION OF THE FIVE STAGES OF GROUP DEVELOPMENT

Goals
1. To help the client achieve insight about his or her interpersonal behavior.
2. To help the client develop a separate identity and increase his or her ability to join with others.

Tools (Process Illumination, Here and Now Activation)
1. Allow the group to form therapeutic norms.
2. Help the group to work through their resistance to change.
3. Give the group a sense of direction that enables them to identify and resolve each step of development.

Outcomes
1. Clients have developed a level of insight about their interpersonal behaviors.
2. Clients have been able to identify each stage of group development with their individual developmental stages.
3. Clients are able to maintain a separate identity while joining with others.
4. Clients have developed new skills and abilities in relating to others.

In our experience, a client's willingness to participate actively in the group sessions and to take responsibility and ownership for his or her problems are the two major criteria for inclusion. These criteria are supported by Yalom (1975), Nash (1957), and Grotjahn (1972). When evaluating prospective group clients, it has been apparent to us that inclusion in the group need not be based on age, sex, marital status, sexual preference, socioeconomic class, or educational background.

Mann (1973) has identified seven factors that are helpful in evaluating a client's level of motivation. If a client has fewer than three of the following characteristics, he or she may be a poor risk for Group Psychotherapy:

1. An ability to recognize that the symptoms are psychological.
2. A tendency to be introspective and to attempt to give an honest account of emotional difficulties.
3. A willingness to participate actively in the treatment situation.
4. A curiosity to understand oneself.
5. A willingness to change, explore, or experiment.
6. A realistic expectation of the results of psychotherapy.
7. A willingness to make reasonable sacrifices.

APPLICATION OF THE INTERVENTION

Stages of Group Development

Each of the five group therapy stages mentioned earlier will be discussed. Discussion of each stage will include purpose, nursing application, and behavioral description, followed by clinical examples of the nursing intervention.

Stage One: Me Centeredness

Purpose. For each client to find a sense of security, trust, and safety as a member of the group.

Nursing Application. The focus of the nurse's interactions with the members is the establishment of norms and expectations for behavior in the group. He or she verbally encourages members to share their commonalities with each other.

Behavioral Description. The first stage is characterized by members groping for the meaning of Group Therapy. There is confusion about the purpose of the group. Statements may emerge such as "I don't really know how this will help me," or "I wish I knew how this was supposed to work."

Members are me centered and self-involved, absorbed with their personal struggles and their image in the group. They are doubtful and skeptical as to how talking with other clients can help them. Because of their feelings of helplessness in solving their personal problems, they have difficulty believing that they can be helpful to others.

At the same time, members are sizing up one another and the group as a whole. They are searching for a role for themselves, often worrying whether they will be liked and respected or ignored and rejected. This search and testing of one another is done through discussing topics in a rational, cognitive manner. The content and communication style are superficial, trite, and stereotyped. In this way clients surmise which members have common viewpoints, ideas, and values. They are intrigued that they are not unique in their distress and may invest much time in sharing their similarities. Responses to each other might be "Yes, I know exactly what you mean," "I thought I was the only one who felt that way," and "I've done that, too."

Giving and asking for advice is another characteristic of the me-centered stage. Members present to the group low-risk problems, such as dealing with employees, children, and neighbors. The group attempts to provide a practical solution. The solution usually has been tried, won't work, or possibly will be tried in the future. The helpfulness is rarely of any functional value, but it is a safe way for members to express mutual concern, interest, and acceptance. In this stage, group members look to the nurse for structure, guidance, answers, approval, and acceptance. Many of the interactions in the group are directed at or through her or him. Members will watch the nurse for nonverbal approval, such as eye contact, head nods, and smiles. His or her comments are examined carefully for directives about desirable and undesirable behavior. Members attempt to discover the leader's expectations, thinking that if they make this discovery they can be cured. Each member unrealistically expects the leader to exhibit special caring toward him; to guard him from being emotionally hurt by other members; to protect him from uncomfortable feelings; and to provide him with an instant cure.

Stage Two: Awful Me

Purpose. To find a place in the group by aggressively seeking approval or establishing individual territory.

Nursing Application. The focus of the nurse's interactions with the members is verbal acceptance of their anger toward and confrontation of him or her. The nurse also assists members in the process of exploration and acceptance of their anger toward her and others.

Behavioral Description. This second stage of Group Therapy is characterized by frustration, conflict, competition, and preoccupation with dominance, power, and control. The conflict and competition occur between members or between members and the leader. Members attempt to establish boundaries for themselves and the group. Through power and control a social pecking order is established.

Members are more critical of each other. They feel that they have the right to judge and analyze problems of other group members. As in the me-centered stage, advice is given, but in a less caring manner. The intent is not to get to know or to help, but to establish territory and position in the group. Social conventions are abandoned. There is increased personal criticism about members' behaviors, values, attitudes, and lifestyles. Advice is given using the words "should" and "ought," indicating judgment. Issues between members become polarized with an absence of choices and an intolerance of a middle ground.

The emergence of hostility and resentment toward the nurse is an inevitable occurrence in the Awful Me stage. The sources of hostility are obvious. They are linked to the unrealistic expectations that group members placed on the leader in the Me-Centered stage. Expectations are too high. Regardless of the nurse's competence, the clients will view him or her as a failure.

Gradually, as the members recognize these limitations, they view the nurse as less magical and powerful. This recognition creates doubts as to the nurse's ability to take care of them and guide them in the proper direction. Other members realize that they never will discover the leader's expectations of them. They will never know what to do to be cured. It is frustrating for members whose past experiences have allowed them to get special treatment from authority figures. They no longer know what expectations to meet.

Resentment toward the nurse grows as each member realizes that he will not be the special, favored one. This realization started in the Me-Centered stage, but now it is more keenly experienced because of the increased rivalry between members.

Group members demonstrate hostility toward the nurse in varied ways. Some members complain that he or she is too authoritarian and say they want more permissiveness. Other members declare that they want more structure. They request specific group exercises and structuring of time. Or members may directly attack the leader's leadership style, a personality trait, a speech mannerism, or nonverbal behavior.

Indirect attacks may be seen by tardiness or absence of members. A change in seating order may occur. The group sits together, distancing themselves from the nurse, or a member may sit in the nurse's chair. Discussion in the group might focus on past useless therapies and hospitalizations. Scapegoating of a group member also may occur.

Stage Three: Very Good Me

Purpose. To sacrifice own needs for safety and individuality in service of group harmony.

Nursing Application. The focus of the nurse's interactions with the members is validation of their support and caring toward each other. He or she encourages this process through role playing, problem solving, and verbal acknowledgment.

Behavioral Description. This third stage is characterized by the group's gradual development into a cohesive unit, with maintenance of group harmony at any cost. This stage is the opposite of the Awful Me stage, in which group members vied for territory. Now cohesiveness is more important than individual boundaries or working through group issues. The group suppresses all expressions of negative affect in order to maintain group amity. Individual differences are minimized or not discussed. Members are polite, smug, sweet, savoring the group's newly discovered unity. Silent members are encouraged to talk. It is important for all members to feel satisfied. Attendance improves and there is considerable concern for missing members. Members may meet after the group sessions.

The main concern of the group is with intimacy, closeness, and acceptance. Members worry about being liked, getting too close, or not getting close enough. It is important for them to show this Very Good Me after having previously demonstrated the Awful Me. They need to give and receive acceptance and approval from each other and the leader. Eventually this harmony and unity seem ritualistic and unrealistic. This necessitates finding a balance between the Awful Me and the Very Good Me.

Stage Four: Union of the Awful Me and the Very Good Me

Purpose. To integrate both "senses of me" in the group by going through the process of legitimizing conflict.

Nursing Application. The focus of the nurse's interactions with members is the identification of a range of conflictual feelings. He or she encourages members to share their anger, sadness, humor, mistrust, and other feelings with each other. The emphasis is on the nurse's ability to help members provide feedback to each other so that they develop insights into their own behaviors.

Behavioral Description. In this stage it has become apparent to the members that the methods of stage three are not proving to be effective. The "Good Me" of stage three has achieved a sense of security and of being liked and nurtured, but these are not sufficient goals in themselves. They are, however, a condition for more effective action to take place. The members who are more willing to compromise recognize the self-defeating behaviors of stage three: its focus limits the members to one aspect of who they are—the Good Me—and negates the more conflicted, ambivalent, angry side—the Awful Me. In stage four, the members begin to talk about this conflict. They attempt to legitimize the feelings and the thoughts that were not positive. This focus creates conflict or forces the group to consider alternative approaches. Stage four has intense periods of conflict, but it also tends to be more effective without being destructive to the individual. Members grow in their ability to participate and to formulate perceptions about group process. They feel less judged by each other. Rapport is experienced by knowing what to expect from others.

The overall focus in this stage is on the "here and now," for members are talking directly to one another about their feelings and thoughts. A sense of trust is experienced by their being more open about expressing their lack of trust. There is a willingness to take risks by sharing meaningful here and now reactions. Most members feel a sense of inclusion, and excluded members are invited to become more active.

Leadership is more shared. Members feel free to initiate exploration of specific areas. Interactions tend to be honest and spontaneous. An emotional bond is present because of the identification with each other's problems and areas of concern. This helps to promote a willingness of members to risk experimental behaviors. Conflict among members and the leader is recognized, discussed, and often resolved.

In the previous stages, when members were confronted or offered feedback, they frequently interpreted it as an attack or gave a defensive response. In stage four, members accept the responsibility for whatever actions they will take to solve their problems. Feedback is given freely and accepted with less defensiveness. Each member seriously reflects on the accuracy of the feedback. Confrontation is viewed as an opportunity to examine one's behavior, not as an uncaring attack.

There is an emphasis on combining feeling and thinking functions. Catharsis and expression of feeling occur, but so does thinking about the meaning of various emotional experiences. This combination of both cognitive and affective components in evaluating themselves helps the members utilize non-group time to work on problems. It will become apparent to the leader that the continuity of work from one session to the next will not be fragmented and lost. The leader will not need to do all the initiation to help the members address unfinished business or leftover concerns from a previous session. There is a strong commitment to work. This attitude has resulted from the unification of the Good Me and the Awful Me. The legitimization of the Awful Me provides a more objective and realistic basis from which to begin the process of change.

Stage Five: Me Letting Go

Purpose. To achieve a sense of separation that promotes self-reliance and a joining with others.

Nursing Application. The focus of the nursing interaction is termination. The nurse helps the members review the past group history and each member's relationship with the leaving members. He or she also helps the members to share their anger, disappointments, frustration, sadness, joy, jealousy, and fears of leaving the group.

Behavioral Description. This final stage of Group Therapy is characterized by members feeling and acknowledging that they have or have not achieved their personal goals. These goals may have changed since the group's beginning. As members gained a more objective perspective of their interpersonal behaviors, their goals may have expanded or become more realistic.

Members have learned how they are viewed by other people. They know with whom they might demonstrate particular behaviors and why. Aloof, wary group members have begun to examine their fears of intimacy. Aggressive, vindictive members understand their need to control in order to protect themselves from feeling vulnerable or rejected. Group members have learned that they can behave in different ways without being destroyed, rejected, or abandoned. They feel less locked into one position because they have learned not to fear their feelings. They have expanded their behavioral choices. Members are talking about these changes. "I never thought I could feel like this when I started the group." "You have helped me a lot." "Did I really act like that?" Clients also talk about healthier behaviors occurring outside the group.

Because members leave at different times they can experience how others leave before they decide to let go of the group. This will be experienced differently by each client, depending upon the relationship of each with the separating member. Experiencing this letting-go of individual members assists remaining clients in their preparation for their own termination with the group. Reactions from each other and the leader are watched closely. Members feel ambivalent about leaving the group and show this in varied ways. Some clients exhibit anger in having to let go of the group's security. Others minimize or deny the group's importance to them. Still others think of reasons to remain in the group.

Through the process of Group Therapy, members have learned to cherish and respect their individual feelings, thoughts, and values. They accept themselves as an important separate identity from others. This self-reliance is strong enough not to be lost when joined with another person. It enables them to develop relationships without sacrificing their identity.

An important outcome of Group Psychotherapy is the client's achievement of a level of insight about himself—about his behavior, motivational system, fantasy life, or unconscious. Clients may obtain "insight" on at least three different levels. Yalom (1975) describes these levels.

1. Insight about interpersonal behavior.
   Clients learn how they are seen by other people and how they manifest themselves interpersonally. Are they tense, warm, aloof, seductive, bitter? Clients learn about their dealings with others over a longer time span. Are they exploiting others, rejecting others, courting constant admiration from others, so needy of others that their effacing behavior elicits the opposite response from others?
2. Insight about motivations.
   Clients learn why they do what they do to and with other people. Aloof, detached clients may begin to learn why they have so much fear about intimacy. Competitive, vindictive, controlling clients may learn about their needs to be taken care of, to be nurtured.
3. Insight about genesis of behavior.
   Clients understand the genesis of present patterns of behavior through an exploration of their developmental history.

CLINICAL EXAMPLES

The group described is composed of eight members. Identifying information for each member is included in Table 16–2. There is one example from each developmental stage. Each one has two components: (1) group process, which comprises the client's discussion and the nurse's interaction, and (2) rationale for the nurse's interaction.

Example from Stage One—Me Centeredness

Bill:	(Looking at nurse) I can't stand reading the paper anymore. Society is unfair. How are people supposed to be creative in society today?
Paula:	It's not just society, it's even right at home.
Marge:	Yeah, I have problems at home, too.

Table 16–2. CHARACTERISTICS OF GROUP MEMBERS

Name	Identifying Data	Client's Description of Problem	Client's History of Interpersonal Relationships and Nursing Diagnosis
Katy	38; married, 2 children, homemaker	Nonassertive, unable to make decisions, procrastinates, lacks self-confidence.	Passivity, hostile dependency, low self-esteem. Nursing Diagnosis: Disturbance in Self-Esteem.
Ed	44; divorced, no children, head of hospital department	Drinks alcohol under stress, uncontrollable temper, doesn't get along with people.	Alcoholism, uses aggression to protect dependency needs; projection of problems onto others. Nursing Diagnosis: Ineffective Individual Coping.
Elaine	24; single, student	Wants to know why can't form a relationship with a man. "No one understands me or gives me what I need."	Narcissistic, unrealistic sense of entitlement, lack of differentiation of self. Nursing Diagnosis: Disturbance in Self-Esteem.
Bill	42; married, 4 children, househusband	Anxiety, panic attacks, lack of motivation, psychosomatic complaints.	Avoidant behavior, intellectualizes and rationalizes problems, alcoholism. Nursing Diagnosis: Ineffective Individual Coping.
Paula	39; divorced 3 times, 1 child, part-time employment Food Service	Problems with marriage, difficulty getting along with people on the job and with roommate.	Hostile aggressive behavior, minimization of problems, compulsivity and rigidity as a way of maintaining control. Nursing Diagnosis: Impaired Interpersonal Relationships.
Marge	28; married, no children, graduate student	Feels isolated, not cared for, cries a lot, has self-doubt about her work and studies.	Passive-aggressive behavior, self-absorption, problems with boundaries, inability to negotiate her needs with the needs of others. Nursing Diagnosis: Disturbance in Personal Image.
Jean	25; divorced, no children, student	Feels misunderstood, lacks friends, wants to know why relationships with men don't work.	Tangential and circumstantial verbal communication as protection for her confusion around sexual identity and early childhood trauma. Nursing Diagnosis: Disturbance in Self-Esteem.
Mike	21; single, full-time clerk	Unhappy with life, uncertain about future plans regarding work, school.	Use of sarcastic humor as way to deflect his difficulty with issues of separation and individuation. Nursing Diagnosis: Impaired Interpersonal Relationships.

Ed to Bill:	Maybe if you didn't read the paper you wouldn't get so upset.
Nurse:	It seems like people feel that society and home don't always treat them fairly. What concerns come to mind when people think about being treated unfairly in the group? (*here and now activation*)
Mike:	Ha! Maybe we need a referee.
Ed:	I hope he will be more fair than the one at the Hawks game last night.
Jean:	I don't known much about sports, but sometimes my art teacher doesn't appreciate my work.
Nurse:	It seems that it is more comortable for members to talk about unfairness outside the group. Are people not knowing what to expect from each other in this group? (*process illumination*)
Rationale:	The nurse recognized that the discussion of unfairness and lack of appreciation reflected the members' concerns for safety and security in the group. She used the tool of *here and now activation* and moved the focus from outside to inside the group. Her second interaction recognized the members' concerns about needing approval and acceptance. She also addressed the issues of structure and expectations. She used the tool of *process illumination* to focus on the members' relationships to each other.

Example from Stage Two—Awful Me

When group members come into the room, Elaine rushes over to a chair that Paula has occupied since the beginning of the group. Members begin to talk.

Bill:	I am so sick of being a househusband. I can never do the things I really want to do. Everything keeps piling up.
Ed:	It doesn't sound too bad to me. I would love to stay home and not work. If you want to do something different you should get a real job.
Bill:	I can't find a job where I can be creative. I like being my own boss.
Ed:	I think you enjoy being a bum.
Nurse:	As soon as the session began, Elaine took Paula's chair and Ed told Bill what he should do to solve his problems. (*process illumination*) Are people concerned about their position in the group? (*here and now activation*)
Elaine:	Paula doesn't need to have the most comfortable chair each week.
Ed:	I'm not that concerned about position. I'm just expressing my feelings like you're always telling us to do.
Marge:	(To nurse) Why aren't you helping us with this? Why isn't the group working on more important issues?
Nurse:	It seems that members are feeling frustrated and angry because all your expectations are not being met in the group. (*process illumination*)
Rationale:	The nurse recognized that the members' aggressive behavior indicated their need to establish their own territory in the group. She used *process illumination* and *here and now activation* to bring this need to the group's attention. In her second interaction she identified the issues of power and feelings of anger and frustration. This focus on group process reflected the significant meaning of the members' communication.

Example from Stage Three—Very Good Me

Marge appears sullen and sad.

Jean:	Marge, what's wrong? Are things going badly?
Kathy:	You're much quieter.
Marge:	Last week I had lots of problems to talk about, but there wasn't enough time. Everyone else was doing all the talking.
Bill:	Why don't you tell us what's bothering you now? Maybe we can make you feel better.
Marge:	Well, that's all right. It doesn't matter so much this week.
Mike:	Come on now, we don't bite. I really want to hear what you have to say.
Marge:	Well, two weeks ago I was at this party. . . (Marge describes her problem)
Nurse:	People seem very caring and concerned about each other. Are people overlooking other feelings or concerns that they are having? (*process illumination*)
Rationale:	The nurse recognized the members' need for group harmony and their willingness to sacrifice their own concerns and feelings for group amity. She used *process illumination* by identifying the members' concern for others and by recognizing their minimizing of individual differences. She gave them the opportunity to explore these issues, a necessary step in order to move into the next group stage of development.

Example from Stage Four—Union of the Awful Me and Very Good Me

Paula:	I'm feeling nervous about going home. Everyone will be there, my brothers, sisters, mother.
Kathy:	What is it that you don't like about going home?
Paula:	I always seem to do all the cooking and cleaning up. I get so sick of it.
Mike:	What is it you want us to do?
Paula:	I don't know. I just needed to tell you that.
Elaine:	It's hard for me to tell what you're really thinking about your problems. You don't show much feeling here. You're always so controlled.
Paula:	(Starts crying) I'm afraid to tell people what I want. No one understands me.
Jean:	At least when you start to cry I know how painful this is for you. I don't know why you always feel that you must take care of everything by yourself.
Nurse:	(Remains silent. The group continues to work.)

Next Session:

Paula:	I went home and for the first time I asked for help with cooking and cleaning. I let the family plan their own activities. I didn't feel I had to do it all.
Nurse:	Between this and the last session, Paula has struggled with some of the feedback that was given to her by group members. She was able to test out some new responses with her family. (*process illumination*).

Example from Stage Five—Me Letting Go

This is the first of the three sessions dealing with Paula's terminating from the group.

Paula:	Every time I think about leaving the group I have so many feelings.
Nurse:	Can you try and identify what you're feeling now? (*here and now activation*)
Paula:	(Becomes teary-eyed) I just feel confused.
Nurse:	How do members feel about Paula leaving the group? She has been a member of the group for a year. (*here and now activation*)
Jean:	Oh, I feel sad and I'm going to miss her. But I also feel happy for her (starts to cry).
Mike:	(Flippantly) Look at it this way. You won't have to sit with a bunch of maladjusted people every week.
Katy:	I would be afraid to leave this security.
Nurse:	It seems that Paula's leaving the group has caused members to express a variety of feelings. Jean talked about feeling sad and missing Paula. Mike seemed angry. And Katy expressed her fear of leaving the group. (*process illumination*)
Paula:	Well, I guess I have some mixed feelings about leaving the group, also.
Elaine:	How do you think the group has helped you?
Paula:	Well, I'm not as afraid of people. I don't need to control them anymore, and I understand more why I had to do that.
Nurse:	Could people share with Paula how they experience her changes in the group? (*here and now activation*)
Rationale:	The nurse's use of *here and now activation* and *process illumination* made explicit the ambivalent feelings involved with the termination. She helped members focus on the components involved in the termination process. She acknowledged the importance of reviewing the client's change and development of insight. This process allows for the client and the remaining members to experience a successful separation that promotes self-reliance and a joining of others.

In the presentation of these five clinical examples, the nurse applied her knowledge of group development in each stage. By utilizing the tools of process illumination and here and now activation, she enabled the group to form therapeutic norms, to work through their resistance to change, and to identify and resolve each stage of development. The effects of this intervention resulted in the clients' developing a level of insight about their interpersonal behaviors and maintaining a separate identity while joining with others.

RECOMMENDATIONS

Psychiatric nurses are being increasingly encouraged and challenged to expand their traditional roles to include Group Psychotherapy. Armstrong and Rouslin (1963) recommended that this training be restricted to nurses with a master's degree in psychiatric nursing. Other qualifications that enable a nurse to practice Group Psychotherapy are a basic foundation in individual and group dynamics, observation and process recording of an ongoing psychotherapy group for a minimum of six months, and supervised experience for a minimum of one year.

Psychiatric nurses can extend their practice of Group Psychotherapy to include a variety of populations: patients with chronic disease, patients and families dealing with death, prisoners with substance abuse problems and mental illness, children of divorce, and school-age children with problems of aggression, peer relationships, abuse, incest, and phobias. The focus of these groups would be the application of the knowledge of the five stages of group development. For example, patients with chronic diseases may have regressed to the individual developmental stage of autonomy versus shame (Erickson, 1968). The major issues in this stage are control, aggressiveness, independence, and self-discipline. This regression can be resolved by the patient identifying with and experiencing the stage of the Awful Me. This process allows the client to work through the remaining stages so that he or she is no longer resistive to the physical and emotional changes accompanying the chronic disease.

A current challenge nurses are facing is how to include research in their clinical practice. Questions for possible research projects are (1) how to use this intervention in a time-limited group; (2) how to correlate the stages of group development with Erickson's developmental stages; (3) how to test the effectiveness of this intervention; (4) how to judge if the effectiveness of the intervention depends on the selection of clients; and (5) determining if the intervention is more effective when all the clients are in the same stage of human development.

The main objective of Group Psychotherapy is not to see how well the nurse can proceed through these five stages; rather, it is to provide the clients with abilities and strengths they can use in interpersonal relationships both within the group and outside of it. By using this intervention the nurse provides the group members with an experience that allows them to develop new skills and abilities in understanding themselves and relating to others. It also provides them with the opportunity to explore and to test out new behaviors.

EDITORS' COMMENTS AND QUESTIONS
The authors identify five stages in this intervention, which the nurse can make use of in assisting the client to develop abilities and strengths that can be used in interpersonal relationships both within and outside the group. The aim is for the client to develop insight about self and behavior. Associated nursing diagnoses related to this intervention appear in Table 16–2.

Questions for Discussion
1. *Distinguish between Group Psychotherapy and Support Groups.*
2. *How do nurses become qualified to conduct Group Psychotherapy?*
3. *How can a mix of clients facilitate this intervention?*
4. *What variables need to be controlled when testing the effectiveness of this intervention?*

References

Armstrong, S. W., and Rouslin, S. *Group psychotherapy in nursing practice.* New York: Macmillan, 1963.

Cathcart, R. S., and Samouar, L. A. *Small group communication.* Dubuque, Iowa: Wm. C. Brown Company, 1979.

Corey, G., and Corey, M. S. *Groups: Process and practice.* Monterey, Calif.: Brooks/Cole Publishing Company, 1977.

Erikson, E. H. *Identity: youth and crisis.* New York: W. W. Norton Company, 1968.

Grotjahn, M. Learning from dropout patients: A clinical view of patients who discontinued group psychotherapy. *International Journal of Group Psychotherapy,* 1972, *22,* 306–319.

Heckel, R. V., Holmes, G., and Salzberg, H. Emergence of distinct verbal phrases in group therapy. *Psychological Reports,* 1967, *21,* 630–632.

Kauff, P. F. The termination process: Its relationship to the separation-individuation phase of development. *International Journal of Group Psychotherapy,* 1977, *27,* 3–18.

Lacousiere, R. *The life cycle of groups.* New York: Human Sciences Press, 1980.

Mann, J. *Time-limited psychotherapy.* Cambridge, Mass.: Harvard University Press, 1973.

Martin, E. A., Jr., and Hill, W. F. Toward a theory of group development. *International Journal of Group Psychotherapy,* 1957, *7,* 20–30.

Misel, L. T. Stages of group treatment. *Transactional Analysis Journal,* 1975, *5,* 385–391.

Moreno, J. L. *Psychodrama* (Vol. 1). Beacon, N.Y.: Beacon House, 1946 (revised, 1964).

Nash, E., Gludman, L., Imber, S., and Stone, A. Some factors related to patients remaining in group psychotherapy. *International Journal of Group Psychotherapy,* 1957, *7,* 264–275.

Smith, A. J. A manual for the training of psychiatric nursing personnel in group psychotherapy. *Perspectives in Psychiatric Care,* 1970, *8,* 106–126.

Sweeney, A., and Drage, E. Group therapy: An analysis of the orientation phase. *Journal of Psychiatric Nursing and Mental Health Nursing,* 1968, *6,* 20–26.

Tuckman, B. W. Developmental sequence in small groups. *Psychological Bulletin,* 1965, *63,* 384–399.

Whitaker, D. S., and Lieberman, M. A. *Psychotherapy through the group process.* New York: Atherton Press, 1964.

Yalom, I. D. *The theory and practice of group psychotherapy.* New York: Basic Books, 1975.

17 ▯▯ ▭ ▭ ▭

ASSERTIVENESS TRAINING

ANNE G. SADLER

Lisa is a 26 year old graduate student at the local university. After completing a stressful examination two days ago, Lisa went to an exclusive women's store and on impulse purchased a silk blouse. She is now aware the blouse is too costly for her to afford comfortably at this time and she must return it. She arrives at the store within the three days required for cash refund of exchanged merchandise and approaches the clerk. After hearing Lisa's request for a refund, the clerk snidely retorts, "You students always buy things you can't afford and then return them. If there's nothing wrong with the blouse, we'll just give you a credit slip."

How could Lisa handle this situation assertively? Take a minute and think how you would respond.

ASSERTIVE BEHAVIOR

What is assertive behavior? Assertiveness and assertion training have been popular terms in today's society, but the concept of assertive behavior is often misunderstood. Assertive behavior can be defined as setting goals, acting on these goals in a clear and consistent manner, and taking responsibility for the consequences of those actions. An important aspect of assertive behavior involves getting in touch with one's own desires, thoughts, and feelings. This involves assessing and owning up to one's strengths and limitations. It also means being able to admit errors and accept compliments with equal ease (Clark, 1978). Assertive behavior "enables a person to act in his or her own best interests, to stand up for herself or himself without undue anxiety, to express honest feelings comfortably, or to exercise personal rights without denying the rights of others" (Alberti and Emmons, 1978, p. 27). Alberti and Emmons further define assertive behavior as:

1. Self-expressive;
2. Honest;
3. Direct and firm;
4. Self-enhancing and relationship-enhancing;
5. Respectful of the rights of others;
6. Partially composed of the content of the message (feelings, rights, facts, opinions, requests, limits);
7. Partially composed of the nonverbal style of the message (eye contact, voice, posture, facial expression, gestures, distance, timing, fluency, listening);
8. Appropriate for the person and the situation, rather than universal;
9. Socially responsible;
10. A combination of learned skills, not an inborn trait. (Alberti and Emmons, 1982, p. 19.)

Assertive behavior is the expression of oneself in a positive and productive manner. It is not necessary to be continually confrontive, boorish, belligerent, or antagonistic to achieve self-assertion (Whiteley and Flowers, 1978). It is likely that no one is completely assertive at all times or in all situations. This can be partly due to choice and partly due to lack of skill or energy (Clark, 1978).

How, then, would Lisa respond assertively in her situation?

> Assertive: Lisa looks the clerk directly in the eyes, holds her posture erect and firmly but pleasantly says, "I appreciate that it is probably frustrating when customers make frequent exchanges. I am, however, returning my purchase within the three day limit for cash refund and cash is what I prefer." The clerk acknowledges the frustrations associated with her job and goes about refunding Lisa's money. Lisa leaves feeling good that she was able to deal with the situation appropriately and effectively.

WHAT IS ASSERTIVENESS TRAINING?

Assertiveness Training was one of the most popular therapeutic approaches of the seventies. Unlike many of the other therapeutic approaches, no universally accepted set of procedures defining Assertivenesss Training has emerged. Even though no two authors seem to completely agree, there is more agreement than disagreement on Assertiveness Training approaches (Cress, 1976). Assertiveness Training, which may be performed in groups or individually, is defined by Alberti and Emmons (1982) as a systematic approach to more effective self-expression, based upon a balance between achieving one's own goals and respecting the needs of others. Rimm and Masters (1975) define Assertiveness Training as any therapeutic procedure that focuses on increasing a person's ability to express feelings openly and honestly in a socially appropriate manner.

Jakobuwski and Lange (1978) characterize Assertiveness Training by four distinct features:

1. People are taught the difference between aggressive, passive, and assertive behavior.

2. People are helped to identify their interpersonal rights and responsibilities as well as those of others.

3. Participants in Assertiveness Training are helped to reduce cognitive and affective obstacles to assertive behavior.

4. Specific assertive skills are developed through active practice methods. These skills can also be acquired through vicarious living. There is variation in the literature worth noting here. Smith (1975) presents Assertiveness

Training as a set of skills rather than a lifestyle. His framework consists of approximately six general assertive skills to be applied routinely, singly or in combination, in situations of daily living. Fensterheim and Baer (1975), conversely, present assertiveness more as a lifestyle than as a set of skills. They do not encourage rote drill, but emphasize how an assertive lifestyle leads to various new strengths in self-control (Cress, 1976). This chapter will integrate these two approaches, stressing improvement in behavioral skills yet working toward the development of an assertive lifestyle.

HISTORICAL OVERVIEW

Assertiveness Training has been shaped by social events, therapy trends, and differing theoretical orientations. One of the original contributors to its formation was Moreno (1946), the founder of psychodrama. Psychodrama and behavior rehearsal are techniques used in Assertiveness Training. Both involve role playing, improvisation, and working through interpersonal conflicts on stage. Psychodrama and behavior rehearsal goals differ, however, as psychodrama aims at insight and catharsis (Cress, 1976), whereas behavior rehearsal aims at behavior modification.

Salter (1949), another major shaper of Assertiveness Training, advocated excitatory behavior as the remedy for every possible psychological deficit. The excitatory behavior consisted of prescribed response styles:

1. "Feeling talk" (saying what you feel).
2. "Facial talk" (corresponding nonverbal expression of feelings).
3. "Contradict and attack" (statements when disagreeing with someone).
4. "I" statements (used frequently).
5. Acceptance of praise and compliments.
6. Praising oneself.
7. Living for the present and being spontaneous.

For several reasons, Salter's work was not well received at the time of his initial writings. Perhaps in the early 1950s therapists were hesitant to accept a learning-based or behavioral approach. Skinner, Dollard, and Miller had not yet published their works, and Slater offended many psychotherapists by vigorously and antagonistically attacking psychodynamic approaches. Finally, he never addressed the issues of dealing with the consequences of his advocated spontaneous, impulsive behavior (Cress, 1976). Salter's book *Conditional Reflex Therapy* (1949) has been recommended to clients and therapists by assertiveness trainers (e.g., Alberti and Emmons, 1975; Lesser, 1967; Wolpe and Lazarus, 1966) as an excellent reading assignment (Cotler and Guerra, 1976).

Kelly (1955) also was a valuable contributor to the Assertiveness Training movement. Kelly developed a fixed-role therapy in which the patient constructs a personality profile of an imaginary person who is entirely free of the shortcomings, anxieties, and inadequacies troubling the patient. The patient is to assume this role to the extent of seeing the world through the eyes of the imaginary person, thinking as the person might, and behaving accordingly. Fixed-role therapy strives for cognitive changes. Assertiveness Training stresses behavioral changes while welcoming any appropriate cognitive and affective changes.

Wolpe and Lazarus (1966) have probably made the greatest impact on the course the assertiveness movement has taken. They demonstrated that Assertiveness Training was firmly rooted in an empirical and widely accepted theory of behavioral change. They did not assume that Assertiveness Training was the treatment of choice in every situation, nor did they support the concept that assertiveness was a generalized trait. They saw assertiveness as a situation-specific phenomenon. Finally, Wolpe and Lazarus were quite concerned about the interpersonal consequences of assertive behavior. This approach was in direct contrast to Salter's work (Cress, 1976).

Between 1966 and 1970, the number of articles on Assertiveness Training and related procedures began to increase dramatically. Cotler and Guerra (1976) provide a detailed listing and description of this period. Cress (1976) emphasizes that although many factors created an ideal atmosphere for the emergence of Assertiveness Training during the 1970s, the most salient factor was the role played by the National Organization for Women (NOW). Consciousness-raising and rap groups accompanied the rapid growth of the NOW and focused on assertive issues from the beginning. Uniting with the common goal of equal rights for women and against the common enemy, repressive and subjugating influences in society, women became more assertive and outspoken. Feelings, opinions, and desires of women began to be articulated. Although some groups were shortsighted and focused their Assertiveness Training primarily on interpersonal relationships with men, most groups saw nonassertiveness as pervasive. Women who were nonassertive with men also tended to be nonassertive with other women. Assertiveness Training was focused on more general areas than male-female interactions. Nurses, being predominantly women, found particular relevance in this movement and began to abandon the handmaiden role for more independent nursing practice.

After nearly 30 years of formation, Assertiveness Training continues to develop. No universally accepted set of procedures or philosophies exists that defines it. Conflicts exist as to whether assertiveness consists of techniques or lifestyle. Because of the broad boundaries, many individuals integrate viewpoints and individualize Assertiveness Training approaches.

ASSESSMENT OF CLIENTS FOR ASSERTIVENESS TRAINING

Although it may generally be stated that Assertiveness Training is likely a treatment of choice for nearly anyone with interpersonal conflicts and difficulties, it is necessary to distinguish carefully appropriate from inappropriate candidates (Cress, 1976). Clients who could potentially benefit from Assertiveness Training have the following nursing diagnoses:

- Impaired Verbal Communication
- Anxiety
- Knowledge Deficit of Assertion Skills
- Ineffectual Individual Coping
- Fear, Secondary to Assertion Deficits
- Social Isolation

Not all clients having these nursing diagnoses are necessarily appropriate candidates for Assertiveness Training, however. The screening process to determine appropriate candidates should therefore include assessment of the following:

1. Assertion deficits.
2. Verbal and nonverbal presentation.
3. Patient motivation.
4. Patient pathology.

Each of these will be explored briefly.

Assertion Deficits

In client assessment, it is important to keep in mind that no one acts assertively all of the time. Determining the need for Assertiveness Training becomes a matter of how often and under what circumstances the individual responds in a nonassertive or an aggressive manner (Cotler and Guerra, 1976). Several assertion assessment inventories have been developed to make this process more consistently precise as well as to assist with patient education and time management. Assessment scales an assertiveness trainer could select include the Wolpe-Lazarus Assertion Questionnaire (1966), the Lawrence Assertive Inventory (1970), the Constriction Scale (Bates and Zimmerman, 1971), the Conflict Resolution Inventory (Gambrill and Richey, 1972), the Behavioral Assertiveness Test (Eisler, Miller, and Heisen, 1973), the Alberti and Emmons Assertive Inventory (1974), Assertiveness Inventory and Uptight Inventory (Fensterheim and Baer, (1975), Assertion Self-Assessment Table (Galassi and Galassi, 1977), Assessment of Assertiveness (Clark, 1978), and Discrimination Test on Assertive, Aggressive, and Nonassertive Behavior (Jakubowski and Lange, 1978; Cotler and Guerra, 1976). In addition to these scales, several others exist that assess specific populations—for example, women, minority groups, the elderly, or nurses. Reviewing the chosen assertion scale with the client promotes further discussion and clarity of the problems at hand. During the discussion the trainer can use questions such as the following: "How do you usually act in this type of situation? How would you like to act? What prevents you from acting in the way you would like to in this situation? What type of emotional response does this situation elicit (anxiety, anger, guilt)?" These questions generate useful information for the trainer not only for assessment but for future treatment plans. This interaction with the client can also be used for initial trust and rapport building.

Verbal and Nonverbal Presentation

It is important to pay close attention to the verbal and nonverbal presentation of the client. There may be harmony or disparity between what a client is saying occurs and what he or she is doing.

During the interview does the client assert himself verbally by demonstrating open self-expression; use of "I" or "you" statements; giving or accepting of compliments; discussion of limitations in a neutral way; expression of goal-directed thoughts; spontaneous speech; use of a clear voice with speech of normal rate and volume; use of awareness, feeling, and want statements?

Does the client assert himself nonverbally by demonstrating calm behavior while being evaluated; good eye contact; good posture; affect appropriate to conversation; open body posture; use of gestures; interactions at appropriate spatial distances from others; good attention to interaction?

Patient Motivation

As Alberti and Emmons (1982) emphasize, Assertiveness Training is not a magic formula, script, or potion that will bring order out of the chaos. It is training that, it is hoped, will help an individual to maximize assertive skills and the capacity to choose for himself how he will act in a given situation. Changing coping behaviors, particularly long-term ones, is a difficult process that requires motivation and commitment. An Assertiveness Training program demands certain expectations of a client, and these should be made clear (i.e., long-term work, self-disclosure, role playing, homework, etc.). If the client is not sincerely interested in changing his behavior, perhaps just wanting to talk about his problem, he is not a good candidate for training.

Patient Pathology

Clients with severe anxiety, aggression or psychiatric problems should seek professional counseling. Assertiveness Training can sometimes be pursued after basic problems have been dealt with or at times concomitantly with therapy. As Assertiveness Training is primarily useful for essentially healthy individuals with interpersonal conflicts or assertion deficits, there is little literature relating Assertiveness Training to specific patient populations. Steinmark (1975) and Cress (1976) addressed this issue. Table 17–1 illustrates an Assertiveness Training guide to assist with selection of clients.

Table 17–1. ASSERTIVENESS TRAINING GUIDE

Disorder	Primary Intervention(s)	Assertiveness Training Goals	Comments
Adjustment Disorders	Counseling Medical management or medication Relaxation training Assertiveness Training	1. Needs to learn new skills to better cope with situation 2. Needs to learn assertive behaviors to reintegrate into social or role functioning	Type of adjustment disorder symptoms (i.e., depressed mood, anxious mood, conduct disturbance) influences intervention
Anxiety Disorders	Relaxation training Assertiveness Training Medical management or medication	1. Needs to learn or improve interpersonal skills 2. Needs to learn new skills to better cope	Assertiveness Training is not the treatment of choice for obsessive-compulsive or phobic types of anxiety disorders Generalized anxiety and panic disorders are more likely to respond to assertiveness and relaxation training
Affective Disorders	Counseling Medical management or medication	1. Needs to learn positive reinforcement through covert role rehearsal (guided imagery) and emphasis of individual rights and responsibilities 2. Structural program approach can increase physical activity and energy levels 3. Irrational thinking will be managed with use of cognitive therapy techniques 4. Needs to learn or improve interpersonal skills	Assertiveness Training appears to be helpful when used jointly with medical management or counseling, particularly with reactive depressions Bipolar disorders best respond to Assertiveness Training when medication has been effective in stabilizing moods Cyclothymic disorders appear to have good response to Assertiveness Training
Psychotic Disorders	Medical management or medication Supportive counseling	1. Requires assertive behaviors to reintegrate into society 2. Needs to learn new skills to better cope with condition	Appropriateness of Assertiveness Training depends on patient's level of wellness as well as the nature of patient's altered thinking and feeling processes
Personality Disorders	Assertiveness Training Counseling	1. Needs to learn appropriate expression of feelings, thoughts, or desires 2. Needs to learn new skills to better cope with condition	Assertiveness Training is often the treatment of choice for sexual deviations and inadequate, schizoid, and passive/aggressive personalities Assertiveness Training can be helpful in treating aggressive, antisocial behavior Insight and motivation must be thoroughly assessed, as hysterical and antisocial personalities often do not respond to Assertiveness Training Obsessive-compulsive, addictive, and explosive personalities likely benefit best from a combination of treatment modalities.

ASSERTIVENESS TRAINING TECHNIQUES

After appropriate candidates have been selected, the process of Assertiveness Training can begin. As previously mentioned, there is no general agreement as to the set of techniques composing Assertiveness Training. The process recommended by this author includes:

    1. Educating clients concerning the differences between passive, assertive, and aggressive behavior.

    2. Identifying barriers to assertive behavior and ways to reduce these barriers.

    3. Helping clients to recognize and reduce cognitive distortions that block assertion.

    4. Educating clients about assertion types and strategies.

1. Passive, Assertive, and Aggressive Behavior

In all interpersonal communications, people choose and differ among three basic behavioral styles: passive (or nonassertive), aggressive, and assertive. Passive and aggressive styles lie at opposite ends of the continuum, with assertive styles somewhere in the middle (Cotler and Guerra, 1976). It is often helpful for assertiveness trainers to clarify and compare each of these styles. The individual responding in inconsistent or exaggerated behaviors may not be adapting comfortably in interpersonal relationships. Freedom of choice and self-control are realized by developing assertiveness responses for situations that have previously produced nonassertive or aggressive behavior (Alberti and Emmons, 1982).

    As assertive behavior has previously been examined, we will now discuss passive and aggressive behaviors. Use of a specific case example, such as Lisa's, can be useful in client education. The client can identify particular situations of his own that he would like to explore in this manner.

Passive or Nonassertive Behavior

The nonassertive person tends to bottle up emotions, ranging from warmth to anger, because of high levels of anxiety, guilt, or social skill deficiencies. As a result, this individual may experience difficulty in satisfying needs; socializing comfortably (socially or at work); expressing feelings or thoughts, positive or negative, to friends, spouse, relatives, or acquaintances; or accepting a compliment without demeaning it. (Cotler and Guerra, 1976). The nonassertive person typically denies self and is inhibited from expressing actual feelings. People behaving nonassertively often feel hurt and anxious since they allow others to choose for them. Their own goals are seldom realized (Alberti and Emmons, 1981). Nonassertive behavior can hurt directly by causing the individual to lose self-respect. The continued nonassertion and acts of chronic self-apology decrease the sense of self-esteem and, in some individuals, can lead to a general sense of worthlessness and depression. The nonassertive behavior invites others to infringe upon and take advantage of the nonassertive individual (Jakubowski and Lange, 1978). The passive person is also called an avoidant personality type because he or she adopts a defensive stance of withdrawal and lack of action. Stressful situations are avoided by the very nature of his lifestyle (Cress, 1976). With this in mind, how would Lisa have acted nonassertively in her situation?

Nonassertive: Typically Lisa would never have attempted to return the blouse, but since her finances are low, she makes an attempt. She stares at the counter, accepts the credit voucher, and thanks the clerk for her service. Internally she feels agitated and deflated. As low as her bank account is, she really needs the cash. The credit voucher cannot be used practically in this expensive shop. Lisa is disappointed and feels badly about herself for not handling the situation more effectively. She is internally angry at the clerk who took charge.

Aggressive Behavior

For the most part, the aggressive person has little difficulty expressing negative feelings. Like the nonassertive person, he or she has an extremely difficult time expressing positive feelings. The aggressive individual has his needs met, but often at the expense of someone else's rights, feelings, dignity, or self-worth. Aggressive behavior can range from nitpicking or criticizing to screaming or physical attack. Some aggressive people develop a behavior pattern in which they vacillate between impassivity and impulsive outbursts of aggression. In this cyclic behavior, the individual withdraws and bottles things up inside. As intrapsychic tension builds, the person explodes at the slightest provocation, losing self-control and engaging in self-defeating behavior (Cress, 1976).

The aggressive individual is similar to the nonassertive counterpart in that he or she may experience concern over poor relationships with others and may be experiencing anxiety, guilt, or deficiencies in social skills. He or she may even be nonassertive in the situations in which he does hide feelings. The nonassertive person is frequently "victimized" by others and may tend to avoid others. The aggressive individual, conversely, is avoided by others who cannot predict or tolerate his behavior (Cotler and Guerra, 1976). If others do not directly confront the individual, he might not fully realize the extent to which he is aggressive. Continued aggression could cheat the individual of the joy of having others trust and value him enough to reveal themselves genuinely to him (Jakubowski and Lange, 1978). Again, the end result is the same as with the nonassertive individual in that the aggressive individual's behavior can leave him with few meaningful relationships (Cotler and Guerra, 1976). In addition, the aggressive behavior may also generate bitterness and frustration, which may later return as vengeance (Alberti and Emmons, 1982).

As noted previously, nonassertive and aggressive behaviors have similarities; they are both reactive instead of goal-directed, they both reflect underlying insecurity, they both represent indirect communication, and they both demonstrate a lack of taking personal responsibility for one's own actions and feelings (Clark, 1978). With this in mind, how would Lisa have acted aggressively in her situation?

Aggressive: Lisa pounds on the counter and in a loud voice berates the "insignificant, stupid, hired help." She creates a scene in which she humiliates the clerk and makes a fool out of herself. Even though she receives her refund she later feels embarrassed and vows never to return to the store. She wishes she had better self-control.

Passive aggression or nondirect aggression refers to indirect and subtle means of getting back at others, a passive resistance. This type of aggression includes sarcastic remarks, catty comments, and malicious gossip. Nonverbal aggressive behaviors include physical gestures performed while the person's attention is directed elsewhere, or physical acts directed toward other persons

242   LIFESTYLE ALTERATION

or objects (Galassi and Galassi, 1977). With this in mind, how would Lisa act in a passive or nondirect aggressive fashion?

> Passive Aggressive: Lisa accepts the credit voucher and inwardly feels like a failure because she has no better control of the situation. She is angry because the clerk "put her in this situation." She passively demonstrates this anger by taking a large armful of clothes she has no intention of purchasing into a fitting room and taking little care to return them to their hangers. Later she gossips with her friends about the poor service and undesirable clothing in this store.

2. Barriers to Assertive Behavior and Ways to Combat These Barriers

Clarification of aggressive, passive , and assertive behaviors further emphasizes the superior benefits of assertive behavior. The next logical step in Assertiveness Training therefore involves exploration of the barriers that make it difficult for the client to be assertive. Alberti and Emmons (1982, p. 2) noted three important barriers to self-assertion: (1) many people do not believe they have the right to be assertive; (2) many people are anxious or fearful about being assertive; (3) many people lack the social skills for effective self-expression. Each of these barriers will be explored further.

The Right to Be Assertive

Responsible assertive behavior is created from an awareness of personal rights and standing up for these rights (Cress, 1976). Keeping in mind that human rights vary somewhat in individuals, families, and cultures, several assertiveness trainers have defined universal human rights. The following list of rights combines those proposed by Smith (1975) and Jakubowski and Lange (1978). It is also important to emphasize that with these rights there are concomitant responsibilities (Smith, 1975; Steinmark, 1975).

I have the right:

1. to judge my own behavior, thoughts, and emotions and to take responsibility for their initiation and consequences upon myself.
2. to offer no reasons or excuses for justifying my behavior.
3. to judge if I am responsible for finding the solutions to other people's problems.
4. to change my mind.
5. to make mistakes and be responsible for them.
6. to say "I don't know."
7. to be independent of the good will of others before coping with them.
8. to be illogical in making decisions.
9. to say "I don't understand."
10. to say "I don't care."
11. to say "No" without feeling guilty.
12. to be treated with respect.
13. to ask for what I want.
14. to act in ways that promote my dignity and self-respect as long as others' rights are not violated in the process.
15. to express my feelings.
16. to slow down and think.
17. to feel good about myself.

I have the responsibility:

1. to allow others to be their own ultimate judge.

2. to allow others to do what they choose, without demanding reasons and excuses.
3. to allow others to express their own opinions.
4. to allow others to express their feelings.
5. to explain myself if I want to be understood.
6. to ask for or work for something that I want.
7. to obey laws, or to work to change them, or to accept the consequences of breaking them.
8. to grant others the same rights I want for myself.

There are many societal or Judeo-Christian norms that make it difficult for individuals to comfortably adopt these human rights identified by the Assertiveness Training movement (Cress, 1976). Jakubowski and Lange (1978) examined some of these messages.

We Should Put Others Before Ourselves. The implication of this norm is that we have no right to place our own needs above those of other people. Selfishness is not a recommended ideal, but neither is selflessness. Our own needs are as valuable as those of another person. If a conflict arises in which it appears that fulfilling one person's needs precludes filling those of another, a compromise is in order.

We Should Be Meek and Humble and Certainly Not Behave as Though We Were Better Than Anyone Else. This message implies that if we can do something better than someone else, then it would be better not to do it at all. If someone inadvertently engages in behavior that leads to outstanding accomplishment, he or she should put down all compliments that might be received. It is indeed undesirable to build oneself up at the direct expense of another; however, it is also true that all of us have the right to demonstrate our strengths and abilities. We also have the right to feel good about them.

We Should Be Understanding, Accepting, and Forgiving. The implication of this message is that we have no right to feel or express anger, which is a sign of weakness. One of the basic tenets of assertiveness theory is that a person has the right to experience the entire range of human feelings. It is important to express angry feelings appropriately when they occur, as they will otherwise build up internally and create inward disintegration or eventually explode externally. This does not promote being a picky complainer.

We Should Always Be Willing to Sacrifice and Help Others, but We Should Not Make Requests of Other People. It can be self-defeating to incessantly make demands and requests of other people. However, it is quite appropriate to make requests if they are helpful in meeting one's needs and they do not violate others' rights. When an individual's rights are being violated, he or she has the right to demand they be honored.

We Should Be Sensitive to Others' Feelings and Never Say or Do Anything that Might Hurt Someone Else's Feeling. The implication here is that we should not act spontaneously because we might hurt someone else. Hurting someone deliberately would entail a violation of his or her rights, but it is impossible to live without hurting someone at some time. Many people become hurt because they are overly sensitive, whereas others are hurt secondary to being manipulated. A person has the right to express thoughts and feelings despite the fact that someone might become hurt.

Identification of global rights, responsibilities, and conflicting norms is particularly helpful as an early Assertiveness Training strategy. This strategy allows clients to further individualize and clarify particular problem areas they may have in asserting themselves in interpersonal relationships with others or in individual self-concept. Ventilation of thoughts and feelings can be promoted, as well as defined problem solving. By clearly identifying personal rights and responsibilities, the client becomes aware of exactly what rights assertive behavior guards and reemphasizes that assertive behavior involves responsibilities toward others.

Anxiety or Fear of Assertion

Alberti and Emmons (1974) identify fear as perhaps the most significant obstacle to assertiveness. Even after individuals know how to express themselves, they may be uptight about doing so. The risks seem overwhelming. A modified list of risks or possible negative outcomes of Assertiveness Training as adopted from Clark (1978) includes the following:

1. Risking new behaviors that may challenge social norms or expectations.
2. Fear of losing familiar coping devices.
3. Fear of losing control.
4. In taking responsibility for own behaviors, others can't be blamed anymore.
5. Takes time, energy, and hard work.
6. Fear of learning the "truth" about self.
7. Does not guarantee you will get what you ask for even though you asked assertively.
8. May result in frustrations, anger, or impatience toward others or toward one's own passive or aggressive behavior.
9. Fear of being too aggressive.
10. For women, fear of being unfeminine.
11. Fear of being rejected, especially since some relationships may not tolerate change.
12. Fear of retaliation or revenge.
13. Fear of being punished by authority figures.

Discussing each of these outcomes with the client is the responsibility of the assertiveness trainer.

It is important to reiterate here that assertion is a choice. Alberti and Emmons state, "If you can act assertively, you are free to choose whether or not you will. If you are unable to act assertively, you have no choices; you will be governed by others, and your well-being will suffer" (1982, p. 123). There are some occasions when the individual's best interests are promoted by choosing not to be assertive. An example would be an interaction that takes place with someone whose good will is vital (e.g., a boss), and the incident does not infringe on the client's self-worth. Or a client may be in a situation in which he could respond assertively but he does not feel that he has the energy to do so effectively at the time. Assertion should be sensitive not only to the occasion but also to the ultimate outcome desired. This choice should obviously not be used as an excuse for indiscriminately avoiding assertive behavior.

In order to deal with fear and stress about assertiveness, it is necessary to determine what causes the reaction. Use of the foregoing list can be helpful in this determination. Alberti and Emmons (1982) recommend narrowing down exactly what stimulates fear or anxiety in the process of assertion. The use of a log to systematically record reactions can be valuable. The Subjective Units of Disturbance Scale (SUDS) developed by Lazarus and Fay (1975) is another helpful and commonly used scale to assess anxiety levels. Both of these tools will be discussed later in this chapter.

Another intervention to combat anxiety is Relaxation Training, which is discussed in Chapter 2. The techniques used for relaxation can be used to create a systematic desensitization, that is, an automatic association of relaxation instead of anxiety with a situation. It is impossible to be relaxed and anxious at the same time.

It is important to reiterate that one of the long-range benefits of Assertiveness Training is decreased anxiety secondary to improved communication skills, self-esteem, and interpersonal relationships. Stress management is a necessary intervention in helping the client make this transition.

Lack of Social Skills

Individuals who benefit from Assertiveness Training usually require some help in improving their social skills. In the social environment they find themselves to be anxious, tongue-tied, and at a loss for words (Smith, 1975). Some report being able to meet new people only under certain ritualistic circumstances, such as introduction by a mutual friend for two or three consecutive times, after having a few drinks, or being in a comfortable setting discussing noncontroversial issues (Cotler and Guerra, 1976). These ways of meeting people are better than none at all; however, the probability of having such requirements met on a regular basis is slim. People who require a set of conditions lack the ability to initiate enjoyable meetings and conversations (Cotler and Guerra, 1976). They often have deficient social networks. Social networks are social relationships in which the person feels secure, and in which other members know and accept him. Fensterheim and Baer (1975) place people with deficient social networks into five categories: the loner who lives in isolation; the person who has no social network but who does have relationships (often sporadic) with other people; the husband and wife or couple who exist in isolation from the rest of the world; the barricaded personality, who easily maintains superficial relationships but who cannot share intimate things; and the undifferentiated person who cannot maintain superficial relationships because of indiscriminate self-disclosure.

In a social sense, being assertive is communicating appropriately to another person about yourself, who you are, what you want from life. If the other person is assertive also, it is possible to discover whether the relationship has great or no potential for each party (Smith, 1975). Social worries that block communication include fear of appearing stupid, looking foolish, rejection, and closeness (Fensterheim and Baer, 1975). The following conversational skills, as defined by Cotler and Guerra (1976), are recommended as Assertiveness Training techniques to improve conversational skills and help combat these fears.

Open-Ended Questions. Open-ended questions are questions that cannot easily be answered by a monosyllabic reply. These questions usually ask who, what, when, where, how, and why. Use of how and why questions generally generates more conversation.

Attending to Free Information. Free information is unsolicited information given beyond the question being answered by another individual—e.g., "The weather is terrible, particularly since the climate was so beautiful on our vacation." Free information is helpful in maintaining ongoing, spontaneous conversation.

Self-Disclosure. Self-disclosure is free information that you give about yourself during the course of a conversation.

Changing Topics. Changing topics involves teaching people to have some control over the direction of the conversation by use of open-ended questions, free information, self-disclosure, or direct request.

Breaking into Ongoing Conversations. This technique involves assessing other individuals' nonverbal cues and utilizing timing in joining into an ongoing conversation with self-disclosure, opinion, free information, or whatever is appropriate.

Silences. Silences are normal parts of conversations. Clients need to be aware of this and learn to utilize the time to think or relax.

Telling Stories. Relating stories, experiences, or jokes indicates greater social comfort. It is important that these be relevant and have a beginning, middle, and end.

Nonverbal Cues. As discussed previously, nonverbal skills are as valuable to practice as verbal content skills. Space, smiling, animation, automation, and so on are all important components of a smooth-flowing conversation.

Terminating Conversations. Training clients how to terminate conversations helps them to avoid anxiety they feel about entering conversations in which they may later feel trapped or imposed upon. Examples of termination techniques include "canned" verbal responses ("It was good to talk to you"), change in verbal content, less self-disclosure, and fewer open-ended questions as well as nonverbal cues, such as increased body distance and decreased eye contact.

Clients trained in the group setting can practice these techniques with others in the group and receive immediate feedback. Those clients in individual training sessions can role play with the trainer and practice the techniques in real world settings for homework assignments. Social skills training is a valuable assertiveness technique in teaching the client to communicate appropriately with others.

3. Cognitive Therapy and Assertiveness Training

Cognitive therapy is a therapeutic approach used to help individuals assess their thinking and identify irrational beliefs and the resulting feelings and behaviors. Assertiveness requires that correct thinking be combined with assertive behavior. Many irrational ideas directly influence guilt feelings resulting from assertive behavior. Conversely, nonassertive behavior is frequently the outcome of irrational and incorrect thinking (Mishel, 1976). A basic introduction to cognitive therapy therefore is the next logical step in Assertiveness Training.

A primary cognitive technique involves recognition of automatic thoughts—i.e., the things you tell yourself. Beck (1976) identified four types of cognitive distortions that can be specified for the client.

1. Drawing a conclusion when evidence is lacking or contradictory.
2. Making unjustified generalizations on the basis of a single incident.
3. Exaggerating the meaning of an event.
4. Disregarding an important aspect of a situation, or not using information form previous experience.

Client and trainer try to identify types of irrational thinking as well as self-defeating thoughts. Continued use of cognitive assessment brings to awareness habitual, automatic cognitive processes (Beck, 1976).

Most individuals accept the validity of their cognitions without subjecting them to any type of critical evaluation. Patients are sometimes surprised to find they have been equating inference with reality. In cognitive therapy sessions, patients are told repeatedly that just because they think something is true does not necessarily mean that it is true. The patient is trained to evaluate cognitions continually to make distinction between thought and extended reality (Beck, 1976).

Rational emotive therapy is a cognitive therapy developed by Ellis (1962). Ellis suggests an A-B-C paradigm. Point A represents an activity, event, or situation that is upsetting to the individual. Point B represents the belief the individual attaches to the situation, rational or irrational. At point C the individual feels the results of the belief chosen at point B. For example, let's go back to Lisa's situation.

How would Lisa respond if she utilized rational thinking? A: Situation, returning purchase to store. B: Rational belief, if return challenged or denied, "This clerk is not honoring store policy." C: Rational consequences, "I'll talk to the manager about this, I feel that I'm in the right here."

How would Lisa respond if she utilized irrational thinking? A: Situation, returning purchase to store. B: Irrational belief, "Everybody thinks I'm stupid and a pushover." C: Irrational consequences, "I feel lousy about myself, it's depressing when everyone gives me a hard time."

Ellis extended the A-B-C theory to include points D and E. Point D represents trainer and client working to determine and dispute irrational beliefs connected with the unassertive behaviors. Point E represents client substitution of more rational ideas for the irrational beliefs.

To continue with the irrational B and C sequence above, at point D the trainer and Lisa would note Lisa's overgeneralized situational cues which cause the irrational belief that she is inadequate. At point E, Lisa would more rationally substitute the idea that perhaps the clerk's behavior was what should be in question. Lisa's positive behavior would be reinforced.

Use of cognitive therapy techniques in Assertiveness Training involves educating the client about these techniques and the continued practice of the techniques. Clients can benefit from the trainer's using the A-B-C approach with individual events, just as we have done with Lisa. Effective Assertiveness Training involves cognitive as well as behavioral interventions.

4. Assertion Types and Strategies

There are several different ways to act assertively. Knowledge of the various assertion forms enables the individual to select the most appropriate assertive response for his or her individual needs and goals in a given situation. Assertion strategies are utilized to facilitate the client's development and maintenance of assertion skills. Educating the client about these differing assertion types and strategies constitutes the final Assertiveness Training technique discussed in this chapter.

Assertion types are most accurately thought of as principles to help guide assertion instead of techniques to manipulate others (Jakubowski and Lange, 1978). The following list of assertion types is modified from the works of Cohen and McQuade (1983), Jakubowski and Lange (1978, p. 157), Smith (1975), and Steinmark (1975).

Basic Assertion. Basic assertion involves standing up for one's rights, beliefs, feelings, or opinions. Other social skills, such as persuasion, empathy, or confrontation, are not utilized. For example, the clerk continues to interrupt Lisa when she speaks. Lisa: "Excuse me, I'd like to complete what I'm saying." Or, the clerk states she will give Lisa 25 per cent more credit if Lisa accepts a voucher instead of cash. Lisa is unprepared and replies, "I'll have to take a few minutes to think that over."

"I" Language Assertion. Using the "I" when giving another individual feedback (positive or negative) demonstrates that the assertor is the "owner" of the thoughts and feelings that he is demonstrating. This shows that the assertor respects himself and anticipates respect from the other person. "I" language assertion consists of the following components:

1. Objectively describing the situation or other person's behavior that interferes with you. Be direct and specific.

2. Describing how this situation or behavior concretely affects your life (e.g., in terms of time, money, energy). Be honest.

3. Describing own feelings (use expressive verbs, such as "feel," "like," "want").

4. Concretely describing what you want the other person to do (e.g., explain, react, change behavior, apologize).

In applying Lisa's situation to "I" language assertion, Lisa might respond: "You are pressing me to take a credit voucher instead of giving me the cash refund allowed by store policy. I don't have enough cash in my checking account to comfortably accept a credit voucher. I also don't have the time to argue this point with you or feel I should need to. I feel angry that you are not honoring store policy and irritated that you are making this exchange unnecessarily difficult. I want a cash refund immediately."

Confrontive Assertion. Confrontive assertion is appropriate when discrepancies occur. Examples are when there is a difference between what someone tells you he did and what he actually did, or when there is a conflict between what your job description reads and what you are required to do at work. Confrontive assertion consists of three parts: (1) describing in an objective fashion what the other said would be done, (2) describing objectively what the other person actually did, and (3) concretely expressing what you want.

An example of Lisa's using confrontive assertion might be "It is the store's policy to provide a cash refund for merchandise returned within three days, as I have done. I see that you are writing out a credit voucher for the returned blouse. I prefer the cash refund." When using confrontive assertion it is important to point out the discrepancy rather than confront the person. Avoid jumping to conclusions and assuming bad motives. Often the problem lies with the original understanding, which may have been unclear, unrealistic, or interpreted differently by both parties.

Empathic Assertion. Often people want to do more than simply express their wants or feelings. At times they also wish to convey some sensitivity to the other person. This assertion type is called empathic assertion. It consists of making a statement of recognition of the other person's feelings or situation and is followed by another statement that stands up for the speaker's rights. In our case example, Lisa demonstrated empathic assertion. "I appreciate that it is probably frustrating when customers make frequent exchanges. I am, however, returning my purchase within the three day limit for cash refund and cash is what I prefer."

Repeated Assertion. This assertion involves calm repetition—saying what you want over and over again. It is also called the broken record technique. It is appropriate when the other person overreacts and ignores or discounts the assertor's thoughts, feeling, or desires. Repetition of the desired point can occur while still responding to legitimate points made by the other person. In our case example, Lisa could have demonstrated repeated assertion in the following way.

Clerk:	If there is nothing wrong with the blouse, we'll just give you a credit slip.
Lisa:	I am returning my purchase within the three day limit for cash refund and cash is what I prefer.

Clerk:	You can sign here for your credit voucher.
Lisa:	I prefer a cash refund for the returned blouse.
Clerk:	We'll have to call the manager if you're going to be so insistent.
Lisa:	I feel angry that you are not honoring store policy and irritated that you are making this exchange unnecessarily difficult. I want a cash refund.

Soft or Caring Assertions. Positive, caring feelings are often more difficult for individuals to express than basic or "standing up" assertions. Soft assertions include expression warm feelings for someone, verbally or nonverbally; giving and accepting compliments; giving and accepting feelings in general, including anger. Lisa might make statements to significant others such as "Good to see you," "Thank you," "I've been thinking about you," "I love you," "You're terrific," Her nonverbal soft assertions might be a smile, prolonged eye contact, touch, handshake, hug, or a homemade gift for someone.

Fogging. Fogging involves the assertor's acceptance of manipulative criticism by calmly agreeing with the critic that there may be some truth to his criticism. Nonetheless, the assertor remains the judge of what he or she does. The goal of this skill is to receive criticism comfortably without anxiety or defensiveness while giving no positive reinforcement to those using manipulative criticism. This passive assertiveness technique was advocated by Smith (1975) but disavowed by other assertiveness trainers, such as Lazarus (1971), Fensterheim and Baer (1975) and Cress (1976). An example of a way Lisa might have used fogging could be as follows:

| Clerk: | You students always buy things you can't afford and then return them. That's immature and inconsiderate. |
| Lisa: | I agree, it's immature and inconsiderate to buy things you can't afford and then return them. Still, I'd like my refund. |

Lisa's internal thoughts are that she has the right to change her mind and she refuses to be manipulated by the clerk's criticism.

Negative Assertion. Negative assertion is another passive assertion type. The assertor accepts his own errors and faults (without apology) by strongly and sympathetically agreeing with hostile or constructive criticism of his negative qualities. This is subtly different from fogging. The assertor using fogging avoids positively reinforcing the critic, whereas the negative assertor focuses on reducing the critic's anger or hostility. The fogger considers the critic's feedback to be manipulative and unacceptable. The negative assertor sees the critic's feedback as potentially, constructive, and worth listening to. A shared goal of both assertion types is to receive criticism without anxiety or defensiveness. In Lisa's situation, it is unlikely she would have accepted the clerk's feedback as other than manipulation. However, if she had, she would have agreed with the clerk that indeed she was immature and inconsiderate. She would let the clerk ventilate her anger, think about the feedback for future occasions, and continue to request a cash refund from the now less angry clerk.

Workable Compromise. It is practical at times to use verbal assertive skills to offer a workable compromise to the other person. An individual can always bargain for material goals unless the compromise affects his or her personal feelings for self-respect. There can be no compromise if the end goal involves a matter of self-worth. In Lisa's situation, if Lisa felt that a material goal was her end goal, she likely would accept the credit voucher with a 25% bonus for the returned blouse. Both she and the clerk would have compromised. If Lisa viewed the interaction in terms of self-worth ("You are not honoring my rights"), she would accept nothing less than her request for cash refund.

TRAINING STRATEGIES

There are several strategies that can be used to assist the client in his or her transition to assertive behavior. Those we will explore here include behavioral rehersal, SUDS scale, mirror exercises, audiotape and videotape replay, assertiveness log, role models, and peer support network.

Behavioral Rehearsal. This refers to the role playing of an experienced or anticipated situation in the individual's life that has created or is expected to create some difficulties. It is hoped that the client is able to acquire additional verbal and nonverbal skills by active role playing of those situations which he or she has avoided or fears. Anxiety levels will be reduced in the process of skill acquisition. Overt rehearsal involves having the client actively role play the situation with a coach or with a recipient for the assertor and a coach. Covert rehearsal involves having the clients mentally visualize (or imagine) scenes in which they respond assertively in situations that are usually anxiety provoking. Clients can imagine an assertive model instead of playing the role themselves if this is more comfortable initially (Cotler and Guerra, 1976; Kazdin, 1979).

SUDS Scale. The Subjective Units of Disturbance Scale (SUDS) is an anxiety self-assessment scale used by most assertiveness trainers. It simply involves the client's rating his or her own physical feelings of anxiety (pulse, muscle tension, perspiration, and so forth) on a scale of 0 to 100. Near 0 represents total relaxation, the way the body feels after a relaxation technique. Near 100 represents almost total anxiety, as a person might visualizing he or she would feel after being involved in a frightening situation, such as a plane crash or tornado. Having calibrated this comfort-discomfort continuum, the client can use it to evaluate how anxious he or she is in any given situation. Every 10 points on the scale represents a "just noticeable difference" in anxiety. Measuring anxiety can help identify life situations that are most troublesome. Once this is known, methods can be learned to eliminate the fear or anxiety. SUDS scores can also be used as positive indications of anxiety reduction when techniques are working successfully (Alberti and Emmons, 1982; Jakubowski and Lange, 1978).

Mirror Exercise. Observing nonverbal behavior (gestures, posture, facial expression) in a mirror can give the client an idea of how he is presenting himself. Practicing an assertive speech in front of the mirror can give the client necessary practice as well as feedback as to whether verbal and nonverbal communications are integrated. Use of the mirror is a good way for the client to get reacquainted with himself (Clark, 1978).

Audiotape Practice. Tape recorders can give helpful, instant feedback to the client about how he or she sounds—i.e., tonality, affect, volume, speed. Practice with the tape recorder can help the client to work with any noted problem areas, as well as to rehearse and get feedback on specific assertiveness exercises (Clark, 1978).

Videotape Replay. Videotape provides the truest representation of how the client represents himself or herself to others verbally and nonverbally.

Interchanges can be stopped for study of assertive aspects or replayed for feedback. Role models can be videotaped and used for training sessions as well (Clark, 1978).

Assertiveness Log. A log is used as a daily record of the client's progress. A daily record of assertiveness can help the client judge where he or she is now, the progress made over time, and problem areas to work on. Log entries include self-examination on situations (which people or situations are troublesome and which can be handled effectively); attitude (how the client feels about his or her right to behave assertively in the situation); behavior (verbal and nonverbal action and integration); and obstacles (barriers which seem to make assertion difficult—i.e., anxiety, lack of skills) (Alberti and Emmons, 1982).

Role Model Observation. Clients should find people in their work and social environment who they believe demonstrate the assertive behaviors they wish to learn. If it is possible, spending time with the role model is recommended. Assertive behavior can be learned by merely being with more assertive people. The client can also praise the role models for their assertion skills and enlist their support in learning to become more assertive. The client should attempt to emulate behaviors they observe and like (Clark, 1978).

Peer Support Network. The client should seek out peers who are also working on improving assertion skills. These peers can meet regularly to give each other support and feedback and to work toward specified goals (Clark, 1978).

IMPLICATIONS FOR NURSING PRACTICE

It is hoped this chapter has provided a basic foundation of assertiveness education. This author concurs with Alberti and Emmons (1982) that the assertive behavior facilitator and potential assertiveness trainers should have personal training before being allowed to practice. General qualifications considered to be a minimum requirement for professional facilitators in all settings and at all levels include the following:

1. Understanding of basic principles of learning and behavior.

2. Understanding of anxiety and its effects upon behavior.

3. Knowledge of limitations, contraindications, and potential dangers of Assertiveness Training.

4. Training as a facilitator under qualified supervision (Alberti and Emmons, 1982, p. 138). At present there exists no formal certification body for assertiveness trainers.

This does not indicate that the reader cannot begin to apply knowledge gained from this chapter personally or to clients. It does imply that the degree to which one incorporates Assertiveness Training into nursing practice must be guided by these recommendations in order to practice ethically.

Assertion skill and nursing outcome are intertwined. "The more assertive a nurse is, the better she can relate to and guide others, and the more she will respect herself and command the respect of others" (Cohen and McQuade, 1983, p. 417). Most nursing literature applies this belief to interactions of the following three types: nurse to patient, nurse to professional staff and physicians, and nurse to nurse. Each of these will be examined briefly.

Nurse to Patient. The current emphasis in nursing is wellness oriented.

This health care orientation requires nurses to actively involve clients in goal-directed activity in which competence and education are the focus. The myth that the nurse should meet all of the needs of all patients and be all things to everyone is no longer thought to be desirable. This health promotional model requires that nurses respect the rights of clients and teach them to respect nurses' rights (Clark, 1978). In addition, patients are often freer to voice their concerns more directly when nurses are more direct and sincere (Herman, 1978).

Obviously, those nurses performing Counseling or Psychotherapy have clients who could benefit from a formal Assertiveness Training program, as described in this chapter. Again, the nurse must be personally trained in assertion interventions to practice effectively in response to nursing diagnoses.

Nurse to Professional Staff and Physicians. Being treated as a professional peer includes presenting yourself as a confident, reasonable professional who can cooperate and collaborate with others (Clark, 1978). Nurses pursuing independent practice must be able to define and stand up for their rights. They must be able to set work priorities and goals and move toward them in consistent ways (Clark, 1978). Relationships between physicians and nurses are too often filled with conflict and competition instead of cooperation. At present 87 per cent of physicians are male and 97 per cent of nurses are female. With such statistics it is easy to see how power struggles between health occupations can often disintegrate into power struggles between men and women (Chenevert, 1983). Conversely, the continued increase in female physicians necessitates a change from sexually stereotyped communication patterns between physicians and nurses. This issue can further be confounded by traditional views of nurses as caring individuals who believe they must reduce tensions. Nurses limited by this belief, therefore, would not create any additional tension by reacting in an assertive manner to disagreements and conflict in health settings (Herman, 1978). Open, nonblaming, and goal-directed communication can, it is hoped, facilitate this relationship between nurses and fellow professionals. Client advocacy by nurses can be improved, consequently, as well as positive regard for the nurse. By respecting his or her own rights, the nurse will more easily be aware of patients and staff rights (Herman, 1978).

Nurse to Nurse. It is necessary for nurses to begin to define and accept each other's rights as nurses and as individuals. It appears that as nursing progress is made among the disciplines, the results are negated or set back by infighting or divisiveness within nursing ranks (Clark, 1978). McCloskey (1974) reported that interpersonal relationships are primarily correlated to job satisfaction for nurses and are more rewarding than salary. The more comfortable nurses become with assertion skills, the greater the chance that they will be able to communicate openly, confronting each other with ideals and issues. The alternative is scapegoating and angry outbursts, resulting in further divisions in nursing (Clark, 1978).

In summary, it is vital that nurses be knowledgeable of assertion skills. Assertive behavior in nursing practice can enhance competent interventions in response to nursing diagnoses; clear and effective communication with patients, other professionals, and fellow nurses; respect of nurses and the profession of nursing; and finally, self-respect and growth as individuals.

EDITORS' COMMENTS AND QUESTIONS

The consumer movement, the various patient's bills of rights, and the increased questioning of doctors and seeking of second opinions have all contributed to the increased consciousness about assertive behavior. Many nurses have learned Assertiveness Training for use in their own lives. The focus in this chapter is on helping the client with development of assertive behavior.

Questions for Discussion

1. *Can nurses teach clients to be assertive if they themselves are nonassertive?*

2. *How has the women's movement influenced this intervention?*

3. *Distinguish between aggressive and assertive behavior.*

4. *Does the patient have the right to choose to be passive?*

5. *Name factors in the hospital that influence passive, aggressive, and assertive behaviors.*

References

Alberti, R. E., and Emmons, M. L. *Your perfect right.* San Luis Obispo, Calif.: Impact Publishers, 1974.

Alberti, R. E., and Emmons, M. L. *Your perfect right* (4th ed.). San Luis Obispo, Calif.: Impact Publishers, 1982.

Bach, G., and Goldberg, H. *Creative aggression: The art of assertive living.* New York: Anchor Press/Doubleday, 1983.

Baldwin, B. A., and Goody Koontz, L. Out of the desk and onto the stage: An experiment in assertive role playing. *Journal of Nursing Education,* 1979, *18*(7), 38–42.

Bandura, A. *Principles of behavior modification.* New York: Holt, Rinehart & Winston, 1969.

Bates, H. D., and Zimmerman, S. F. Toward the development of a screening scale for Assertive Training. *Psychological Reports,* 1971, *28*, 99–107.

Beck, A. T. *Cognitive therapy and the emotional disorders.* New York: International Universities Press, 1976.

Berne, E. *Games people play.* New York: Grove Press, 1964.

Bloom, L., Coburn, K., and Pearlman, J. *The new assertive women.* New York: Delacorte Press, 1975.

Brown, S. D., and Brown, L. W. Trends in assertion training research and practice: A content analysis of the published literature. *Journal of Clinical Psychology.* 1980, *36*(1), 265–269.

Chenevert, M. *STAT, special techniques in assertiveness training.* St. Louis: C. V. Mosby Company, 1983.

Clark, C. C. *Assertive skills for nurses.* Rockville, Md.: Aspen Systems, 1978.

Cohen, S., and McQuade, K. Assertiveness in nursing. Part I. *American Journal of Nursing,* 1983, *83*(3), 417–434.

Cohen, S., and McQuade, K. Assertiveness in nursing. Part II. *American Journal of Nursing,* 1983, *83*(4), 911–928.

Cotler, S. B., and Guerra, J. J. *Assertive training, a humanistic-behavioral guide to self-dignity.* Champaign, Ill.: Research Press, 1976.

Cress, J. N. *An introduction to assertion training: Objectives, procedures, and clinical applications.* Paper presented at the Behavior Therapy Seminar, Reykjavik, Iceland, September 27–28, 1976.

Donnelly, G. F. Assertiveness: Freeing the nurse to practice. *Topics In Clinical Nursing,* 1979, *1*(1), 67–75.

Ellis, A. *Reason and emotion in psychotherapy.* New York: Lyle Stuart, 1962.

Ellis, A., and Harper R. A. *A guide to rational living.* North Hollywood, Calif.: Wilshire Book Company, 1975.

Eisler, R. M., Miller, P. M., and Hessen, M. Components of assertive behavior. *Journal of Clinical Psychology*, 1973, *29*, 295–299.

Fensterheim, H., Baer, J. *Don't say yes when you want to say no.* New York: Dell Publishing Company, 1975.

Galassi, M. D., and Galassi, J. P. *Assert yourself! How to be your own person.* New York: Human Sciences Press, 1977.

Gambrill, E. D., and Richey, C. A. In assertion inventory for use in assessment and research. *Behavior Therapy*, 1975, *6*, 550–561.

Hayman, P. M., and Cope C. S. Effects of assertion training on depression. *Journal of Clinical Psychology*, 1980, *36*(2), 534–543.

Herman, S. J. *Recoming Assertive: A guide for nurses.* New York: D. Van Nostrand Company, 1978.

Jakubowski-Spector, P. Facilitating the growth of women through assertive training. *Counseling Psychologist*, 1973, *4*(1), 75–86.

Jakubowski, P., and Lange, A. J. *The assertive option, your rights and responsibilities.* Champaign, Ill.: Research Press Company, 1978.

Jampolsky, G. G. *Love is letting go of fear.* Toronto: Bantam Books, 1979.

Jette, N., and Logan, B. *Assertive training through movement.* Springfield, Ill.: Charles C Thomas, 1981.

Kazdin, A. E. Imagery elaboration and self-efficacy in the covert modeling treatment of unassertive behavior. *Journal of Consulting and Clinical Psychology*, 1979, *47*(4), 725–733.

Kelly, G. A. *The psychology of personal constructs.* New York: Norton, 1955.

Lange, A. J., and Jakubowski, P. *Responsible assertive behavior: Cognitive/behavioral procedures for trainers.* Champaign, Ill.: Research Press, 1976.

Lawrence, P. S. The assessment and modification of assertive behavior. Doctoral dissertation, Arizona State University, 1970. *Dissertation Abstracts International*, 31, 1B-1601B and University Microfilms No. 70-11, 888.

Lazarus, A. A. *Behavior therapy and beyond.* New York: McGraw-Hill Book Company, 1971.

Lazarus, A., and Fay, A. *I can if I want to.* New York: Warner Books, 1975.

McCloskey, J. Influence of rewards and incentives on staff nurse turnover rate. *Nursing Research*, *23*, 1974, 239–247.

Mishel, M. H. *Assertion training techniques for nurses.* Los Angeles, Calif.: California State University Press, 1976.

Moreno, J. L. *Psychodrama* (Vol. I). New York: Beacon House, 1946.

Osborn, S. M., and Harris, G. G. *Assertive training for women.* Springfield, Ill.: Charles C Thomas, 1975.

Phelps, S., and Austin, N. *The assertive women.* Fredericksburg, Va.: Impact Publishers, 1975.

Rathus, S. A 30 item schedule for assessing assertive behavior. *Behavioral Therapy*, 1973, 4, 398–406.

Rimm, D. C., and Masters, J. C. *Behavior therapy: Techniques and empirical findings.* New York: Academic Press, 1974.

Rogers, C. R. *On becoming a person.* Boston: Houghton Mifflin Company, 1961.

Salter, A. *Contitioned reflex therapy.* New York: Farrar, Straus, 1949.

Smith, M. J. *When I say no, I feel guilty.* New York: Bantam Books, 1975.

Steinmark, S. W. *Assertive behavior training: a preliminary manual for the helping professions.* Iowa City, Ia.: The University of Iowa Clinical Psychology Service and Group Psychotherapy Clinic, 1975.

Whiteley, J. M., and Flowers, J. U. *Approaches to assertion training.* Monterey, Calif.: Brooks/Cole Publishing Company, 1978.

Wolpe, J., and Lazarus, A. A. *Behavior therapy techniques: A guide to the treatment of neuroses.* Oxford: Pergamon, 1966.

ACUTE CARE MANAGEMENT

Overview: The Challenge of Nursing in the Acute Care Setting

GLORIA M. BULECHEK
JOANNE C. McCLOSKEY

Most acute care occurs in hospitals, and hospitals are where most nurses work. In the past few decades hospitals have undergone some dramatic changes: more technology, an increased number of intensive care units, reorganization with more short-term beds, increased use of outpatient clinics and emergency rooms, a shift in payment mechanisms with more health care costs now assumed by the federal government, an influx of new workers, and an increase in specialization. Patients in hospitals are sicker than before and the care they require is more complex and intensive. To hold down escalating costs, today's patients are discharged quickly. In such an atmosphere, the challenge to deliver quality nursing care is greater than ever.

Although the interventions included in other sections are often used by nurses working in hospitals and other acute care settings, the interventions listed and described in this section are *essential* for competent care in the acute setting.

The first intervention discussed in this section has a strong research base, although none of the research was conducted earlier than 1970. Preparatory Sensory Information (Chapter 18), is a "description of the typical sensory experiences a patient may expect to have during a potentially threatening health care event." This intervention is uniquely nursing in that all of the studies have been done by nurses, notably by Johnson and her colleagues. In

255

their chapter, Christman and Kirchhoff carefully and fully described all of the studies and then delineate four areas for further research. They conclude, "the beneficial effects of Sensory Information have been replicated in a wide variety of clinical settings and patient groups and with different types of threatening events." Although the exact mechanism for its effectiveness is unclear, Preparatory Sensory Information in a short-term diagnostic situation (e.g., nasogastric tube insertion, barium enema, cast removal) reduces the emotional responses to the threatening procedure. In a long-term situation (surgery has been the one tested) Preparatory Sensory Information promotes the patient's ability to use existing coping behaviors.

Christman and Kirchhoff identify three potential diagnoses that might call for the intervention of Preparatory Sensory Information: Potential Anxiety or Fear, Potential Ineffective Individual Coping, and Potential Powerlessness. They point out that the intervention is *not* appropriate for the diagnosis of Knowledge Deficit, for its purpose is not to teach. Preparatory Sensory Information has, however, been used in combination with Preoperative Teaching and with Discharge Planning (see next section) with successful results.

Unlike some other interventions, Preparatory Sensory Information has low risk for the patient and takes little time of the nurse and is easy to do. Based on a sound research base, it should be an intervention that all nurses in acute care settings should know about.

Crisis Intervention (Chapter 19) is frequently required in emergency rooms and psychiatric units but should be applied in any setting where there are individuals in crisis. As Kus points out in his chapter, crises are normal events for all people. Thus, Crisis Intervention is a psychosocial, not a psychiatric, intervention. In Crisis Intervention, the nurse assists the client through the steps of problem solving. The goal is to achieve at least the same level of psychological comfort as experienced before the crisis. The process, however, of marshalling their support systems enables many clients to be able to cope *more* effectively. Thus the intervention is a form of preventive mental health.

As Kus points out, Crisis Intervention is not a 9-to-5 activity, and people in crisis need immediate attention. A nurse who implements this intervention has to be flexible and has to work in a system that provides for unpredictable and irregular time periods. Kus's case study of a gay alcoholic client in crisis demonstrates that a nurse implementing Crisis Intervention needs good understanding of how to do the intervention but also needs to have good knowledge of the crisis situation. Sometimes, as in the case study, the nurse must educate others about the situation. A reading of Kus's chapter will help all nurses who work with clients in crisis.

Acute care patients often require surgery, and nurses have long been helping patients recover from surgery by doing Preoperative Teaching. In Chapter 20, Felton defines Preoperative Teaching as "the gamut of supportive-educational actions the nurse engages in to assist surgical patients to act responsibly in their own interests before and after surgery." Using Seligman's theory of learned helplessness, Felton explains how Preoperative Teaching helps the patient to maintain control in a threatening situation.

While research on Preoperative Teaching is extensive, there is, says Felton, no clear identification of what aspects of the intervention are responsible for the effects. Nor is there a singular pattern that emerges for implementation. In the future, Felton maintains that nurses should concentrate their efforts on evaluation of the intervention. Preoperative Teaching programs should be evaluated for their patient outcomes (e.g., improved ventilatory function, decreased length of stay, decreased frequency of complication) and their effects on the staff and the organization. Felton points out that little is accomplished with ad hoc unstructured preoperative teaching. She says that Preoperative Teaching needs to be structured for particular patient populations and needs to be supported by nursing administration. Using the example of planning a Preoperative Teaching program for ostomy patients, Felton demonstrates how the nurse should first spell out expected patient outcomes. These are derived from the current research base and dictate the content of the intervention. An evaluation tool constructed before teaching begins ensures that there will be postoperative follow-up and evaluation. With such systematic implementation, the intervention of Preoperative Teaching can benefit large numbers of patients and demonstrate to others the value of nursing care.

The last two interventions in this section, Surveillance (Chapter 21) and Presence (Chapter 22), have long been practiced by nurses but have little or no research base. While nurses do the interventions they have little understanding of them as interventions. The last two chapters open up important new areas of study for nurses and articulate important aspects of the nurse's role that have previously been assumed but not described.

The intervention of Surveillance is practiced by critical care nurses in life-threatening situations. Dougherty and Molen define Surveillance as "the application of behavioral and cognitive processes in the systematic collection of information used to make judgments and predictions about a person's life status." The purpose of Surveillance is no less than to save the person's life. Thus, it is an appropriate intervention for the nursing diagnoses of Ineffective Breathing Patterns, Decreased Cardiac Output, and Potential for Injury. Surveillance encompasses observation but is much more. Drawing on literature from the field of espionage, Dougherty and Molen point out that a nurse using Surveillance must know when to look, what to look for, and why to look. Surveillance requires a data collection tool that lists the types of information to observe and the frequency of the observations. Surveillance is intensive assessment, but it is not to be confused with the initial assessment all nurses do in order to arrive at a nursing diagnosis. Surveillance is a focused, detailed assessment done after a diagnosis is made, with the data continually evaluated in order to prevent the patient's death. The rich case study of the critically ill patient with the nursing diagnosis of Decreased Cardiac Output demonstrates well the importance of this intervention and the skills necessary for the nurse to implement it.

The presence of the nurse as central to a patient's recovery has long been understood (at least by nurses), but Presence, as a conceptualized, described, and tested intervention, is missing from the nursing literature. While several nursing theorists, most notably Patterson and Zderad, have included the presence of the nurse as a key aspect of successful therapy, little has been done to describe this important intervention.

Presence, as delineated by Gardner, has two aspects: the physical ("being there") and the psychological ("being with"). The nurse uses herself as the intervention through such techniques as listening, reassurance, and communication. In her chapter, Gardner describes how Presence is closely aligned with such related concepts as empathy, support, physical closeness, and caring. The fact that Gardner is not clear on whether these concepts are the same or different, or merely parts of the intervention Presence, is due to the scarcity of literature in the area. Through two case studies, both involving patients with Fear and Anxiety, Gardner demonstrates the value of this important nursing intervention.

While all five interventions listed in this section are important for the nurse who works in an acute care setting, they will not be effective unless the setting supports their use. The implication for many settings is a system change. Hospitals and other acute care settings need to be supportive of nursing interventions. Unless the system allows time for Preoperative Teaching and Crisis Intervention, the nurse cannot do these interventions; unless the system provides the equipment and personnel to monitor the acutely ill patient, the nurse cannot implement Surveillance; unless the system recognizes the importance of preparing patients for threatening events and having the nurse stay with threatened patients, Preparatory Sensory Information and Presence will not be done.

Thus, nurses must demonstrate the effectiveness of these interventions in order to win needed system changes. The ability to deliver quality nursing care in the acute care setting depends on them.

18

PREPARATORY SENSORY INFORMATION

NORMA J. CHRISTMAN
KARIN T. KIRCHHOFF

Preparing patients for threatening or stressful health care events has long been a traditional part of nursing practice. Generally, patients have been given information that nurses thought would be useful. Intuition suggested that such information would be beneficial in reducing the patient's stress during or following a health care procedure. Most often such preparatory information included description of the sequence of events or activities to which the patient would be subjected and, in some instances, behaviors that the patient would be expected to perform. Nursing textbooks are replete with examples where it is suggested that patients would benefit from receiving such preparation. Yet, the textbooks provide little evidence of clear delineation of the goal to be achieved by giving such preparatory information beyond that of decreasing the patient's experienced stress. Without a clearly delineated goal, the outcome criteria to use in evaluating the effectiveness of the intervention are also not explicit.

When preparatory information is grounded in intuitive knowledge, little guidance is provided to the practitioner for making clinical decisions involving (1) selection of patients who would benefit from the information; (2) the goal to be achieved by providing the information; and (3) the criteria that indicate a positive patient response to the information. Intuitive knowledge rarely gives rise to questions such as the following: Why is preparatory information helpful? What particular types of information are helpful? Are some types of information more helpful than others? These questions arise from the quest for scientific knowledge, which is gained through the research process.

An example of asking questions about the specific effects of differing types of information on patient responses and the knowledge generated thereby is evident in the research of the effects of Preparatory Sensory Information. Johnson and her colleagues have been involved in this research over a period of nearly 15 years. Their work has also led others to work in this area. Thus, this chapter focuses on discussion of sensory information; its nature—what it is and what it is not; its scientific basis; tests of its effects in varying health care situations; and guidelines for its use in clinical practice.

SENSORY INFORMATION: WHAT IT IS; WHAT IT IS NOT

Judgments about and responses to an event are based on information acquired from the environment through our senses. Schema, or mental images of past experiences, are used to interpret new experiences and guide responses (Neisser, 1976). When sensory input does not fit an existing schema or no schema is available to aid in interpreting the newly acquired sensory input, accurate judgments about the event, and responses to it, may be inappropriate or slowed. Sensory Information assists patients to form a schema of the experience by describing the typical sensory input to be anticipated during the event; it describes what will be felt, heard, seen, tasted, and smelled during the experience (McHugh, Christman, and Johnson, 1982). Then, while undergoing the procedure, the patients can use the schema to interpret their experiences and to guide their behavior.

Sensory Information describes both the subjective and objective experiences associated with the health care event (McHugh et al., 1982). Subjective experiences are those known only to the experiencing person, the typical physical sensations. These sensations are described in objective terms; evaluative or qualitative adjectives are not attached to the descriptors of the sensations. With any sensation or experience, one person may label it "very intense" or "terrible," while another may label it as "mild" or "not so bad." The cause of the sensation and its timing, or temporal features, are also described. For example, Sensory Information for a surgical patient would include not only sensations associated with the surgical incision but also the changes in these sensations that occur with movement and the changes in the sensations as the incision heals.

By definition, the objective experiences that are described as part of Sensory Information are those aspects of the experience that can be observed and verified by someone other than the experiencing person (McHugh et al., 1982). These aspects of the experience include the timing of events associated with the procedure as well as the spatial characteristics of the environment in which the procedure takes place. Again using the experience of surgery as an example, description of the objective experiences might include information about the anesthesiologist's visit and when it will occur, the preoperative skin preparation and when it will be done, waiting in the operating suite hallway before entering the operating room, and waking up in the recovery room. In other instances, preoperative Sensory Information might include description of the timing of transfer to a preoperative holding area. It can be seen, therefore, that the exact content of the objective aspects of the experience will vary with the specific practices and policies of the institution in which the health care event takes place.

Other features of Sensory Information should be noted. First, omitting some of the physical sensations will not negate the beneficial effects of the information. Partial sensory description has been found to be as effective as a full sensory description (Johnson and Rice, 1974). Second, the effects of providing Sensory Information are not a function of the power of suggestion.

Subjects given false Sensory Information did not report experiencing those sensations (Johnson and Rice, 1974), and cholecystectomy patients who were given sensory information as well as those who were not reported experiencing similar sensations (McHugh et al., 1982).

Finally, it is reemphasized that only the *typical* sensory experiences are included as part of the preparatory information. Descriptions of the typical subjective sensory experiences must be obtained from interviews with patients who have undergone the procedure. Only those sensations reported as experienced by at least 50% of the patients interviewed are included in preparatory information for future patients (McHugh et al., 1982).

EFFECTS OF SENSORY INFORMATION: EMPIRICAL EVIDENCE

The effects of providing Sensory Information were studied initially in an experimental laboratory and then in a wide variety of clinical situations. In some of the early studies, the effects of the subjective aspects of sensory information were tested against the effects of the objective aspects. In other words, the experimental messages tested were composed of either the typical physical sensations or the objective procedural aspects of the threatening event. In discussion of the research, the term "sensation" is used to denote strictly the typical physical sensation, whereas "sensory information" is used to denote both the physical sensations and the objective aspects of the experience.

In the first study, Johnson (1973) proposed that the degree of distress associated with painful stimuli was related to the congruency between expected and experienced physical sensations. More specifically, it was predicted that accurate expectations would be related to lower levels of distress. Normal, healthy subjects were exposed to ischemic pain induced by the application of a blood pressure cuff. Prior to experiencing the induced ischemic pain, one half of the subjects were given information about the sensations that would accompany the painful experience; the other half received information about the procedure used to induce the pain. The congruency hypothesis was supported. Subjects given sensation information reported less distress during the painful experience than did subjects not so prepared.

In a second laboratory experiment using ischemic pain as the aversive stimulus, Johnson and Rice (1974) examined the effects of full sensation description, partial sensation description, false sensation description, and procedural information. Subjects prepared with either full or partial sensation description reported less distress during the painful experience than did subjects given either false or procedural information. Because subjects given either full or partial sensation information responded similarly, the congruency hypothesis as the explanation for the effects of the information was questioned. Expectation of atypical sensations led to higher levels of emotional response than the varying degrees of accuracy in expectations. Even though the results of this study cause one to question the theoretical explanation for the effects of sensation information, its pragmatic value is clear. As indicated earlier, omission of some sensations should not decrease the effectiveness of the information. In clinical practice it is reasonable to expect situations to occur in which not all of the sensations a specific patient might experience can be described. These findings should also ease the practitioner's concern about inadvertently omitting one or more of the sensations even in situations in which all of them can be described.

Clinical investigations of the effects of sensory information may be divided into two categories, short-term and long-term threatening experiences. The short-term experiences include a wide variety of diagnostic and therapeutic procedures. Undergoing a surgical procedure has been the major long-term threat experience used for the study of sensory information.

Short-Term Threat Experiences

Gastroendoscopic examination was the first clinical procedure used to study the effects of sensory information. Johnson, Morrissey, and Leventhal (1973) provided patients who had had no more than two previous gastroendoscopic examinations one of two types of preparatory information, description of the physical sensation or description of the procedure. A third group of patients received no experimental information. Measures of fear and distress were obtained as the patients underwent the procedure. These measures included (1) amount of diazepam (Valium) taken, (2) heart rate changes, (3) hand and arm movements, (4) gagging during the tube insertion, and (5) restlessness during the first 15 minutes of the procedure. Patients who received either type of experimental information required significantly less diazepam than patients who received no information. Patients in the sensation-informed group evidenced less tension during the procedure by displaying significantly fewer hand and arm movements during tube insertion than did patients in either of the other two groups. Sensation-informed patients were also found to be less restless during the procedure than patients given procedural information, even though both groups required comparable amounts of diazepam. Although the results were not statistically significant, uninformed patients—who received about 6 mg more diazepam than the sensation-informed patients—evidenced more restlessness than the sensation-informed patients. There were no significant differences among the groups for changes in heart rate, although the sensation-informed group evidenced the least heart rate acceleration.

A second study, with patients who were undergoing gastroendoscopic examination for the first time (Johnson and Leventhal, 1974), supports the benefit of the two components of sensory information. The subjective sensation information was combined with the objective procedural information and tested against (1) instruction in behaviors that would ease insertion of the tube and (2) no information or instruction. The findings indicated that for patients under 50 years of age, those who were given sensory information required less diazepam than those who received no information or instruction. There were no significant effects for patients over 50 years of age. As in the previous study, sensory-informed patients tended to evidence fewer heart rate changes, but there were no significant differences between the groups. Patients who received either sensory information or a combination of sensory information and instruction in behaviors experienced significantly less gagging than those in the control group. Those who received instruction alone also experienced less gagging than those not informed or instructed (control group), but the difference was not statistically significant. It was concluded, therefore, that sensory information contributed more to this effect than did behavioral instruction.

One difference in these two studies should be noted. The first provided a test of informing patients of the sensations, the subjective aspects of the experience, versus the objective or procedural aspects of the experience. The second study combined the subjective and objective experiences that were tested against instruction in coping behaviors to use during the event. These differences may be responsible for some of the variations in the findings of the two studies.

The effects of sensory information have also been studied in another situation clinically similar to gastroendoscopy, the experience of undergoing nasogastric tube insertion for gastric analysis (Padilla et al., 1981). In this complex study, 90 per cent of the patients had previously had a tube passed. Filmstrips were used to inform patients of the following: (1) procedure (P); (2) procedure and sensations (PS); (3) procedure and behaviors to decrease discomfort during and after intubation (PB); or (4) a combination of procedure, sensations, and behaviors (PSB). Patients were also classified as to their preference for control (C) or for no control (NC). Measures of patient responses included self-reports of pain, discomfort, and anxiety.

Overall, the combination of procedural and sensation information and instruction in behaviors was most effective in decreasing discomfort both during and after intubation. Procedural information alone was not found effective in alleviating discomfort. Procedural plus sensation information increased discomfort for NC patients but decreased discomfort during and after the procedure in C patients. Procedural information plus behaviors decreased discomfort during the procedure for C and NC patients. The combination of all three types of information (PSB) decreased discomfort both during and after intubation in both C and NC patients. For NC patients who received PS, anxiety during intubation was increased, yet postintubation anxiety was decreased for both C and NC patients who received PS. For those C patients receiving PB, anxiety increased during intubation, then decreased post intubation. A similar pattern was reported for NC patients. Anxiety was also found to decrease both during and after intubation in NC patients given PSB.

Although further study is needed, these findings suggest that preference for control may modify responses to sensory information. Even though sensation information increased the indicators of distress in some patients during the intubation, postintubation distress decreased. These findings further suggest that, in some instances, giving instruction in coping behaviors to employ during a stressful experience in combination with sensory information may facilitate the patient's positive response. This additive effect was also evident in the second gastroendoscopic study (Johnson and Leventhal, 1974), in which patients given sensory information and behavioral instructions experienced less gagging during tube insertion.

The common stressful experience of undergoing pelvic examination has also been used to study the effects of sensory information (Fuller, Endress, and Johnson, 1978). Women, all of whom reported having undergone previous pelvic examination, were given (1) sensory information; (2) health education information; (3) sensory information and instruction in a relaxation technique to use during the examination; or (4) health education information and relaxation instruction. Both behavioral and physiological measures of distress during the examination were obtained. Women who received sensory information displayed fewer distress behaviors and less increase in pulse rate from before to during examination than those who received the general but relevant health education information. Instruction in the relaxation technique produced no significant effects. Thus, sensory information may benefit patients who have had previous experience with the health care event.

Two investigations have focused on the event of undergoing a barium enema in studying the effects of sensation information. In the first study, Hartfield and Cason (1981) gave patients who had never before had a barium enema (1) sensation information; (2) procedural information; or (3) no information. While controlling for predisposition to anxiety, these investigators found that patients given sensation information reported significantly less anxiety following the x-ray procedure than patients given procedural information. Yet the anxiety level of patients given sensation information was not significantly different from that found in patients given no information.

In the second study using barium enema as the stressful event, Hartfield, Cason, and Cason (1982) gave either sensation information or procedural information to patients who had never before had a barium enema. Again controlling for predisposition to anxiety, sensation-informed patients reported less anxiety following the examination than did procedure-informed patients. There was no control or uninformed group in this study; therefore, the results of the two studies are not directly comparable. These two studies also raise the question of how the findings might have differed had the two components of sensory information been combined and tested against the separate components as well as against a control group. Separating the two components in most situations would prevent relating the sensations to their cause and could influence accurate description of their temporal qualities. Such a situation may have occurred in the barium enema studies, for the particular sensations should make more sense to the experiencing person when related to the aspect of the event creating the sensation. Complexity of the event may also be a crucial factor. In the less complex situation—for example, induced ischemic pain—the source of the sensation is readily apparent. In more complex clinical situations, especially those never before experienced, identification of the exact stimulus producing the sensation as well as the ability to judge its normalcy may be impeded or nonexistent.

All of the studies discussed thus far have involved the effects of the information on adults experiencing threatening health care events. There is one study in which the effects of sensation information were tested with children who were undergoing cast removal following on orthopedic injury and who had not had a cast removed within the previous three months (Johnson, Kirchhoff, and Endress, 1975).

Children of ages 6 through 11 years were given (1) sensation information, (2) information describing the procedure, or (3) no information. Both pre–cast removal fear and information were found to affect the indicators of distress during cast removal. Children who indicated they had no fear before cast removal were found to have lower distress than children who reported at least some fear. Children given sensation information experienced significantly less distress than those given no information, whereas the distress level of those given procedural information fell between that of the other two groups. Pulse rate increases from before the procedure to 15 to 30 seconds into the procedure were also found to differ significantly in the three groups. Children in both the no information and procedural information groups experienced significant increases in pulse rate, whereas those who received sensation information did not. Although children reported sensation information to be more frightening than the procedural information, this difference was not significant. Thus, sensation information has been found to decrease emotional responses to threatening experiences in groups of patients of a wide age range.

To summarize, in these short-term threatening events, description of the subjective sensations alone as well as when combined with the objective aspects of the event has been found to reduce the subjects' emotional response during or immediately following the event. Lessened emotional response seemed to enable patients to be more cooperative during the event. Indicators of emotional response have included self-reports and behavioral and physiological measures. In some instances combining sensation information with the objective procedural information and instruction in behaviors to decrease the distress was more effective than either sensation or sensory information alone (Johnson and Leventhal, 1974; Padilla et al., 1981). Yet, in another situation, pelvic examination (Fuller et al., 1978), instruction in a coping behavior did not enhance the effects of the combined components of sensory information.

Even though the exact mechanism by which sensory information produces beneficial effects is unclear, it has consistently reduced patients' emotional responses in a wide variety of short-term threatening health care events. A possible explanation for the conflicting results obtained when combining sensory information with instruction in a coping behavior will become more evident following discussion of the effects of sensory information in long-term threat situations.

Long-Term Threat Experiences

The experience of having surgery is the major long-term threat used to study sensory information. The majority of these studies have investigated patients who were undergoing elective abdominal surgery and have tested the effects of sensory information alone and combined with other interventions.

In the first surgical study, Johnson, Rice, Fuller, and Endress (1978b) tested the effects of sensory information against instruction in a coping behavior with patients who were hospitalized for a cholecystectomy. Patients were randomly assigned to one of six experimental conditions: (1) information about the usual events involved in having a surgical procedure (procedural); (2) description of the typical sensations and the usual events (sensory); (3) instruction in deep breathing, coughing, leg exercises, turning, and ambulating (instruction); (4) procedural information combined with instruction; (5) sensory information combined with instruction; or (6) no information or instruction. Indicators of postoperative recovery served as measures of the effects of the interventions and included (1) self-reports of postoperative pain, (2) doses of parenteral analgesics, (3) amount of ambulation, (4) mood states, (5) length of postoperative hospitalization, and (6) length of time from discharge to first time venturing out of home.

Patients who received instruction in coping behaviors to aid recovery tended to receive fewer doses of analgesics and ambulate more frequently. For patients who reported low preoperative fear, neither information nor instruction affected postoperative mood states. In those who reported high preoperative fear, instruction as well as both procedural and sensory information lowered reports of postoperative anger. Patients who received sensory information had a significantly shorter postoperative hospital stay and tended to leave their homes earlier after discharge than patients who did not receive this information. When the length of postoperative stay for all groups was examined, the group given no information or instruction had the longest postoperative stay. Patients who received the combination of sensory information and instruction had the shortest postoperative hospital stay.

With surgery as the threatening event, sensory information did not affect emotion to any greater or lesser extent than did the other interventions, procedural information and instruction. All three interventions decreased reports of postoperative anger in those patients who were relatively fearful before surgery. Johnson and her colleagues (1978b) suggested that sensory information resulted in earlier recovery because it enabled patients to use coping strategies already in their behavioral repertoire. Because the combination of sensory information and instruction led to the shortest postoperative stay, they further suggested that the instruction gave patients an additional effective coping strategy.

The design used with the sample of cholecystectomy patients was repeated with patients having a herniorrhaphy (Johnson et al., 1978b). With this sample of patients, there were few effects either for type of information or for instruction. Patients who received instruction reported higher distress from the painful incisional sensations than did patients not instructed. Age was the only variable that affected length of postoperative hospitalization; older patients were hospitalized longer than the younger patients.

Possible explanations for the lack of effects in this group may be related to three general issues (Johnson et al., 1978b). First, the experiences associated with a herniorrhaphy are of much shorter duration than those associated with a cholecystectomy. Thus, the interventions may not have seemed as relevant to these patients. Second, the relatively rapid recovery rate following herniorrhaphy may have interfered with adequate measurement of patient responses. Measurements may have been obtained at the wrong time and, therefore, may not accurately reflect the patients' responses to the interventions. Third, sex differences may have been a factor; patients in cholecystectomy sample were primarily female, whereas in the herniorrhaphy sample they were predominantly male.

A second study involving patients undergoing either a cholecystectomy or herniorrhaphy (Johnson, Fuller, Endress, and Rice, 1978a) again tested the effects of sensory information and instruction in postoperative exercises. In addition, the effects of (1) giving specific preadmission preparation, (2) restatement of preoperative sensory information, and (3) temporal orientation were examined.

Preadmission preparation included booklets that were mailed to patients prior to admission. Specific preadmission information described postoperative exercises, i.e., deep breathing, coughing, leg exercises, turning in bed, and getting out of bed; it also gave specific information concerning the preadmission procedures, items to bring to the hospital, admission procedures, visiting hours, and services of the hospital. In contrast, nonspecific preadmission preparation included information on postoperative exercises but did not include detailed instructions for learning the exercises and gave very general information about hospital policies and procedures. On their first postoperative day, patients in the restatement of information group listened to the portion of the sensory information message that described the postoperative period. To test the effects of temporal orientation, additional detail was added to the sensory information to describe when, for how long, and how frequently an event would occur. Approximate length of stay in the recovery room and approximate time of first getting out of bed following surgery are examples of the added temporal detail.

As in the first study, there were no significant effects found in patients having a herniorrhaphy. For patients having a cholecystectomy, however, several effects were found. Patients who had been given specific preadmission preparation reported more anger than patients who did not receive this preparation. It should be noted that although these patients reported more postoperative anger, the specific preadmission preparation did not affect any other indicator of postoperative recovery. Patients who listened to the relevant part of the sensory information a second time required fewer analgesics than those patients who did not have the information repeated. Patients who received sensory information with additional temporal orientation reported less postoperative helplessness than those who received sensory information without this added detail. Also, as in the first study, patients who received sensory information had shorter postoperative hospital stays and, following discharge, ventured from their homes earlier than patients who had not received sensory information.

The beneficial effects of sensory information on indicators of postoperative recovery were replicated. Detailed temporal orienting information was found to reduce postoperative feelings of helplessness. This study also provided additional information to guide clinical use of these interventions. First, providing exercise instruction before hospital admission does not seem to influence postoperative recovery. Second, reminding patients of the typical sensory experiences early in their postoperative course may increase their ability to deal with incisional pain.

Wilson (1981) compared the effects of sensory information and instruction in a systematic relaxation technique in a sample of patients having either a cholecystetomy or a total abdominal hysterectomy. These patients were assigned to one of four conditions: (1) usual hospital care, (2) sensory information, (3 relaxation instruction, or (4) information plus instruction. For all three experimental groups, postoperative stay was essentially the same and significantly shorter than for the control group. Sensory information did not include the detailed temporal orienting information, nor was helplessness measured directly. There were no effects for sensory information on the postoperative moods measured. Relaxation instruction was associated with receiving less parenteral analgesics postoperatively. The combination of information and instruction did not increase recovery rate beyond that produced by each intervention alone, as was found in the first surgical study (Johnson et al., 1978b).

The effects of sensory information have also been studied in surgical patients other than those undergoing abdominal surgery. Hill (1982) used a sample of patients having cataract extractions to study the effects of sensory information and behavioral instruction. Behavioral instruction included ways for the patient to reduce discomfort in the eye and self-care skills that included how to get out of bed. Patients were assigned to one of four groups: (1) general information, (2) behavioral instruction, (3) sensory information or, (4) instruction and sensory information. Patients who received both sensory information and behavioral instruction ventured from their homes after discharge earlier than did those given general information. Although the effect was not significant, patients given sensory information reported less postoperative anxiety, less depression, and shorter time before venturing from home after discharge. Thus, these results tend to confirm the additive effect of sensory information and activity instruction on recovery.

In the last surgical study to be discussed, the effects of preoperative preparation as well as discharge preparation were investigated (Johnson, Christman, and Stitt, in press). Preoperative sensory information alone or combined with one of two types of preoperative instruction was tested. The first type of instruction was an ambulation technique, that is, how to turn in bed and get out with minimal strain on the incision. The second type of instruction was a distraction technique, which guided the patient to focus on the positive rather than the negative aspects of the surgical experience. Prior to discharge from the hospital, all patients were given either information describing the typical recovery period sensory experiences or general health information.

The results of the study are divided into the two phases of recovery, hospitalization and post discharge. In the hospital phase the expected effects of sensory information on recovery were not found. Patients given sensory information did report an increased perception of ability to deal with the experience and a belief that the experience would be less difficult for them. Instruction in an ambulation technique was again found to decrease analgesic requirements. Although patients given the distraction instruction reported greater physical recovery on their third postoperative day, this group had the longest postoperative hospitalization.

For the postdischarge phase of recovery, both the long-term effects of the preoperative interventions and the effects of the discharge preparation were examined. Data were collected by mail at 1, 4, and 12 weeks postdischarge. The effects of the discharge interventions were interpreted with caution. A greater number of patients who received sensory discharge preparation than those who received the control preparation failed to return the postdischarge data and could not be reached by telephone. Thus, sensory-informed patients' resumption of activities outside the home may have affected the return rate (Johnson et al., in press).

At one week postdischarge, patients given preoperative ambulation instruction and sensory information either prior to surgery or prior to discharge reported higher levels of physical recovery. Sensory information either before surgery or before discharge, combined with preoperative instruction in the distraction technique, was related to reports of lower physical recovery at one week postdischarge. Patients who received the sensory preparation both before surgery and before discharge reported less anxiety and confusion, more vigor, and feeling closer to their normal selves than patients who did not receive this combination of sensory preparation. The effect of sensory information on the measure of first venturing from home following discharge was not replicated.

At four weeks postdischarge, no significant effects were found. For the data collected at 12 weeks postdischarge, patients given the preoperative distraction technique reported more anxiety and confusion, less physical recovery, and feeling less like their normal selves than patients not instructed in this technique.

Although this study failed to replicate the previously reported effects of sensory information on recovery indicators, the information produced no negative effects. There was some evidence to support cognitive processes proposed as associated with use of sensory information. There was also some evidence of positive effects for the combination of preoperative and discharge sensory information at one week following discharge. The ambulation instruction produced the same effect on use of postoperative analgesics as the more complex exercise instruction of previous studies (Johnson et al., 1978a, b). Although the distraction technique produced positive effects on the third postoperative day, these effects declined prior to discharge. Then, during the post-discharge phase of recovery, patients given the distraction technique experienced greater negative emotions and a slower physical recovery. Even though the distraction technique was useful to patients during the early postoperative period, its effectiveness did not continue and may have decreased the patient's ability to deal with the rest of the recovery period.

TOWARD CLINICAL APPLICATION

So that appropriate application of the research findings may be achieved in clinical practice, three issues derived from review of the investigations of sensory information require clarification and elaboration. These three issues are: (1) differential effects in short-term and long-term threatening events; (2) efficacy of combining sensory information with instruction in a coping strategy; and (3) the long-term effects of interventions.

Review of all the research findings makes evident the differences in effects of sensory information in short-term and long-term threatening health care events. In the short-term diagnostic or therapeutic situation, sensory information produces its effect on the patient's emotional response. On the other hand, in the more long-term event of surgery, sensory information promotes the patient's ability to use existing coping behaviors that in turn speed recovery (Johnson et al., 1978a, b, in press). These apparent contradictory results are not so troublesome when placed in the context of what is known about how people cope with threat.

Life itself involves continuous transactions with our internal and external environments. Some of these transactions are more taxing than others, eliciting internal feeling states and behaviors aimed at controlling or altering the situation. It is in those taxing situations that persons are said to be coping. Coping involves attempts to regulate internal feelings or emotions and to initiate behaviors that alter the transaction with the evironment toward the desired end (Lazarus and Launier, 1978). More explicitly, coping involves two distinct components, emotional responses and goal-directed behavior.

These two components of coping can be independent (Johnson, Leventhal, and Dabbs, 1971; Leventhal, 1970; Sime, 1976). In other words, high levels of emotion are not consistently related to lack of goal-directed behavior, and neither are low levels of emotion related to increased initiation of effective behavior. In a given situation, it cannot be predicted that a certain level of emotion will lead to either effective or ineffective behavioral responses. Behavior is not directly dependent on the level of the emotional response. Sensory information has affected emotion in one type of situation without altering behavior; yet, in another situation, behavioral responses were altered without affecting emotion. Recognition of the potential independence of emotion and behavior makes this apparent paradox more understandable.

Both the potential independence of emotion and behavior and the differential effects of sensory information in short- and long-term threats are important to the practitioner establishing goals and outcome criteria for patient care. For example, expecting sensory information to be effective in reducing the surgical patient's postoperative emotional response measured by indicators of level of anxiety could lead to the conclusion that the information was ineffective. If, however, the practitioner establishes the goal of increased recovery rate with appropriate outcome criteria, conclusions regarding the effectiveness of the intervention would more likely be positive.

The combination of sensory information and instruction in a coping behavior has not been found to be consistently effective. Examination of the type of instruction and its intended behavioral outcome, target behavior, will help to clarify situations in which the combination of sensory information and instruction may be beneficial. From review of the effects of combining sensory information and instruction, those instances in which the combination was effective occurred when the instruction provided a behavior that did not already exist in the patient's repertoire of coping strategies (Johnson et al., 1978b). In these situations, the learned technique added a new strategy that increased the effectiveness of sensory information (Hill, 1982; Johnson and Leventhal, 1974; Johnson et al., 1978a, b; Padilla et al., 1981). The target behavior of the new strategy was also compatible with the major effect of sensory information. For example, teaching ambulation techniques is intended to increase ambulation and thereby speed recovery, the same end result that sensory information produced.

Those instances in which combining sensory information and instruction did not produce additive effects (Fuller et al., 1978; Johnson et al., in press; Wilson, 191) may be related to (1) incompatible target responses, (2) the presence of an existing and effective coping strategy, or (3) the need to use competing cognitive processes. A newly learned technique may not seem relevant because of the existence of a previously used strategy; or the response elicited by the newly learned technique may differ from the response elicited by sensory information. For example, systematic relaxation is intended to decrease activity, whereas other strategies such as ambulation and exercise techniques increase activity that aids recovery. In other instances, such as pelvic examination (Fuller et al., 1978), the patient may have well-established behaviors that are used in preference to, or are incompatible with, the newly taught technique. Finally, some combinations of information and instruction may not be effective because they require patients to use competing cognitive processes. Combining sensory information and distraction may be one of these combinations. Sensory information draws attention to unpleasant stimuli and the distraction technique requires avoidance of unpleasant stimuli (Johnson et al., in press). Selective attention to only certain unpleasant stimuli may not be easily achieved.

For the practitioner these research findings indicate a need to determine whether intruction will provide a new technique for the patient's use. There is also need to recognize the intended target behavior of the instruction and select evaluation criteria accordingly. Giving instruction in a technique to reduce emotional response is required only when emotional response is a problem and does not guarantee a corresponding behavioral response. Once more recognition of the independence of emotion and behavior (Johnson et al., 1971; Leventhal, 1970; Sime, 1976) becomes important.

There is some evidence that sensory information may have long-term as well as short-term effects. Patients given sensory information resumed their usual activities earlier, presumably by relying on existing coping strategies while guided by the recognition that their experiences during recovery are normal (Johnson et al., 1978a, b). There is tentative evidence that instruction may have negative long-term effects. Giving instruction in coping strategies to use during hospitalization may suggest to patients that new coping strategies are also required to deal with the stress of recovery once discharged from the hospital (Johnson et al., in press). Thus, patients may slow their recovery by searching for new strategies rather than relying on existing strategies. While more study of the long-term effects of interventions used during hospitalization is required, the practitioner's awareness of the potential for sustained effects is important. It is to be hoped that the future will bring clarification of these potentials through the efforts of both practitioners and researchers.

IMPLICATIONS FOR PRACTICE AND RESEARCH

Prior to clinical use, it is necessary to evaluate the research findings carefully (Haller, Reynolds, and Horsley, 1979). Points to consider in evaluating research for clinical use include (1) replication of the findings; (2) the contribution of the investigations to the understanding of relationships between variables; (3) the degree of risk to the patient if the findings are used; (4) the benefit to the patient; (5) nurses' ability to control use of the findings; (6) feasibility of their use; and (7) the cost-benefit ratio associated with use of the findings.

The beneficial effects of sensory information have been replicated in a wide variety of clinical settings and patient groups and with differing types of threatening events. Replication has also led to the differentiation of the intervention's effects in short-term versus long-term threatening health care situations. Through replication, these investigations have contributed to the development of nursing knowledge; their scientific merit is evident. The use of sensory information involves little or no risk to patients, and its beneficial effects on coping with threatening experiences have been demonstrated. Nurses have clinical control of preparing patients for diagnostic and therapeutic procedures, and providing sensory information is feasible. Nurses who have cared for unprepared patients postoperatively frequently wish that the patients had been prepared. The cost-benefit ratio is more heavily weighted toward benefit than cost, since only time is required. If many patients need similar preparation and time requirements prove costly, sensory information could be delivered by use of a group or audiovisual approach.

Selecting Appropriate Patients

Sensory information should be given to healthy or hospitalized adults who are to undergo diagnostic or therapeutic procedures. Children 6 years of age and older may also benefit as long as they are able to understand verbal description of future events. Although younger children need to be prepared for threatening events, sensory information may not be the most appropriate type of preparation because of their level of cognitive development.

Those patients who have never experienced the anticipated threatening event are the most likely to benefit from sensory information (McHugh et al., 1982). Even when patients have had previous experience with the event, they may benefit because the information provided may be more accurate than their memories. Patients' previous experience with the particular threatening event varied across the studies. Yet none of the theatening events used in these studies may be characterized as frequent or regularly recurring. With health care events that occur frequently, such as daily or weekly venipuncture, the patients' past experiences dominates the formation of expectations about the experience. Because of the event's frequency, these patients may not experience fear or anxiety and may have developed effective coping strategies.

The nursing diagnoses for which providing sensory information is an appropriate intervention are potential ones. Since the intervention is of a preventive or facilitative nature, the need for its use is frequently based on the possibility that a particular problem may occur rather than on evidence that it is occurring. Even so, it is safe to assume that all patients experience at least some degree of threat when faced with diagnostic or therapeutic procedures. Their responses to the threat will vary in degree (and timing.) It is also possible that the timing of these responses in relation to the occurrence of the event will vary. Some patients may evidence negative responses prior to an event, whereas others do not dislay such difficulty until during or after the event. Thus, whether the nursing diagnosis is actual or potential will differ from patient to patient. Using sensory information with a potential diagnosis is just as important as using it with an actual diagnosis.

The first nursing diagnosis for which Sensory Information may be an appropriate intervention is *Potential Anxiety or Fear* due to uncertainty about a short-term diagnostic or therapeutic procedure. Fear of the unknown may lead to anxiety in these situations. These procedures, usually unfamiliar to patients, often involve strange noises, uncomfortable sensations, strangers, and a new environment. Attempting to interpret and give meaning to the sensory stimuli in such an experience is difficult when no schema is available. Providing sensory information permits patients to anticipate and label the usual experience as normal and, thereby, to experience less distress. In short-term events, sensory information is used to achieve the goal of decreasing the patients' distress response, which can occur during or after the event; therefore, outcome criteria should include measures of distress appropriate to the particular health care event.

A second nursing diagnosis for which Sensory Information may be used is *Potential Ineffective Individual Coping Behavior* due to the uncertainty of a long-term threat, such as major abdominal surgery. With this type of event, the purpose of using sensory information is to help patients use their existing coping strategies to facilitate recovery (Johnson et al., 1978a, b). Outcome criteria should include indicators of rate of recovery.

Combining sensory information with instruction in a coping behavior should be based on consideration of two factors. First, assessment should be made of whether the patient is likely to already possess a relevant coping behavior. Postoperative exercises and ambulation techniques are probably not a part of most patients' coping repertoire. Thus, this type of instruction should provide added benefit for the patients' recovery (Johnson et al., 1978b). Second, the purpose of the instruction in a coping behavior should be clearly identified. Since the purpose of some coping techniques—for example, relaxation—is to decrease stress, these should be used and evaluated accordingly. Even though relaxation may decrease distress, a lower level of distress may not necessarily speed the rate of recovery. Expecting cumulative effects from combining sensory information with a technique to reduce distress is unreliable; evaluation of the outcome of this combination may be best done on an individual patient basis.

A third nursing diagnosis for which Sensory Information may be appropriate is *Potential Powerlessness* due to uncertainty about the duration and timing of events associated with a threatening experience. Giving time-related sensory information should lessen feelings of helplessness (Johnson et al., 1978a). Helping patients to know when, for how long, and how frequently a specific event will occur may foster patients' sense of control over the experience and add to their ability to use existing coping strategies.

It should be noted that Sensory Information is not an appropriate intervention to use for the nursing diagnosis of Knowledge Deficit. The intent of providing sensory information is not to teach. Determination of whether learning has occurred is unnecessary. Although patients who have been given sensory information report their expectations and actual experience to be more closely aligned than do other patients (Johnson et al., in press), they rarely relate this to the information intervention.

Preparing Sensory Information Messages

Although many of the points to be considered in developing sensory information were discussed in the description of the intervention, they are repeated here for emphasis and clarity. Development of a preparatory message begins with gathering the appropriate information about the two components of the message (McHugh et al., 1982).

The subjective sensation information is obtained by interviewing at least 15 patients who have undergone the experience for which the intervention is being developed. It should be remembered that patients may initially tend to describe their experience in general or evaluative terms. It may be necessary to guide the patients to use more specific and descriptive terms. Once these data are collected, they are reviewed for similarities and only those sensations reported by at least 50 per cent of the patients are incorporated into the message. Sensations should be described in objective terms; evaluative connotations such as "awful" or "intense" should be omitted. The sensation descriptions already developed because of their use in the research studies are presented in Table 18–1.

The objective component of the message will vary from setting to setting because of variations in practices and policies. Nursing staff observing the event can readily note the sequential elements and environmental changes as they occur.

Combining the information gathered about the two components involves linking the sensations to their causes and ensuring that the temporal qualities, frequency and duration, are linked to appropriate sensations and events. This process includes description of changes in sensations over time when appropriate. Once the message has been developed, it should be reviewed to make sure that it portrays a clear picture of the event and the experiences a patient

Table 18–1. SENSATIONS DOCUMENTED IN LITERATURE FOR SELECTED PROCEDURES

Threatening Event	Sensations
Gastroendoscopic examination (Johnson et al., 1973, 1974)	Intravenous medication: needle stick, drowsiness As air pumped into stomach: feeling of fullness like after eating a large meal Physician's finger in mouth to guide tube insertion
Nasogastric tube insertion (Padilla et al., 1981)	Feeling passage of tube Tearing Gagging Discomforts in nose, throat, mouth Limited mobility
Cast removal (Johnson, Kirchhoff, and Endress, 1976)	Buzz of saw Feel vibrations or tingling See chalky dust Feel warmth on arm or leg as saw cuts cast; will not hurt or burn Skin under padding will be scaly and look dirty Arm or leg may be a little stiff when first trying to move it Arm or leg may seem light because cast was heavy
Barium enema (Hartfield and Cason, 1981)	Lying on hard table Fullness Pressure Bloating Uncomfortable Feeling as if might have a bowel movement
Abdominal surgery (Johnson et al., 1978b; McHugh et al., 1982)	Preoperative medications: sleepy, lightheaded, relaxed, free from worry, not bothered by most things, dryness of mouth Incision: tenderness, sensitivity, pressure, smarting, burning, aching, sore Sensations might become sharp and seem to travel along incision when moving Arm with intravenous tube will seem awkward and restricted but will feel no discomfort or pain Tiredness after physical effort Bloating of abdomen Cramping due to gas pains Pulling and pinching when stitches are removed

may anticipate. An example of a sensory message may be found in a report by Johnson, Kirchhoff, and Endress, 1976.

FUTURE DIRECTIONS FOR RESEARCH

Although the beneficial effects of Sensory Information have been clearly demonstrated, there are still areas to be clarified through future research. One issue that requires further investigation is the nature of the process by which sensory information produces positive effects. There is some evidence that sensory information works by increasing the accuracy of expectations (Johnson, 1973; Johnson et al., in press). Yet, because partial and full sensation descriptions were found to be equally effective (Johnson and Rice, 1974), variables other than accuracy may be affecting the positive patient responses. However accomplished, sensory information affects patients' cognitive processing of information in a threatening situation. At best, thought processes are difficult to measure and quantify if, indeed, people are sufficiently aware of these processes to be able to give verbal descriptions of them (Nisbett and Wilson, 1977). Different and creative ways of trying to obtain this information are necessary in future reseach endeavors.

A second area for further study centers on the issue of event complexity. Sensory information has produced differential effects in events of differing complexity. Since the short-term threats used in the studies were variable and multiple, confidence can be placed in expecting the obtained results to be effective in other diagnostic and therapeutic procedures of the same general nature. With long-term threats, whether the results will generalize to other health care threats of equal or greater compexity is less certain. Because of the replication of effects of sensory information with patients undergoing cholecystectomy (Johnson et al., 1978a, b), the research findings should be applicable to patients having other types of major abdominal surgery. It would be interesting to know, however, whether sensory information produces the same effects with patients having surgical procedures that represent a greater risk—for example, open heart surgery. Heart surgery also introduces another variable, a thoracic incision, to be considered in such an investigation.

There is a third area for future study that is somewhat related to the issue of event complexity. In events of greater complexity there are situations in which the patient's subjective sensation experience is less discrete, more diffuse, and less attributable to a specific cause. Movement from one level of nursing care to another or to self-care may be examples of such an experience. Situations involving loss or disfigurement may be other examples of this type of experience. In these situations, the sensations patients experience are diffuse, vague, and primarily due to their own emotional response to the event. These responses are generally normal and unavoidable. Whether providing information to patients about this type of sensory experience is beneficial awaits future study (Christman, 1981).

The last area for further study is clarification of the long-term effects of sensory information, especially when combined with additional sensory description or instruction in various coping behaviors. Giving sensory information prior to hospital discharge as well as preoperatively may produce additional benefits (Johnson et al., in press). Because these findings were only suggestive, further replication is required before confidence can be placed in the benefit of additional sensory preparation prior to hospital discharge. There was also evidence that combining sensory information with instruction in a cognitive distraction technique led to long-term negative effects (Johnson et al., in press). Further study is required to clarify the long-term outcomes produced by combining sensory information with a distraction technique as well as with instruction in other coping behaviors.

CONCLUSION

Clearly, Preparatory Sensory Information is an intervention useful to patients and may be considered appropriate for use with more than one nursing diagnosis. The development and testing of Sensory Information provides an example of how nursing knowledge is developed, refined, retested, and expanded through research. The fact that further research is necessary does not negate its clinical value. Need for further study illustrates an essential part of knowledge development. Knowledge is ever expanding as new questions are posed and answers are sought through systematic study. Development of scientific knowledge is a cyclic process. Answers to questions generate new questions. As nurse practitioners and researchers increase their contributions to the process of knowledge generation by asking questions and seeking answers, the base for nursing practice will continue to expand and be grounded in the scientific process rather than intuition.

EDITORS' COMMENTS AND QUESTIONS

Preparatory Sensory Information is a well-developed intervention with a strong research base. It is based on theory that has been developed and tested by nurses in several client populations. There are strong implications for practice. This chapter does not include a case study, as the strong research base is rich with clinical data.

Questions for Discussion

1. *Give an example of how Preparatory Sensory Information could be used in your practice.*

2. *Identify populations, other than those cited in the text, with whom this intervention should be tested.*

3. *How widely are you willing to generalize the positive results of the testing of this intervention?*

References

Christman, N. J. Predictability and coping with CCU transfer (Abstract). In Proceedings of 1981 Conference of the Western Society for Research in Nursing. *Western Journal of Nursing Research*, 1981, 3(3), 62.

Fuller, S. S., Endress, M. P., and Johnson, J. E. The effects of cognitive and behavioral control on coping with an aversive health examination. *Journal of Human Stress*, 1978, 4(4), 18–25.

Haller, K. B., Reynolds, M. A., and Horsley, J. A. Developing research-based innovation protocols: Process, criteria, and issues. *Research in Nursing and Health*, 1979, 2, 45–51.

Hartfield, M. J., and Cason, C. L. Effect of information on emotional responses during barium enema. *Nursing Research*, 1981, 30,151–155.

Hartfield, M. J., Cason, C. L., and Cason, G. J. Effects of information about a threatening procedure on patients' expectations and emotional distress. *Nursing Research*, 1982, 31, 202–206.

Hill, B. J. Sensory information, behavioral instructions and coping with sensory alteration surgery. *Nursing Research*, 1982, 31, 17–21.

Johnson, J. E. Effects of accurate expectations about sensations on the sensory and distress components of pain. *Journal of Personality and Social Psychology*, 1973, 27, 261–275.

Johnson, J. E., and Leventhal, H. Effects of accurate expectations and behavioral instructions on reactions during a noxious medical examination. *Journal of Personality and Social Psychology*, 1974, *29*, 710–718.

Johnson, J. E., and Rice, V. H. Sensory and distress components of pain: Implications for the study of clinical pain. *Nursing Research*, 1974, *23*, 203–209.

Johnson, J. E., Christman, N. J., and Stitt, C. Personal control interventions: Short and long term effects on surgical patients. *Research in Nursing and Health* (in press).

Johnson, J. E., Kirchhoff, K. T., and Endress, M. P. Altering children's distress behavior during orthopedic cast removal. *Nursing Research*, 1975, *24*, 404–410.

Johnson, J. E., Kirchhoff, K. T., and Endress, M. P. Easing children's fright during health care procedures. *American Journal of Maternal-Child Nursing*, 1976, *1*, 206–210.

Johnson, J. E., Leventhal, H., and Dabbs, J. M., Jr. Contribution of emotional and instrumental response processes in adaptation to surgery. *Journal of Personality and Social Psychology*, 1971, *20*, 55–64.

Johnson, J. E., Morrissey, J. F., and Leventhal, H. Psychological preparation for endoscopic examination. *Gastrointestinal Endoscopy*, 1973, *19*, 180–182.

Johnson, J. E., Fuller, S. S., Endress, M. P., and Rice, V. H. Altering patients' responses to surgery: An extension and replication. *Research in Nusing and Health*, 1978a, *1*, 111–121.

Johnson, J. E., Rice, V. H., Fuller, S. S., and Endress, M. P. Sensory information, instruction in a coping strategy and recovery from surgery. *Research in Nursing and Health*, 1978b, *1*, 4–17.

Lazarus, R. S., and Launier, R. Stress-related transactions between person and enviroment. In L. C. Pervin and M. Lewis (Eds.), *Perspectives in Interactional Psychology*. New York: Plenum Press, 1978.

Leventhal, H. Findings and theory in the study of fear communications. In L. Berkowitz (Ed.), *Advances in Experimental Social Psychology* (Vol. 5). New York: Academic Press, 1970.

McHugh, N. G., Christman, N. J., and Johnson, J. E. Preparatory information: What helps and why. *American Journal of Nursing*, 1982, *82*, 780–782.

Neisser, U. *Cognition and Reality*. San Francisco: W. H. Freeman and Co., 1976.

Nisbett, R. E., and Wilson, T. D.: Telling more than we can know: Verbal reports on mental processes. *Psychological Review*, 1977, *84*, 231–259.

Padilla, G. V., Grant, M. M., Rains, B. L., Hansen, B. C., Bergstrom, N., Wong, H. L., Hanson, R., and Kubo, W. Distress reduction and the effects of preparatory teaching films and patient control. *Research in Nursing and Health*, 1981, *4*, 375–387.

Sime, A. M. Relationship of preoperative fear, type of coping, and information received about surgery to recovery from surgery. *Journal of Personality and Social Psychology*, 1976, *34*, 716–724.

Wilson, J. F. Behavioral preparation for surgery: Benefit or harm? *Journal of Behavioral Medicine*, 1981, *4*(1), 79–102.

19

CRISIS INTERVENTION

ROBERT J. KUS

Wilma S., a 40 year old unskilled laborer and struggling single mother of three, has just learned that the company where she's been employed for the past six years is closing its plant. "I don't know what to do! Who'd buy my house? This is a one-company town! I just don't know where to turn!"

Juan M., a 23 year old student working on his master's degree in fine arts, was awarded a fellowship to study for his doctorate with the stipulation that his master's project be completed by June. In April, flash floods destroyed the paintings he had labored over for the past year and a half. "All that work for nothing! I feel like giving up! Just when things looked so rosy, they collapse. What's the use!"

Lance R., a 28 year old gay high school teacher, is brought to the hospital emergency room. His blood alcohol level is dangerously high, and he has overdosed on "downers." "It's too much! I just can't seem to cope any more. I wish I were dead."

These three people are all faced with life situations for which they are unprepared. While all have led productive lives and until now have solved the usual life problems that have come their way, all are currently experiencing psychological crises.

How each story will end may depend on what help is available. In this chapter, the treatment of Crisis Intervention, applicable in each of the examples cited, is explored. The discussion here focuses on Crisis Intervention with the individual client rather than with families or other groups.

DEFINITION AND DESCRIPTION

The Concept of Crisis. *A crisis is a state of psychological emergency rendering one's usually effective problem-solving skills useless or greatly diminished.*

Walkup (1974) offers a more elaborate definition. She uses the process or "serial operational" definition advocated by nursing theorist Peplau. In so doing, she assumes the client to be a "system." By doing this, nursing can use Crisis Intervention to treat any type of client—an individual, family, social organization, or community. Crisis, in Walkup's view, is defined in this way:

1. A change occurs to a system in a dynamic equilibrium.

2. The system perceives the change as a disruption of intersystem balance between internal needs and external demands.

3. The system mobilizes its habitual problem-solving energies (internal resources) and desires situational support (external resources) to attempt to resolve the imbalance.

4. The internal and external resources fail to resolve the problem.

5. Feelings of helplessness and ineffectiveness result in behavior disorganization (Walkup, 1974, pp. 152–153).

Types of Crises. Crises are classified on the basis of their origins. Some writers, such as Hoff (1978) and Riley (1980), classify crises as either maturational or situational. Others add a third type, called "social" crises by Haber (1982) or "adventitious" crises by Benter (1979).

Maturational or *developmental crises* are those that occur "in responses to stresses inherent in predictable life transitions and events" (Haber, 1982, p. 309). Specific life span periods, such as childhood, adolescence, and old age, and major social role changes, such as marriage, menopause, and retirement, are examples. Usually, maturational crises can be anticipated. Some crises that may be termed developmental can be unanticipated. For example, there exists a process called "coming out," which is unique to gay and lesbian individuals. Kus (1980) states that because gay and lesbian children do not usually recognize their sexual orientation until the teen years or later, and because the early stages of the coming out process are often fraught with a bewildering array of problems, unanticipated crises can occur.

Situational crises occur when "unanticipated events threaten a person's biological, social, or psychological integrity" (Haber, 1982, p. 309). Examples include losing one's job, getting divorced, or losing a loved one.

The *social* or *adventitious crisis* is a special type of situational crisis resulting from uncommon events that cause multiple losses or severe environmental changes (Haber, 1982, p. 309). Examples include being in fires, riots, or earthquakes.

Clinical Picture. According to Powell and Lively (1981), the individual in crisis often exhibits certain signs and symptoms. Both objective and subjective data are used to help the nurse in assessing the client in crisis.

Objective data include inefficient cognition and motor-behavioral responses. Cognitive responses often seen include decreased perceptual ability, narrowing of focus, thought disorganization, changed ability to solve problems, and decreased ability to perform adequately on the job and in decision-making. Objective motor-behavioral responses can be seen in skeletal muscle tension, which includes jerky or rigid movement, restlessness, or constant movement of a body part, or in smooth muscle tension, such as urinary frequency, diarrhea, and vomiting.

Subjective data include alterations in both affective and motor-behavioral responses. Affective responses include feelings of being overwhelmed by one's problem, helplessness, loss of control, anxiety, guilt, anger, and low self-esteem. Subjective motor-behavioral responses include nausea, insomnia or extreme fatigue and sleep, anorexia or overeating, gastrointestinal pains, headache, backache, neck pain, and chest pain.

Crisis Intervention. *Crisis Intervention is the systematic application of problem-solving techniques, based on crisis theory, designed to help the client in crisis move through the crisis process as swiftly and painlessly as possible* *and thereby achieve at least the same level of psychological comfort as experienced before the crisis.*

The minimum goal of Crisis Intervention is that the client will function as well after the crisis as before. His or her emotional equilibrium and coping capacity will be restored.

But successful Crisis Intervention can also help the client grow beyond the pre-crisis coping level. During the Crisis Intervention process, the client may learn to focus more effectively on factors that lead to crisis, eliminate expendable life stresses, adopt healthier ways of living, recognize personal strengths and weaknesses, and gain ways of solving problems. Further, when the client's significant others become involved in assisting the client through the crisis, closer bonds may develop, thus lessening the likelihood of recurrent crises. Therefore, Crisis Intervention can also be seen as a form of primary or preventative mental health care, a future-oriented phenomenon.

According to Jacobson, Strickler, and Morley (1968), there are two main types of Crisis Intervention: generic and individual.

The *generic approach* emphasizes the common patterns found in specific crisis events and focuses the intervention on these commonalities. The therapist does not focus on the individual psychodynamics. For example, Lindemann (1944) found that the grief process is composed of fairly predictable stages. Therefore, to help the person do grief work, the nurse need only know the dynamics of this specific type of crisis to be effective. Thus, doing Crisis Intervention with a widow would be essentially the same as doing Crisis Intervention with a widower. This approach has the advantage of being practiced on a large scale by both professional and nonprofessional helpers. The disadvantage is that a therapist may be extremely knowledgeable and effective in one type of crisis pattern while being ignorant and ineffective in other types of crises.

The *individual approach* focuses on the specific individual in crisis and his or her psychodynamics rather than on a specific type of crisis (Aquilera and Messick, 1974, p. 18). This approach is useful when the generic approach fails to help the individual in crisis. Because it is more complex than the generic approach, it is limited to professionals knowledgeable in psychotherapy, such as psychiatrists, psychosocial clinical nurse specialists, psychiatric social workers, and psychologists.

From the nursing perspective, both approaches are valuable. In actual clinical nursing practice, perhaps the most common approach is a combination of the generic and individual approaches. Certainly nurses recognize many crisis patterns and act accordingly. On the other hand, nurses also focus on the uniqueness of the individual and on his or her perception of reality as well as the host of intervening variables impinging on a client's life. In this chapter, a problem-solving approach to Crisis Intervention will be presented to help the nurse assist the maximum number of clients in crisis. This approach, although it is a blend of the generic and individual approaches, focuses more heavily on the generic approach.

A BACKGROUND OF CRISIS INTERVENTION

A Brief History. The two pioneers in the field of Crisis Intervention are Lindemann and Caplan.

Lindemann formulated his ideas of Crisis Intervention by interviewing persons in bereavement. In his now classic study (1944), he observed surviving friends and relatives of the hundreds of people killed in the 1943 Coconut Grove nightclub fire in Boston. He noted that there were common patterns or stages in grieving. Furthermore, he noted that while some individuals went through the grieving process with relative ease, others had many more difficulties.

From his studies, Lindemann concluded that besides the loss of loved ones, other life crises, such as marriage, might also have predictable patterns. If a helper could intervene early in the crisis, the individual would stand a better chance of getting through the crisis in good mental health. In addition, he believed that mental health workers could intervene in life crises on a community level to help many people as opposed to the traditional method of intensive one-to-one psychotherapy. In 1946, he and Gerald Caplan established just such a Crisis Intervention program, called the Wellesley Project, in the Harvard area.

Caplan, in his *Principles of Preventative Psychiatry* (1964), advocated Crisis Intervention as a primary tool to prevent mental illness on a community-wide level. His work has been vitally important in both its emphasis on preventative care mental health and its emphasis on a cost-effective strategy to help the population with everyday life crises.

In this work, Caplan noted that most often crises are self-limiting; usually they last from 4 to 6 weeks. During the time of crisis, the individual is vulnerable. On the other hand, it is a time for the possibility of new growth. Much depends on whether or not the intervention occurs in time. Therefore, Crisis Intervention is most effective when it occurs in the beginning of the process.

In 1961, a report issued by the Joint Commission on Mental Illness and Health advocated Crisis Intervention. The report showed that too often people in crisis were placed on long waiting lists rather than receiving the immediate help they needed. Following the Commission's recommendations, the United States funded the establishment of community-based Crisis Intervention projects. Today, crisis clinics and crisis hotlines are found in even the smallest towns in America.

The Benefits of Crisis Intervention. As a mental health strategy, Crisis Intervention is relatively noncontroversial. In fact, its popularity arises out of its many benefits.

First, Crisis Intervention is both easy to teach and easy to learn. Besides health care professionals, Crisis Intervention can be and has been taught and effectively used by a wide range of people, such as the police, alcohol counselors, and crisis hotline workers.

Second, it is very cost-effective. Not only does it eliminate costly and time-consuming psychotherapy, but also, when used effectively, it helps prevent crisis coping from becoming an entrenched life pattern leading the individual to require hospitalization.

Third, Crisis Intervention can be applied in any setting rather than being limited to a therapist's office or a hospital ward.

Fourth, Crisis Intervention can help the individual in crisis learn new ways of coping with or preventing crisis events in the future.

Fifth, this intervention can save lives. The suicidal client, by being assisted through the problem-solving process, often finds alternatives to self-destruction and gains rekindled hope.

Sixth, because Crisis Intervention often involves the marshaling of a person's support system, frequently the bonds between the client in crisis and significant others are strengthened. The increased sharing, communication, and understanding often leave the client with a stronger support system after the crisis than existed before.

Finally, because Crisis Intervention is an intervention geared for all persons, it does not carry the same stigma as other forms of mental health therapy.

Guiding Principles. To do successful Crisis Intervention, certain guiding principles should be adopted by the nurse therapist. Borrowing from and building on recommendations by Morley, Messick, and Aquilera (1967), the following points are offered for consideration and adoption by the nurse implementing Crisis Intervention:

1. Crisis Intervention is the treatment of choice for persons in crisis. Any idea that Crisis Intervention is merely a "Band-Aid" type of strategy done to tide the client over until the "real" therapy can be had should be promptly discarded.

2. The nurse clinician who is a novice in Crisis Intervention should have adequate supervision by skilled crisis intervention therapists. Crisis Intervention is a clinical skill that requires training and practice, just as such traditional nursing skills as catheterization or suctioning do.

3. The client in crisis should be viewed as a healthy person who is temporarily unable to cope effectively because of overwhelming life stresses. Crises are normal events. Thus, Crisis Intervention is a form of psychosocial—not "psychiatric"—nursing.

4. Unlike in traditional nursing practice, client assessment is more focused. Rather than delving into all the usual nursing history categories, the nurse focuses only on the client's crisis problem and related information, such as support systems.

5. Both nurse and client must realize that the treatment is sharply time-limited and, therefore, keep their energies focused on solving the current crisis.

6. The nurse deals only with the crisis issue. Extraneous material is not suitable in Crisis Intervention.

7. The therapist is assertive in intervening. Because crises are self-limiting, time is very valuable.

8. The nurse must be flexible. He or she should be able to play any role that will help the client. For example, the nurse might become a resource person, consultant, teacher, message-bearer to loved ones, and the like.

9. The goal of Crisis Intervention is always known: to help the client return to a level of coping that is at least as good as his or her pre-crisis level of coping.

10. The nurse—or any other Crisis Intervention therapist—should never hesitate to ask for outside consultation if confronted with a crisis situation for which he or she is unprepared. For example, the nurse not familiar with the emotional stress associated with the coming out process of gay people might consult a gay therapist or a therapist or agency knowledgeable about this process.

PROBLEM SOLVING

One of the greatest strengths of Crisis Intervention is that it can be effectively used by nurses and other therapists regardless of their therapeutic orientation or clinical field.

Unlike many other nursing interventions, Crisis Intervention has no concrete tools or instruments. However, the crisis interventionist should understand well the stages of the problem-solving process.

The Problem-Solving Process. Expanding on Dewey's classic *How We Think* (1910), the problem-solving process may be viewed as a series of six steps. The job of the nurse is to assist the client through this process to completion to resolve the crisis.

First, the nurse must help the client identify and describe the problem. Because the client in crisis often is overwhelmed, he or she often cannot focus clearly enough to identify the specific problem or problems. In short, he or she cannot see the forest for the trees.

Second, once the problem is identified by nurse and client, the nurse can then assist the client to generate possible solutions. The nurse may make suggestions at this point, if he or she is familiar with alternatives that have helped others in similar crises in the past.

Third, the nurse assists the client in evaluating the possible outcomes or consequences of the alternative solutions. For example, a client in marital crisis might be considering staying with her mate or divorcing him. The nurse might suggest that the client make lists of the positive and negative aspects of each decision.

Fourth, the client decides which alternative will be chosen. It is crucial to remember that it is the client, not the nurse, who must live with this decision. Therefore, it must be the client who makes the decision to act. This is critical to remember as the client is often so vulnerable that any suggestion, no matter how inappropriate for his or her life, is liable to be grasped.

The nurse may, however, offer his or her support for whatever decision is made, but he or she must reassure the client that support will be forthcoming if the client changes his or her mind. This is easier said than done. For example, in working with abused spouses, it is most difficult to support the client's decision to return home to the same setting where repeated batterings have occurred in the past and most likely will occur in the future. Nevertheless, each person must travel his or her own path through life.

Fifth, the client implements the decision.

And finally, the nurse helps the client evaluate the implementation. Did this solution resolve the crisis? Is the client better off now? If not, the client may have to try another solution.

By going through the problem-solving process with guidance, the client is often better able to do problem solving independently in the future, thus lessening the likelihood of similar crises occurring later.

THE CRISIS INTERVENTION CANDIDATE

Who can benefit from Crisis Intervention? What types of nursing diagnoses are likely to be encountered in the person in crisis?

Simply put, any person experiencing life crisis is a candidate for Crisis Intervention. And although some persons have more effective coping and problem-solving skills than others—and are less likely to suffer crisis—life stresses can overwhelm even the strongest among us. Therefore, it is safe to say that all of us are potential candidates for Crisis Intervention.

Some of the more common nursing diagnoses are the following:

- Anticipatory and Dysfunctional Grieving
- Fear
- Ineffectual Individual or Family Coping
- Feelings of Powerlessness
- Disturbances in Self-Concept
- Distress of the Human Spirit, especially Hopelessness
- Alterations in Thought Processes

○ Potential for Self-Injury
○ Rape-Trauma Syndrome

Any conditions in which a person's problem-solving strategies are found to be ineffective may require Crisis Intervention. For a more comprehensive listing of the types of people with whom Crisis Intervention has been successfully used, the reader is directed to the works of Parad, Resnik, and Parad (1976), Ewing (1978), and others for similar anthologies on Crisis Intervention.

DOING CRISIS INTERVENTION

To successfully do Crisis Intervention, the nurse must first recall the principles of crisis theory. An excellent sourcebook for nurses in this area is the book by Infante (1982).

A Synopsis of Crisis Theory. Caplan (1964) identified four phases of a typical crisis.

1. The individual experiences a problem that threatens basic needs. The individual tries to relieve the tension by resorting to traditional problem-solving strategies to end the crisis and thus restore emotional equilibrium.

2. If the individual's usual methods fail, increased tension occurs. He or she becomes disorganized and resorts to a trial-and-error type of solving the problem.

3. If these problem-solving measures fail, the individual experiences an increase in tension, which leads him or her to redefine the problem to fit past experience or to give up certain of the goals as unattainable. The individual now uses novel or emergency ways of trying to solve the problem.

4. If these measures fail, tension rises to the "breaking point," resulting in major personality disorganization.

There are other points in crisis theory to keep in mind. First, crisis isn't pathological. Rather, it's a struggle of the individual to achieve pre-crisis equilibrium. Whether or not the crisis will be a growth process or an avenue into genuine pathology often depends on the intervention of the therapist. Also, the individual in crisis is more amenable to outside intervention than when not experiencing crisis. Furthermore, persons experiencing crisis usually send out signals to others calling for help. Therefore, the crisis interventionist has an excellent opportunity to help the individual learn and grow from this crisis.

With this in mind, we now turn to the actual "doing" of Crisis Intervention.

Assessment. As noted earlier, the assessment in Crisis Intervention is a shorter, more focused form of the traditional nursing assessment. Crisis Intervention is often conducted in 48 to 72 hours, with the client being referred to a more specialized therapist or agency, or it is done in a series of six to eight intense sessions. In addition, because it focuses on the immediate crisis problem and its resolution, many aspects of the usual nursing history are irrelevant.

If the nurse is seeing the client on the first day of the crisis, the client should be assessed for basic physical safety. For example, is the client verbalizing suicidal thoughts? If the client is seen in the community and has to travel after the interview, is he or she in enough control to drive safely?

Besides this basic safety assessment, the nurse assesses three other areas: (1) the precipitating event leading to the crisis and the client's perception of the problem; (2) the client's strengths and previous coping skills; and (3) the extent and quality of the client's support system (Haber, 1982, p. 313).

To discern the precipitating event and the client's perception of the problem, the nurse would ask questions, such as why is the client seeking help at this time, what led to the current crisis, how is the client feeling right now, and how is the problem affecting his or her life and those of people around him or her? Is the client able to function effectively in his or her basic social roles, such as parent, worker, or student?

In assessing the client's strengths and coping skills, the nurse explores the client's previous ways of dealing with crises and the methods he or she has used in attempting to reduce the current tension. In addition, the nurse also looks for particular strengths the client may possess. This is crucial in the intervention, as the client often feels ashamed or has low self-esteem for being "out of control" of life. By cataloguing the client's strengths—such as a sense of humor, past resiliency, articulateness, seeking help—the nurse will later be able to use these to reinforce the client's sense of self-worth.

Finally, the nurse assesses the client's support system and the client's use of this system in the present crisis. It is helpful to know, for example, who, if anyone, the client is close to, if there are friends who could help out in this crisis, and the names of clergy or other helping professionals the client would like to call on.

Planning. Through assessment, the client has already achieved the first step of the problem-solving process, i.e., identifying and describing the problem.

From the assessment data, the nurse is able to plan specific strategies related to (1) the client's coping abilities; (2) the client's support system and his or her willingness to marshal these forces to help resolve the crisis; (3) the severity or complexity of the crisis; and (4) the nurse's knowledge of this particular type of crisis event.

Intervention. By assessing adequately, it is expected that the nurse has established a trusting and therapeutic relationship with the client. The nurse assures the client that he or she will not abandon the client and will be available until the crisis is resolved; Crisis Intervention is not a 9 to 5 activity. Therefore, the client should have some way of reaching the therapist when not in a formal session.

If the client is in physical danger, the nurse must initiate steps to ensure physical safety. For example, a distraught client may need a ride home or a safe refuge from an abusive spouse. Again, the client with suicidal ideation may need to stay with a friend rather than be alone at home. Often getting the client to promise not to harm self provides enough motivation to help the client from carrying out harmful actions.

The nurse then assists the client through steps 2, 3, and 4 of the problem-solving process, i.e., generating possible solutions to the problem, listing the possible consequences of the various solutions, and offering support for the client's decision.

In the fifth step of the problem-solving process, the client implements his or her chosen solution. At this point it is wise for the nurse to be "on call" in case the client's actions end in failure.

Evaluation. Having carried out the client-chosen plan, the client is assisted by the nurse in evaluating the effectiveness of the solution. The basic question to answer is this: "Are you now at the same level of psychological comfort and coping as you were before the crisis?" Often the nurse will find the client better off now than before, as he or she may have deepened friendships and family bonds, found support in self-help community groups not previously known about, or made significant life alterations leading to better mental health.

Furthermore, the nurse is able to evaluate the effectiveness of the intervention on the basis of objective data. For example, is the client exhibiting a brighter affect than at the first session, less motor restlessness, better grooming?

Whether the client will be able to solve problems more effectively in the future is usually known only to the client. Because Crisis Intervention is so time-limited, the nurse does not usually learn this information.

CASE STUDY

Although Crisis Intervention has its roots in the community, it is often effectively used in acute inpatient settings. Following is the story of one such successful crisis intervention. Although the story is true, the client's name has been changed to ensure anonymity.

The Situation. L.R., a 28 year old high school teacher, was brought to the emergency room of a large southern general hospital via ambulance. On arrival, he was barely conscious. His blood alcohol level was dangerously high, and he stated he had overdosed on "downers" but didn't know what kind. He stated, "It's too much! I just can't seem to cope any more. I wish I were dead."

After his medical condition was stabilized L.R. was transferred to the acute psychiatric unit. His medical diagnosis was "depression and suicide attempt," and his nursing diagnosis was *Psychological Crisis related to feelings of Hopelessness and Powerlessness.*

The Assessment. Initially, L.R. was both angry at himself for ending up in the hospital and very ashamed of his suicide attempt. While still semiconscious, he told the admitting nurse on the unit that she couldn't possibly understand him or help him because she wasn't a gay man. This unit had a gay clinical nurse specialist, an expert in gay mental health, who was called to see L.R.

The assessment revealed that L.R. was a high school drama teacher in a small-to-medium-sized southern town. Although he accepted being gay as a positive force in his life, he had not disclosed this to his family or colleagues. He was afraid of family rejection, of losing his teaching job if those in authority knew he was gay, and of possible anti-gay bigotry of the townspeople if his sexual orientation were known. Furthermore, his only gay support system consisted of persons outside of his town, many of them living in coastal states many hundreds of miles from where he lived.

Initially, L.R. defined his problem very globally: "I'm just too stressed at work. I've gotten so many assignments at school that I'm doing the work of four people."

With some probing, however, it was learned that L.R. had a severe drinking problem resulting in past "driving while under the influence" citations, alcoholic blackouts, and overdosing on pills.

He denied now having suicidal ideation, and he signed a pledge promising not to harm himself while in the hospital. This document, also containing the promise to tell the nursing staff if he felt suicidal at a later time, was put in his chart. Such action is standard psychosocial nursing practice in acute inpatient settings.

After two hour and a half sessions, L.R. defined his crisis as a three-pronged problem: (1) alcoholism; (2) lack of freedom to share self, related to being "in the closet"; and (3) lack of assertiveness in the workplace.

The Plan. From the data gathered, the priority problem seemed to be alcoholism and alcohol abuse. Fortunately, L.R. was in a very suggestible state, and the usual denial stage found in alcoholics was quickly overcome. I decided to introduce L.R. to gay-related alcoholism literature and to some Alcoholics Anonymous readings, especially *Alcoholics Anonymous,* called the "Big Book" by AA members, and to explore options with him, such as joining AA. Furthermore, I planned to teach him about alcoholism as needed. Finally, I planned to supply him with positive gay literature while he was in the hospital.

His lack of freedom to share his gay identity, and his lack of assertion in telling the school when he had too much work to do, were crucial, although secondary, aspects of the problem. Alcoholism is in itself a primary disease, not merely a "symptom" of some other problem. Furthermore, it is always terminal if not arrested.

Finally, my plan called for conducting a miniseminar for the nursing staff related to the gay coming-out process and some of the health problems often experienced in the various stages of coming out.

The Intervention. L.R. was faced with three main choices to solve the primary problem. He could continue drinking, cut down on drinking, or abstain from all alcohol. The first choice was readily discarded; drinking is what led him to the crisis in the first place. The second option was also discarded, as controlled drinking has been shown to be ineffective in helping the alcoholic. This led L.R. to choose abstinence as the solution.

With his permission, I contacted the local gay AA group. Several men from this group took turns coming to visit L.R. in the hospital. Also, his psychiatrist gave her permission for L.R. to attend the gay AA meetings outside of the hospital and to go out for coffee with the members after meetings.

During this time, L.R. called on his gay friends for support, and the result was overwhelming. Friends began arriving from both coasts and points in between. And because both L.R. and his friends were extremely popular with both patients and staff, visiting hours on the unit became a time of great joy, laughing, and sharing even for patients who had no visitors of their own. No one was untouched by L.R. and his friends.

A miniseminar was conducted for the nursing staff. All indicated a great willingness to learn and be as helpful as possible. Following this in-service program, the staff felt freer and more knowledgeable to help L.R. Also, L.R. began being more open with the staff.

Evaluation. When L.R. first arrived on the unit, he had been intoxicated and reported problems with eating, sleeping, concentrating, and relaxing. Then, after the 4 weeks of Crisis Intervention, his sleeping, eating, and concentration were back to normal. He did have some trouble relaxing, however, as he was a high energy type of individual. His affect was bright and his outlook on life became extremely positive. He became very committed to AA and became an active member of the gay AA group. He was also very proud of the fact that his psychiatrist gave him a big hug and told him that she wished all her patients could be like him.

But L.R. went much further than successfully dealing with his alcoholism. With his new-found lease on life, he decided to tackle the other two aspects of his self-defined problem.

First, he told his family and peer teachers that he was gay after deciding that, whatever their reactions to his being gay would be, dealing with these reactions could not be worse than living an "uptight life." Fortunately, his family, his teacher colleagues, and the school principal all accepted his disclosure with solid support. In addition, his workload, which the principal agreed had gotten out of hand, was reduced.

In 1983, L.R. celebrated his first AA birthday, the first anniversary of his sobriety. Today he describes himself as "really grateful for this second chance at life."

EDITORS' COMMENTS AND QUESTIONS

Crisis Intervention is a well-established intervention that is utilized by many professional groups. Nurses are in a unique position to implement this intervention, as they so frequently encounter clients who are in crises. Nurses are well qualified to do the intervention because they are adequately prepared with communication and problem-solving skills. The case study in this chapter describes a complicated crisis, involving alcohol abuse, lack of social support, and work-related stress, and is a good example of how to apply the intervention. The case study deals with a cultural minority group that for the most part has been ignored by health care providers.

Questions for Discussion

1. Cite other clinical examples for which Crisis Intervention would be appropriate.

2. Is Crisis Intervention a necessity or a luxury in clinical settings where physiological variables need constant and careful monitoring?

3. Can all nurses be expected to do Crisis Intervention or is this a treatment to be referred to the clinical specialist?

References

Aquilera, D. C., and Messick, J. M. *Crisis intervention: Theory and Methodology (2nd ed.)*. St. Louis: C. V. Mosby, 1974.

Benter, S. E. Crisis therapy. In S. J. Sundeen and G. W. Stuart (Eds.), *Principles and practice of psychiatric nursing*. St. Louis: C. V. Mosby, 1979, pp. 368–386.

Caplan, G. *Principles of preventative psychiatry*. New York: Basic Books, 1964.

Dewey, J. *How we think*. Boston: Heath, 1910.

Ewing, C. P. *Crisis intervention as psychotherapy*. New York: Oxford University Press, 1978.

Haber, J. Crisis theory and application. In J. Haber, A. M. Leach, S. M. Schudy, and B. F. Sideleau (Eds.), *Comprehensive psychiatric nursing (2nd ed.)*. New York: McGraw-Hill Book Company, 1982, pp. 305–319.

Hoff, L. A. *People in crisis: Understanding and helping*. Menlo Park, Calif.: Addison-Wesley, 1978.

Infante, M. S. (Ed.). *Crisis theory: A framework for nursing practice*. Reston, Va.: Reston Publishing Company, 1982.

Jacobson, G., Strickler, M., and Morley, W. E. Generic and individual approaches to crisis intervention. *American Journal of Public Health*, 1968, *58*, 339–342.

Kus, R. J. *Gay freedom: An ethnography of coming out* (unpublished doctoral dissertation). Department of Sociology, University of Montana, Missoula, 1980.

Lieb, J., Lipsitch, I. I., and Slaby, A. E. *The crisis team: A handbook for the mental health professional*. Hagerstown, Md.: Harper & Row, 1973.

Lindemann, E. Symptomatology and management of acute grief. *American Journal of Psychiatry.*, 1944, *101*, 101–148.

Morley, W. E., Messick, J. M., and Aquilera, D. C. Crisis: Paradigms of intervention. *Journal of Psychiatric Nursing*, 1967, *5*, 531–544.

Parad, H. J., Resnick, H. L. P., and Parad, L. G. (Eds.). *Emergency and disaster management: A mental health sourcebook*. Bowie, Md.: Charles Press, 1976.

Powell, S., and Lively, S. Psychological crisis. In L. K. Hart, J. L. Reese, and M. O. Fearing (Eds.), *Concepts common to acute illness: Identification and management*. St. Louis: C. V. Mosby, 1981, pp. 340–353.

Riley, B. Crisis intervention. In J. Lancaster (Ed.), *Adult psychiatric nursing*. Garden City, N.Y.: Medical Examination Publishing Company, 1980, pp. 528–548.

Walkup, L. L. A concept of crisis. In J. E. Hall, and B. R. Weaver (Eds.), *Nursing of families in crisis*. Philadelphia: J. B. Lippincott, 1974, pp. 151–157.

20

PREOPERATIVE TEACHING

GERALDENE FELTON

DESCRIPTION AND DEFINITION

Preoperative Teaching is defined as *the supportive and educational actions the nurse takes to assist surgical patients in promoting their own health before and after surgery*. The patient's requirements for nursing assistance lie in the areas of decision making, acquisition of knowledge and skills, and behavior changes.

Using a nursing intervention label such as "Preoperative Teaching" means that there is a category of information—clues and evidence—that can help understand patient responses to surgery. These clues and evidence are associated with nursing diagnoses and involve a process of clinical inference based on theoretical knowledge. The process requires identification of the patient problem (or potential problem) based on observation of change or the potential for change in the patient's physiological or psychological condition; recognition of the cause of the problem; and acceptance that the responsibility for nursing intervention can be assumed by the professional nurse. Furthermore, the label "Preoperative Teaching" implies that there will be an accompanying statement of behavior (nursing goal) that the nurse expects the individual, family, or group to demonstrate as a result of the teaching. The goal statement also includes the condition under which the behavior will be expected to occur and the criteria that will provide evidence that the behavior has been demonstrated. Lastly, there will be some way to measure progress or lack of progress toward achievement of the goal. Thus, the cyclical aspect of nursing process is completed as we examine the efficacy of the intervention.

ASSOCIATED NURSING DIAGNOSES

The following represents one way of organizing nursing diagnoses related to the nursing intervention Preoperative Teaching. These diagnoses are not the only possible or valid ones. But whatever the modifications and interrelationships, the identification of nursing diagnoses associated with nursing interventions offers an exciting way to evaluate and administer responsive nursing services that aspire to the ideal of accountability.

Using the nursing diagnosis nomenclature, the actual and potential problems most applicable to the supportive educational intervention of Preoperative Teaching are the following:

- Anxiety
- Ineffective Individual or Family Coping
- Ineffective Breathing Patterns
- Alterations in Comfort
- Fear
- Impaired Gas Exchange
- Knowledge Deficit
- Sensory Perceptual Alterations
- Alteration in Tissue Perfusion
- Potential for Deep Vein Thrombosis

This list is not exhaustive but does serve to demonstrate the common and frequently encountered nursing diagnoses that would require the nursing and self-care practices implied in Preoperative Teaching, where the intervention is administered preoperatively and followed up postoperatively.

RESEARCH-RELATED LITERATURE

Preoperative Teaching has traditionally been treated in nursing as one aspect of medical-surgical nursing. But notwithstanding design, methodological, and conceptual problems, research on Preoperative Teaching does not deserve the label of "hodgepodge" assigned to it by de Tornyay (1976). Good research in the area of Preoperative Teaching provides direction for action in clinical practice.

Seligman's theory of "learned helplessness" (1975) is useful in considering the effects of surgery on the patient's sense of independence, self-control, and the development of postoperative depression and in understanding some of the behaviors that have been described by Gross (1977), Lenneberg and Rowbotham (1970), and Morrow (1976). The theory states that when an individual experiences inescapable, painful, or shocking events that occur independently of any responses he is able to make, he learns that his usual response patterns are useless and may react to future events with a sense of helplessness, futility, passivity, and depression.

Seligman identifies three stages of this type of learning. The first occurs as the individual receives information about his or her ability to control or probability of controlling outcomes in a given situation. The second stage occurs when the expectation is formed that outcomes in the situation occur independently of any of the responses the individual may make. The third stage encompasses the behavioral manifestations of motivational and emotional disturbance. As the individual accepts the concept of response-outcome independence, the incentive to respond or attempt to affect the outcomes for self is diminished or lost. When confronted with traumatic events, the individual then responds with anxious, fearful, passive behavior. If the outcomes of such events are controlled, the anxiety and fear experienced by the individual are reduced. If, however, control is not achieved, the individual may become increasingly depressed.

The major objectives of Preoperative Teaching are (1) to ensure the best possible physiological and psychological condition for an individual undergoing an operation; (2) to ensure the avoidance or reduction of postoperative discomfort and complications; and (3) to enhance wound healing and encourage activity and psychological well-being. On the basis of current research findings, it can be said that, within the nursing domain, Preoperative Teaching is psychologically and physiologically beneficial.

Research on Preoperative Teaching has been extensive. However, on examining studies published over the past decade and designed to test particular preoperative and postoperative follow-up nursing teaching strategies, there is no clear identification of the characteristics of the various physiological, psychological, sociosupportive, and educational components of the intervention that can be associated with greater and lesser effects. Rather, the studies define the nurse's actions through which the patient is assisted to modify attitudes and to develop the necessary knowledge and behaviors that aid health promotion and maintenance, enhance the quality of life, and reduce morbidity.

Of the ten areas for which Horsley and colleagues uncovered sufficient research to recommend use of the findings for protocols for implementation into nursing practice (CURN Project, 1981, 1982), three areas related to Preoperative Teaching: *Structured Preoperative Teaching; Distress Reduction through Sensory Preparation;* and *Preoperative Sensory Preparation to Promote Recovery.* In the CURN Project, the investigators first synthesized multiple research studies in a common conceptual area, then prepared and evaluated clinical protocols and specific nursing actions based on the knowledge derived from the research. The authors determined the specific merits of the research studies before transforming the individual studies into the synthesis of the *clinical protocol.*

Subsequently, Hinshaw and colleagues (1983) used earlier studies to explicate nursing interventions involved in the delivery of care, patient outcomes, and their relationships to test the impact of a preoperative teaching program on coping, anxiety, recovery pattern, pain, and patient satisfaction. Other studies, including those evaluated by the CURN investigators, may appropriately be said to offer research-based solutions for the adoption into practice of those activities involved in "Preoperative Teaching."

Table 20–1 presents useful examples of some methodologically sound, clinical experimental studies published in the years since 1971, the content of the carefully structured preoperative teaching programs and postoperative follow-up, and the composite outcomes reported by the investigators. The teaching and follow-up strategies represent the gamut of approaches used in all the studies. The outcomes represent the range of the impact of the nursing intervention. The approaches used can reasonably be expected to be equally applicable to one-to-one teaching or to group teaching. It is recommended that interested practitioners seek out these scientifically sound reports of related studies and research-based solutions, whose efficacy has been demonstrated.

FACTORS THAT INFLUENCE IMPLEMENTATION OF PREOPERATIVE TEACHING

Nursing service administration is the organizational means by which nursing is planned and implemented; nursing service administration is responsible for the forms, content, and systems of nursing care, as well as the qualitative and quantitative appraisal of the worth of the care achieved through the application of explicit criteria. Thus, nursing service administrators must

Table 20–1. EXAMPLES OF CLINICAL EXPERIMENTAL STUDIES OF OUTCOMES
OF PREOPERATIVE TEACHING PROGRAMS IN PATIENT RESPONSES
POSTOPERATIVELY

Representative Research Sources
Lindeman and Van Aernam (1971)*
Lindeman (1972)*
Minkley (1974)
Wolfer and Visintainer (1975, 1979)
Felton et al. (1976a)*
Johnson, Rice, Fuller, Eidrell (1978)*
Fortin and Kerouac (1979)
Silva (1979)
Hinshaw et al. (1983)

Content of Structured Systematic Preoperative Teaching
Diaphragmatic breathing
Effective coughing
Turning, leg exercises, and active body movement
Orientation information
Sensory information
Procedural information
Relaxation techniques
Emotional support
Pain control

Postoperative Influence (Outcomes) on Patient and Family
Improved ventilatory function
Improved physical functional capacity
Sense of well-being
Decreased length of hospital stay
Knowledge about self-care
Decreased number of analgesics
Positive postoperative mood
Decreased postoperative anxiety
Increased comfort
Satisfaction with care
Decreased frequency of complications
Decreased distress
Increased coping capability

*CURN Project personnel found sufficient research quantity and quality to recommend using the findings for protocols for nursing practice.

accept the responsibility for increasing the quality of nursing care by enhancing the quality of the climate in which nurses work. Guidance, education, research, change, and evaluation of the quality of nursing care delivered are required. Moreover, nursing care cannot be examined without considering the manner in which the entire nursing department is organized, since the social structure of care is highly predictive of the behavior patterns of the persons who occupy the various positions in the structure. Nursing administrators, then, must set in motion a plan by which nursing is assessed, planned, implemented, and evaluated.

As with any expectation for performance based on standards, the introduction and maintenance of the nursing intervention Preoperative Teaching has to be an accepted goal of the nursing staff and the nursing service administration. Here is implied both initiative and shared responsibility.

The process of implementing or extending Preoperative Teaching activities is systematic and deliberate. It begins with the philosophy of the nursing service administration and extends to the quality of the working relationships, the objectives for Preoperative Teaching, necessary equipment and supplies appropriate to the setting, and nursing assignment staffing patterns to handle the multidimensional clinical situation and allow time for Preoperative Teaching and postoperative follow-up.

Shukla (1981) posits that it is likely there is a significant interaction effect between the structure of the support systems and nurse competency. Effective Preoperative Teaching may require that opportunities be provided for nurses to acquire or maintain knowledge and skills applicable to a variety of patient populations. Staff members need to know what is expected of them and what will be rewarded. Feedback to the staff on acceptable performance can be a major motivational tool to ensure quality work. Monetary incentives, tied to clear performance objectives, have been found to be effective in motivation, particularly when the nurse has control of job quality. The nurse manager can use pay to motivate by writing fair objective standards for evaluation, by making performance checks, and by giving positive praise and reinforcement as well as monetary rewards. Finally, the new practice needs to be implemented on a pilot unit and evaluated on the basis of objectives previously decided on. Extension of the new practice to other hospital units awaits successful outcome of the pilot testing. Successful implementation of Preoperative Teaching should make the nursing process more visible and more important.

No clear and singular pattern for the implementation of Preoperative Teaching is reported in the research literature. For example, the time duration in which a nurse plans and carries out preoperative nursing may span hospital admission to discharge and beyond, or cover only the time immediately before surgery to 24 to 48 hours after surgery. One nurse may be responsible for all Preoperative Teaching, or all nurses on a unit may share responsibilities. Patients may be taught and supervised individually or in groups. It is clear, however, that the approaches chosen for use (i.e., one-to-one, group teaching, slide tape series, demonstrations, pictures, audiotapes, lecture-discussions) must be appropriate to the particular setting and the client in the setting. Furthermore, the literature indicates those aspects associated with effective Preoperative Teaching.

1. An orientation to Preoperative Teaching is necessary so that the full range of behaviors can be modeled.

2. Nurses who want to be responsible for managing nursing practice and who are able to work with other professionals in the joint planning of care must be available.

3. Staffing patterns must promote the concept of accountability and support and complement expected behaviors.

4. The organization must desire Preoperative Teaching.

5. A strong and knowledgeable chief nurse manager is needed to act as a buffer in a hostile system.

6. The system must monitor standards of care and quality, effectiveness, and efficiency of service. Reflected in the list are components of professionalization, accountability, autonomy, coordination of services, continuity, and adequate administrative support to ensure that high standards can be met and quality care delivered (Task Force on Nursing Practice in Hospitals, 1983).

INTERVENTION AND EVALUATION TOOLS

The nursing research literature on Preoperative Teaching appropriate for adoption in practice recommends prescriptions for practice that vary in content, time of implementation, and delivery methods. However, since attribution of cause-and-effect relationships is not easy to make, tools to measure results have appeared.

For instance, for a group of elective surgical patients, Fortin and Kerouac (1977) developed a questionnaire to evaluate a structured preoperative educational program. The effectiveness of the preoperative teaching program was measured by improved physical functional capacity of patients following surgery. Questions used by Fortin and Kerouac asked about assistance in washing the face, shaving, dressing, undressing, combing the hair, using the toilet, preparing food, and feeding oneself. When the patient reported difficulty, other questions were asked that sought to elicit the kind of assistance required, such as having food specially prepared, having food placed in containers, or supervision when eating.

The Fortin and Kerouac instrument was determined to have both content validity and concurrent validity. Other tools to evaluate the outcomes of Preoperative Teaching are described elsewhere (Johnson et al., 1975). Moreover, the practice protocols developed by CURN project personnel also have an evaluation procedure that includes the effect on staff and the organization as well as the effect on the patient.

A second example of an evaluation tool appears in Table 20–2. The Ostomy Outcome Questionnaire (Felton et al., 1983) was designed to evaluate preoperative teaching programs for clients undergoing ostomy surgery. Measures are taken at discharge and again at 6 months after discharge.

Table 20–2. OSTOMY OUTCOME QUESTIONNAIRE*

Yes	No	Outcomes at Discharge
		1. Has skills necessary for ostomy care Will demonstrate a. Performing his irrigation
		b. Care of the skin
		c. Management of skin breakdown
		d. Care of the pouch
		e. Application of stomal appliance
		2. Has information necessary for ostomy management Can describe
		a. Methods of managing odor
		b. Relationship of diet to gas formation
		c. Early signs and symptoms of complications
		d. One method of managing skin breakdown
		e. One method of managing diarrhea
		f. One method of managing constipation
		g. Signs and symptoms that require assistance from professional source
		h. One method of managing spillage
		3. Has information about available resources Can identify a. One community group that deals with problems of ostomates
		b. Two sources by which to obtain ostomy supplies
		c. A self-help group for ostomates
		d. Another person able to perform ostomy care for him/her in the event he/she cannot

Table continued on following page

Table 20–2. OSTOMY OUTCOME QUESTIONNAIRE* (*Continued*)

Yes	No	Outcomes at Discharge
		4. Has information for health maintenance Can describe a. The nature of her/his surgery in own words
		b. Own plans for resumption of activities to include: 1) Self care
		2) Recreation
		3) Sexual activity
		4) Work
		c. Time of follow-up appointments (clinic, physician)
		5. Demonstrates coping behaviors Is able to a. Look at the stoma without grimacing
		b. Handle ostomy equipment
		c. Manage ostomy independently
		d. Talk about ostomy and its management
		e. Verbalize feelings about way ostomy looks
		f. Verbalize feelings about diagnosis
		g. Resume grooming behavior
		h. Talk about events other than those related to self and own illness
		i. Allow spouse (significant others) to view stoma
		6. Has achieved an optimal health status On inspection a. Abdominal wound is dry
		b. Perineal wound is clean although sero-sanguinous drainage may be present
		c. Peristomal skin is intact
		d. Weight is within 10 lbs of pre-op level
		e. Bowel evacuations are predictable once a day with less than 30 ml spillage
		f. Odor is not detectable within proximity of patient
		g. Pulse rate is 60 to 90 beats per minute
		h. Respiratory rate is 12 to 22 beats per minute
		i. Temperature is not more than 100.0 degrees Fahrenheit orally
		j. There are no complaints of discomfort, i.e., pain, insomnia
		k. Diet is tolerated. Note: Mild distress—any discomfort reported which does interfere with adequate nourishment. Includes patients whose discomfort is relieved or prevented by antiemetics. Includes nausea, gas pains, small emesis. Severe distress—any discomfort which interferes with adequate nourishment. Includes vomiting, severe anorexia, diarrhea.

Table 20–2. OSTOMY OUTCOME QUESTIONNAIRE* (*Continued*)

Yes	No	Outcomes at Six Months
		Has achieved an optimal health state 1. Skin is intact
		2. Weight is within normal range
		3. Evacuations are predictable
		4. Odor not detectable
		5. No complaints of discomfort
		6. Can identify those foods that cause distress (diarrhea, con-stipation, gaseous upset)
		7. Time for stoma care takes no longer than one hour
		8. Utilizes two available resources
		9. Has kept follow-up appointment(s)
		10. Has resumed pre-operative level of social and recreational activity
		11. Has resumed pre-operative level of sexual activity (barring physical impairment)
		12. Has resumed pre-operative level of physical activity
		13. Experimented with no more than three types of skin bar-riers and appliances until appropriate equipment was found
		14. No report of use of emergency medical services for non-urgent care
		15. Has successfully adapted home environment to ostomy care

*From Felton, G., Lotas, M., and Eastman, D. A tool for research in the clinical setting: Outcomes for educational programs for stoma clients. In G. Felton and M. Albert (Eds.), *Nursing research: A monograph for non-nurse researchers.* Iowa City: University of Iowa, 1983, pp. 6–27.

Tools such as these are particularly useful because they document the effectiveness of nursing care. A major thrust within the health care delivery system over the past several years has been the development of comprehensive quality assurance programs. Agencies have increasingly felt the need to evaluate and document the effectiveness of the full range of services they provide. Evaluation refers to making judgments about merit, success, excellence, or quality. For nursing administrators, evaluation applied to direct clinical practice is represented as the foundation for ensuring quality of nursing services.

In evaluation, whether outcome or process is emphasized depends on the nature of agency responsibility and the questions that the agency believes must be asked. The most direct answer to a question such as, "Does Preoperative Teaching indicate that the patient receives good care?" would seem to derive from an examination of the process of the Preoperative Teaching. If the question is, "What good, if any, are we doing?", the answer is obviously to be found in the outcomes of the Preoperative Teaching. However, the distinction between process and outcome is, to some extent, an abstraction. Between the initiation of care and its termination are a number of completed tasks and states of the patient that can be used as indicators of the quality of care. A well-founded system of quality appraisal must include assessments of structure, process, and end results, to the extent that each of these is observable and measurable under the constraints inherent in any given setting.

Quality control in Preoperative Teaching means the purposeful structure of an organizational system. Within this system can be found a constellation of standards, measures, laws, policies, procedures, and individual commitments to ensure the delivery of services that are consistent with predicted anticipated outcomes. The major step in the evaluation of quality is the formulation of criteria or yardsticks against which judgments can be made. Criteria are descriptive statements of performance, behavior, circumstances, or clinical status that represent a satisfactory, positive, or excellent state of affairs. In evaluating Preoperative Teaching, criteria explicitly describe the assessable elements of the care process that can be used to measure quality. They are stated in the form of desired or expected manifestations and they will require assessment of the health status of the patient, the health knowledge of the patient, and the patient's readiness to assume responsibility for self-care.

The evaluation of existing and proposed preoperative nursing regimens to determine their effects on patient health outcome status and how their implementation affects the quality of the delivery of health services is crucial. Consumers not only demand answers to questions about the health care they receive, but also view health education as a right. Providing appropriate information and making it meaningful to the patient or significant other enhance the ability of the patient to gain a necessary sense of control and competence in relation to his or her own health care.

Evaluation of Preoperative Teaching programs is needed not only to broaden perceptions of the value of nursing intervention, but also to determine what logically goes into the costs of nursing services that affect patient outcomes of uneventful convalescence and self-care. Self-care is an emerging concept of health care and is composed of several components. These components include patients developing their own definitions of health and identifying their priorities, options, and risk indices; developing abilities for living a healthful life; preventing and managing disease; assessing and intervening in health and illness; and using the health care system. Self-care emphasizes growth and health as the goals for the services professional nursing offers.

GROUP CASE STUDY

Research on the needs of the ostomy patient provides a good example of the basis for the intervention of Preoperative Teaching and resulted in the tool presented in Table 20–2. For greater clarity, the rationale for the research and a description of the development of the tool are given in considerable detail.

The literature suggests that the problems facing ostomy patients have not been well handled by medicine and nursing. The impact that the creation of a permanent stoma will have on the individual's ability to function as a member of society for the remainder of his or her life is seldom considered when planning and implementing hospital care. Much of the information that is available focuses primarily on identification of problems of individuals with permanent colostomies, even though patients with other kinds of ostomies and temporary colostomies may have more problems in management.

Physiological responses of the ostomy subject have been described as major and minor. Review of the literature indicates the major complications found among colostomates and ileostomates include stenosis, herniation, prolapse, retraction, fistulas, perforation, and bleeding. Minor complications (which can lead to major complications) have also been described by Sterling and McIlrath (1970) and Lenneberg and Mendelssohn (1971). They include skin irritation (caused by a poorly fitting appliance or improper cleaning), constipation, abdominal distention, pain, nausea, vomiting, diarrhea, gas, and odor. Many minor complications are diet and fluid related.

Psychological responses to ostomy surgery have been well documented. Initially, responses of depression, altered perception of body image, and lowered self-esteem were identified as common among colostomates; these lasted as long as 5 to 15 years beyond the operation. Other responses in the immediate postoperative period include fear of spillage; fear of loss of sexual attractiveness; feelings of weakness, fragility, passivity, vulnerability, and inferiority; and preoccupation with, involvement in, and resentment of long, ritualistic care of the ostomy. These responses have also been described as reasons for later restriction in social activities (Druss, O'Connor, and Stein, 1968; Lenneberg and Rowbotham, 1970; Orbach and Tallent, 1965).

Ostomates' patterns of sexual withdrawal were reported by Sutherland in 1968. In 1975, Wirsching, Druner, and Herman studied 214 colostomates and found a significant number showed a decrease in sexual activity, with almost half (48 per cent) indicating no sexual activity at all. In addition, the finding that colostomates visit friends and attend the theater significantly less often than noncolostomates led them to conclude that colostomates are less active both in seeking out social contact and in initiating close contact. The Wirsching group labeled these phenomena "social impotence" and "negative social resonance."

Even before the study by Wirsching and colleagues, Lenneberg and Rowbotham (1970) posed questions to 1425 ileostomates one year postoperatively to determine the impact of an ileostomy on the person's vocational activities. The findings showed that individuals with ileostomies suffer from disability and discrimination.

As indicated previously, Seligman's theory appears generally applicable to persons having major surgery and to the ostomy patients in particular. In the ostomate, two experiential phases have been identified. The stoma patient first experiences uncontrollable outcomes with the impact of the diagnosis itself. Whatever the diagnosis, the effect is that once the diagnosis is made no response by the patient can significantly affect the medical outcome or the need for surgery. The surgery must be accepted passively.

The second experience of uncontrollable outcomes occurs in relation to the subsequent loss of the ability to control the process of elimination. In varying degrees, elimination occurs independently of any efforts to control it; since the process cannot be controlled, it must therefore be accepted. The passivity of Seligman's theory of learned helplessness is accompanied by decreased energy, inability to accomplish tasks, difficulty in concentration, and erosion of motivation and ambition, all combining to impair efficient functioning. It is this constellation of psychological responses that militate against the development of desirable self-care behaviors. The effect of ostomy surgery is to create in the individual a sense of loss of the ability to control aspects of his or her life. The purpose of the nursing intervention of Preoperative Teaching is to provide the information necessary for the patient to regain a sense of control.

On the basis of this theoretical formulation, Felton, Lotas, and Eastman (1983) developed the Ostomy Outcome Questionnaire in Table 20–2. The questionnaire identifies the patient's performance behaviors, knowledge, and self-care skills to be expected as an outcome of Preoperative Teaching and postoperative follow-up. Thus, the content of the tool is representative of the domain of behaviors that define the knowledge, psychological status, and performance requirements of one classification of patients, the ostomy subject. The evidence for content validity of the Ostomy Outcome Questionnaire consisted of expert opinions provided by teachers, practitioners, and subject matter experts with extensive knowledge in professional practice. Such a general consensus approach to content validity is as useful to the practitioner as to the researcher.

This tool dictates the content of the nursing intervention with the typical ostomate. However, it is to be remembered that the tool is not refined to the extent that it can elicit all the information every expert would consider indispensable for every population of ostomates. For example, questions about irrigations would not be appropriate for the ileostomate or the urostomate who does not irrigate. Questions that do not apply to a particular subject may simply be marked "not applicable". Subsequent use of the Questionnaire may require some modifications in the questions, or different editions of the Questionnaire may be used to make clear exactly what information is wanted or to test other possible ways to present some questions. Since the tool is a guide for the content of the Preoperative Teaching, scoring involves simply counting the number of "yes" answers. "Yes" responses give indication of the attainment of skills necessary for care and management, coping, and optimal health status.

Use of this tool in one study (Felton et al., 1983) reaffirmed the boundless opportunities to demonstrate how the efficacy of Preoperative Teaching can be measured by patient outcomes. A tool similar to the Questionnaire could be designed and tested for other groups of patients in such a way as to guide Preoperative Teaching for other classifications of surgical patients and their families and allow a mechanism to systematically and critically evaluate effects.

CONCLUSION

The accretion of knowledge from research on Preoperative Patient Teaching mandates attention to its efficacy as a nursing intervention. Unfortunately, the widespread use of unstructured Preoperative Teaching with little postoperative evaluation masks its significance as an effective, reliable, and objective method of monitoring and eventually altering undesirable patient responses. Preoperative Teaching is an intervention to be applied judiciously by professionals who treat, and serve, and understand the whole person. By acquiring sound knowledge, nurses and other professionals can ensure the use of Preoperative Teaching as a legitimate nursing intervention for helping patients in a scientifically correct and ethical manner.

EDITORS' COMMENTS AND QUESTIONS

This chapter has presented a theoretical discussion of the intervention of Preoperative Teaching. Emphasis has been placed upon the research base and recommendations concerning evaluation of the intervention. Structured Preoperative Teaching has been shown to be more effective than Unstructured Preoperative Teaching. In order to implement Structured Preoperative Teaching there must be organizational support of the nursing efforts. Beginning readers who are looking for specific steps to implement Preoperative Teaching are referred to the CURN protocol entitled "Structured Preoperative Teaching" cited in the references.

Questions for Discussion

1. What are the benefits of Preoperative Teaching?

2. Is Sensory Preparation a part of Preoperative Teaching or a separate intervention? How can Sensory Preparation and Preoperative Teaching be used together?

3. What are the commonalities and the differences between Preoperative Teaching and Patient Teaching, which is discussed in Chapter 12?

4. The author points out several barriers in the system that prevent good Preoperative Teaching. Identify other barriers that impede successful implementation of this intervention.

References

CURN Project (J. Horsley, Ed.). Using research to improve nursing practice. New York: Grune & Stratton. Series of Clinical Protocols: Clean Intermittent Catheterization (1982), Closed Urinary Drainage Systems (1981), Distress Reduction Through Sensory Preparation (1981), Intravenous Cannula Change (1981), Mutual Goal Setting in Patient Care (1982), Pain: Deliberative Nursing Interventions (1982), Preoperative Sensory Preparation to Promote Recovery (1981), Preventing Decubitus Ulcers (1981), Reducing Diarrhea in Tube-Fed Patients (1981), Structured Preoperative Teaching (1981).

Druss, R. G., O'Connor, J. G., and Stein, L. Psychological response to colostomy. Archives of General Psychiatry, 1968, 18, 53–58.

Felton, G., Huss, K., Payne, E., and Srsic, K. Preoperative nursing intervention with the patient for surgery: Outcomes of three alternative approaches. International Journal of Nursing Studies, 1976a, 13, 84–96.

Felton, G., Frevert, E., Galligan, K., Neill, M., and Williams, L. Pathway to accountability: Implementation of a quality assurance program. Journal of Nursing Administration, January, 1976b.

Felton, G., Lotas, M., and Eastman, D. A tool for for research in the clinical setting: Outcomes of educational programs for stoma clients In G. Felton amd M. Albert (Eds.), Nursing research: A monograph for non-nurse researchers. Iowa City: University of Iowa, 1983, pp. 6–27.

Flaherty, G. G., and Fitzpatrick, J. J. Relaxation: Technique to increase comfort level of postoperative patients. A preliminary study. Nursing Research, 1977, 27, 352–355.

Fortin, F., and Kerouac, S. Validation of questionnaires on physical function. Nursing Research, 1977, 26(2), 128–135.

Gross, L. Enterostomal therapy and ostomy rehabilitation programs. Alabama Journal of Medical Sciences, 1977, 14(1), 50–55.

Hinshaw, A. S., et al. The use of predictive modeling to test nursing practice outcomes. Nursing Research, 1983, 32, 35–42.

Johnson, J. E. Sensory information, instruction in coping strategy and recovery from surgery. Research in Nursing and Health, 1978, 1, 4–17.

Johnson, J. E., Rice, V. H., Fuller, S. S., and Endress, M. P. Sensory information, instruction in a coping strategy, and recovery from surgery. *Research in Nursing and Health*, 1978, *1*, 4–7.

Johnson, J. E., et al. Altering children's distress behavior during orthopedic cast removal. *Nursing Research*, 1975, *24*, 404–410.

Johnson, J. E., Fuller, S. S., Endress, M. P., and Rice, V. H. Altering patients' responses to surgery: An extension and replication. *Research in Nursing and Health*, 1978, *1*, 111–121.

Kinney, M. R. Effects of preoperative teaching upon patients with differing modes of response to threatening stimuli. *International Journal of Nursing Studies*, 1977, *14*(1), 49–59.

Lenneburg, E., and Mendelssohn, A. *Colostomies: A guide.* Los Angeles: United Ostomy Association, 1971.

Lenneburg, E., and Rowbotham, J. L. *The ileostomy patient.* Springfield, Ill.: Charles C Thomas, 1970.

Lindeman, C. Nursing intervention with the presurgical patient: Effectiveness and efficiency of group and individual preoperative teaching--phase two. *Nursing Research*, 1972, *21*, 196–209.

Lindeman, C., and Van Aernam, B. Nursing intervention with the presurgical patient: The effects of structured and unstructured preoperative teaching. *Nursing Research*, 1971, *20*, 319–322.

Minkley, B. B. Physiologic and psychologic responses of elective surgery patients. *Nursing Research*, 1974, *23*, 392–401.

Morrow, L. Psychological problems following ileostomy and colostomy. *Mt. Sinai Journal of Medicine*, 1976, *43*(4), 368–370.

Orbach, C. E., and Tallent, M. Modification of perceived body and of body concepts. *Archives of General Psychiatry*, 1965, *12*, 126–135.

Seligman, M. *Helplessness.* San Francisco: W. H. Freeman, 1975.

Shukla, R. K. Structure vs. people in primary nursing: An inquiry. *Nursing Research*, 1981, *30*(4), 236–241.

Silva, M. C. Effects of orientation information on spouses' anxieties and attitudes toward hospitalization and surgery. *Research in Nursing and Health*, 1979, *2*, 127–136.

Sterling, W., and McIlrath, O. A normal life with a colostomy. *Postgraduate Medicine*, February 1970.

Sutherland, A. Psychological responses to colostomy. *Psychological impact of cancer.* American Cancer Society, 1968.

Task Force on Nursing Practice in Hospitals. *Magnet hospitals: Attraction and retention of professional nurses.* Kansas City, Mo.: American Nurses' Association, 1983.

Tornyay, R. *Nursing research in the bicentennial year.* Boulder, Colo.: Western Interstate Commission for Higher Education, 1976.

Visintainer, M. A., and Wolfer, J. A. Psychological preparation for surgical pediatric patients: The effects on children's and parents' stress responses and adjustment. *Pediatrics*, 1975, *56*, 187.

Wirching, M., Druner, H. U., and Hermann, G. Results of psychosocial adjustment to long-term colostomy. *Psychotherapy and Psychomatics*, 1975, *26*(5), 245–246.

Wolfer, J. A., and Visintainer, M. A. Pediatric surgical patients' and parents' stress responses and adjustment as a function of psychologic preparation and stress-point nursing care. *Nursing Research*, 1975, *24*, 244–255.

Wolfer, J. A., and Visintainer, M. A. Prehospital psychological preparation for tonsillectomy patients: Effects on children's and parents' adjustment. *Pediatrics*, 1979, *64*(5), 646–655.

21

SURVEILLANCE

CYNTHIA M. DOUGHERTY
MARILYN T. MOLEN

B. S. is a 27 year old construction worker who developed congestive cardio-myopathy following a viral infection. He contracted a subsequent respiratory infection, which resulted in an exacerbation of his congestive heart failure, placing him in a life-threatening condition. In order to save his life, he was hospitalized in the coronary care unit and intra-aortic balloon pumping (IABP) was instituted in an attempt to reverse his impending cardiogenic shock.

B. S. is typical of the critical care patient who, in a life-threatening situation, may require the nursing intervention of Surveillance.

DEFINITION AND DESCRIPTION

Surveillance in the critical care situation is defined as *the application of behavioral and cognitive processes in the systematic collection of information used to make judgments and predictions about a person's life status.*

Webster's dictionary (second college edition, 1970) defines surveillance as: "to watch over, a close watch, a vigil, to look over and examine closely, or to view or study as a whole." Surveillance is similar to observation, which is defined by Webster as: "an act or the power of seeing or fixing the mind upon something; gathering information by noting facts or occurrences."

Surveillance encompasses observation, in that the gathering of information through watching, feeling, or touching is part of this intervention. Both observation and surveillance are oriented toward collecting as much information as necessary to achieve a particular purpose. But Surveillance extends beyond observation in two ways. It utilizes more and different types of methods to gather the data, and it includes an evaluative or judgment component. This evaluation component is essential to establishing a nursing diagnosis and in predicting patient outcomes.

Thus, Surveillance is both a behavioral and a cognitive process. Information is gathered to determine how to deal with future developments, to make estimates about knowable things that are not obvious, and to make judgments about things that are unknowable. Estimates are made because a

301

certain situation requires close scrutiny (Dulles, 1963). In this instance, Surveillance is the primary nursing intervention in a critical care, life-threatening situation.

The behavioral component of Surveillance involves the collection of information from both primary and secondary sources. Direct data collection will include inspection, palpation, percussion, and auscultation (Papenhausen, 1981; Sedlock, 1981). Secondary sources of information may involve the use of several types of highly technical equipment.

The cognitive component of Surveillance includes studying, interpreting, analyzing, evaluating, and intercepting data to indicate a range of probabilities and isolating those factors that are influencing a given situation (Dulles, 1963). The process of Surveillance involves knowing both where to look, or remembering how frequently certain observations are required, and when to expect a change in response to a treatment (Karch, 1976). A basic understanding of normal and abnormal findings is essential, since we see only what we know (Winslow, 1976). Perception and the ability to relate sensory stimuli to some relevant knowledge or previous experience are two important elements of Surveillance. From direct study, and from a theoretical orientation, we accumulate factual information that gives relevance to what we see (Winslow, 1976). The nurse is responsible, in the critical care situation, for interpreting signs and symptoms with a high degree of accuracy and for reporting abnormalities to those responsible for decision making (Pool, 1976). It is vital to know what to look for because, in Surveillance, the most obvious sign may not be the most important one to monitor.

Knowing when to look, what to look for, and why to look, are basic characteristics of Surveillance. Establishing baseline data and preparing a systematic method for Surveillance techniques are also essential components of this nursing intervention. Successful Surveillance is derived from the piecing together of tiny items of information, which, taken by themselves, may appear to be unimportant (Seth, 1957). It involves the utilization of facts to make conclusions, decisions, and predictions; therefore, the act of gathering data within specified parameters must be a reliable process (Seth, 1963).

Because of the critical nature of the situation, Surveillance involves continuous recording and reporting of data. In Surveillance, both the time for data collection and the parameters used for information gathering must be determined carefully. Surveillance of the critically ill patient becomes legitimate when information that is obtained through observation is evaluated and used to take actions directed toward saving the patient's life.

The purpose of most intensive care units is to carefully watch or monitor specific signs or symptoms in order to intervene quickly or prevent a disaster from occurring (Griffin, 1976). With complex organ dysfunction in a life-threatening condition, many aspects of the patient's signs and symptoms and response to treatment are monitored closely and frequently (Hayward, 1977). Thus, time and the acuteness of the situation are the structural components of Surveillance.

Relatively minor changes in the critically ill patient are often very important, and if detected quickly enough may make it possible to avoid further complications or death (Chalmers, 1977). To do this, the ordering of priorities in critical care needs to be systematic and routinized. Treatments need to be set into motion without delay, and data must be extracted as rapidly as possible, analyzed speedily, and acted upon (Weil and Carlson, 1976).

RELATED LITERATURE REVIEW

The concept of surveillance has been abstracted from literature primarily in the field of intelligence related to espionage. In this field, surveillance suggests that a judgment has been made by some governmental unit that the behavior being monitored is outside the range of legitimate political power. In the case of the person being watched, the events under surveillance are categorized as potentially threatening and the individual functions appropriately in terms of his or her own well-being to avoid or minimize the perceived possible negative consequences.

In Eastern Europe, the Soviet Union, and Nazi Germany, surveillance has been used as an intrinsic control to maintain the governmental structure. Political surveillance has been used as a term to describe a set of techniques employed in the collection of political information about a "subject." These activities have been used to produce a set of political assumptions (Askin, 1973). Blum (1972, p. 98) has defined surveillance as "watching, recording, and compiling information about another person's activities and movements, for whatever purposes such information can be used by the person for whom it is gathered." Thus, surveillance has an open-ended meaning with control of the information clearly left to the one who has undertaken the surveillance.

In American society, surveillance also has had a negative connotation, but is less threatening. In the United States surveillance implies that some actor or entity has subjected another actor or entity to being watched because of the probability that he or she has been doing something contrary to established practice (Askin, 1973, p. 74).

Intelligence, which is a synonym of surveillance, involves the process of information gathering followed by evaluation, judgment, or prediction, and then reporting the findings to some organization or group that is participating in the policy-making process (Blum, 1972).

In 1955, a task force on intelligence activities of the Second Herbert Hoover Commission, in an advisory report to the government, stated: "Intelligence deals with all the things which should be known in advance of initiating a course of action" (Dulles, 1963, p. 9). Again, the implication of surveillance or intelligence is that information is used to predict consequences as a basis for action.

As stated earlier, information is gathered about an individual or group to determine how to deal with future developments and to make estimates about knowable things that may not be obvious or about things that may not be knowable. Estimates are made because some member of the intelligence community thinks that a particular situation requires attention. Generally, in the political sphere, this situation has had negative or threatening implications.

The very nature of information evokes power in any decision-making situation. In the intelligence literature, it is apparent that the decision to place a subject under surveillance is made by some agency or some level of government. The usual justification for the surveillance is the likelihood or actuality that certain acts planned by the subject are either criminal in nature or detrimental to the national security. The subsequent gathering of data implies a rather strong indication that the information collected will be used for a specific purpose (Askin, 1973).

The process of surveillance has involved an ongoing "development" of information about events, persons, groups, and even attitudes of large segments of the population (Blum, 1972). Surveillance must have planning and structure. Objectives are outlined, priorities are established, and obstacles are examined.

Information that is gathered is of little use unless it reaches the hands of the decision-maker. In priority cases, someone has to decide what constitutes important information. Special watch is kept to scan incoming data for anything of a critical nature, clues are sorted, and ideas are exchanged as to the development of an impending crisis. Because there is not time to submit every item for detailed analysis, "raw" intelligence can become a dangerous thing without an understanding of the circumstances under which it was gathered. Therefore, information must be interpreted within these circumstances (Dulles, 1963).

Because the concept of surveillance has emerged in the field of intelligence or espionage, implications of deviance and secrecy have been associated with it. Espionage is chiefly a matter of circumventing obstacles in order to reach the objective of gathering data secretly. It uses agents, sources, and informants to gain access to a person, place, or thing to discover the facts without arousing the attention of those who might want to protect the information (Dulles, 1963). With espionage, gaining access to the information is as important as the knowledge gained from the secret activity. It is not uncommon for the agent to "plant" himself or herself into the office or circle of another power in order to elicit desired information from those who are trusting and unaware of the agent's role (Seth, 1963). Continuous reporting of the information obtained is obviously difficult in these situations, where the agent's presence is either secret or illegal.

When viewed in the light of police operations, criminal investigations, or political or intelligence activities, surveillance stigmatizes or labels those behaviors under close watch as deviant. When applied to a hospital situation in which patients have voluntarily placed themselves in the care of professionals for the purpose of remedying a health problem, the act of Surveillance is legitimate and appropriate. In this instance, information gathering is the basis for establishing a diagnosis and making prompt intervention in order to resolve the problem. Therefore, in the hospital setting, Surveillance is both legitimate and necessary for the patient in a life-threatening situation. The specific purpose for collecting information in this situation is to save the patient's life.

Surveillance of the critically ill patient is important because the information gathered is utilized to either benefit the patient or prevent his death. Patients in critical care settings receive more frequent and more detailed Surveillance activities than patients with less acute health problems. In complex organ dysfunction or life-threatening conditions, many aspects of the patient's symptoms and response to treatment are carefully monitored in order to quickly intervene when necessary (Hayward, 1977).

For the acutely ill patient, systematic observing and recording will increase the nurse's ability to predict disasters (Karch, 1976). Because complications can occur rapidly, a baseline from which to recognize changes in the patient's condition is needed. In these situations, systematic assessment of vital signs and symptoms can save lives (Karch, 1976). Without Surveillance in the critical care situation, important information is likely to be overlooked; and as a result, problems of life-threatening proportion may either be missed altogether or be misidentified.

We have already stated that in nursing the process of Surveillance involves knowing what to look for, where to look, remembering how frequently certain observations are required, and knowing when to expect certain changes as a result of treatment. In Surveillance, the more obvious signs and symptoms may not always be the most essential ones to be watching. Thus, the nurse must have a good understanding of normal and abnormal findings as well as their significance to the prognosis of the patient. In the critical care situation, the nurse frequently monitors certain patient parameters, signs and symptoms, laboratory values, x-ray reports, and responses to medication, in reference to a particular medical and nursing diagnosis. Any abnormality that is detected is promptly evaluated for the purpose of instituting interventions to save the patient's life.

The cognitive and behavioral aspects of Surveillance will be described separately.

BEHAVIORAL COMPONENT

The behavioral component of Surveillance involves collecting information by physical observations and, according to the literature on surveillance, may encompass familiar as well as some strange forms and activities (Blum, 1972).

In the intelligence field, information may be obtained from both primary and secondary sources, such as governmental records, and people, including neighbors, business associates, acquaintances, family, and relatives. Watching and listening are basic behavioral activities of surveillance. Information may also be gathered by means of examining letters, notes, bills, memoranda, newspapers, security indexes, books, codes, and journals or by checking garbage can contents or traffic routes (Askin, 1973; Blum, 1972; Seth, 1957). Surveillance may be carried out by physically following another person's actions for a specific period of time or by collecting data through the use of electronic devices, such as wiretaps, listening devices, tape recorders, video-tapes, cameras, and closed circuit television (Blum, 1972; Dulles, 1963).

In the critical care situation, the behavioral component of Surveillance includes direct observation of the patient to survey mental and physical status. Methods include checking pupils, observing eyes, checking color of skin and mucous membranes, noting external jugular veins for distention, taking vital signs, auscultating heart and lung sounds, palpating pedal pulses, noting edema and temperature of extremities, and recording reactions to medications (Hayward, 1977; Owen, 1982; Pool, 1976; Weil, 1976; Winslow, 1976).

It also includes indirect observation with the use of several kinds of technical or electronic equipment, such as cardiac output computers, venti-lators, fluoroscope equipment, intravenous pumps, and laboratory facilities (Weil and Carlson, 1976).

COGNITIVE COMPONENT

As stated earlier, the cognitive aspect of Surveillance involves the collection and evaluation of data to draw conclusions and make predictions. In order to do this, the act of gathering information must be a reliable process. All observations should be tailored to suit the individual patient. Recognition of inappropriate signs becomes easier when the exact nature of what is being looked for is known. Thus, a theoretical knowledge base underlying the information collection is an essential part of the cognitive component of Surveillance. Establishing baseline data for future comparison is part of this cognitive process. A systematic head-to-toe assessment includes looking, seeing, understanding, recording, and reporting (Karch, 1976). However, with-out an understanding of the significance of changes as they occur, the value of close surveillance of a patient is lost.

The cognitive component of Surveillance requires the agent—in this case the nurse—to have certain attributes or skills. Among these are the theoretical base and clinical skill to implement the behavioral components of Surveillance.

The attributes required of the nurse using Surveillance in the critical care area are similar to those of an effective intelligence officer identified in the basic surveillance literature. They include the ability to be perceptive about people; to work well with others in difficult conditions; to distinguish between essentials and nonessentials; to be ingenious, inquisitive, and intelligent; to pay attention to detail; to express ideas clearly and briefly; to make rapid decisions; and to be nonjudgmental (Dulles, 1963; Pool, 1976; Seth, 1963; Winslow, 1976). In addition, Surveillance by the nurse in the critical care setting requires certain technical skills necessary for operating the monitoring equipment and for performing the physical assessment. Although these attributes cannot always be observed by another person watching the nurse carry out Surveillance, they are nonetheless very important aspects of this intervention.

SUMMARY

The concept of Surveillance has been abstracted from the field of intelligence, or espionage, where it is initiated by the agent because of some expected deviation from an expected practice. In this context secrecy is used to gain information without arousing the attention of those who might want to protect the information.

When applied to the critical care situation, Surveillance is determined to be a legitimate nursing intervention because of the dependency status of the patient, who is in a life-threatening circumstance. In this case the secrecy implies an unawareness by the patient of this intervention. Although his or her life depends on the process of the surveillance, he or she may not be consciously aware of the intervention at the time it is being utilized. Part of the "secrecy" surrounding Surveillance is that it is conducted in an unobtrusive manner in order that it may not generate anxiety in the patient or family during this critical period.

In both the intelligence field and the critical care setting, Surveillance has behavioral and cognitive aspects. Surveillance is more than observation in that it includes the collection of vast amounts of relatively minute pieces of information from primary and secondary sources. This information is evaluated in order to predict certain actions and outcomes. Successful Surveillance involves putting together these small amounts of information in some meaningful way. Time and the life status of the patient are at stake in the critical care situation, in which Surveillance may be the only appropriate intervention of the moment. Thus, the cognitive and behavioral requirements of the nurse are particularly significant since the patient's life depends on the success of this intervention.

INTERVENTION TOOLS

From our experience and a review of the literature, we have concluded that there are two basic elements to any Surveillance tool. These are (1) time, measured in seconds, minutes, or hours; and (2) parameters of interest, such as vital signs or blood gas levels. Several examples of Surveillance tools exist in the form of flow sheets used in critical care areas.

The medical and nursing diagnoses will help to determine both the frequency of data collection and the types of information needed during the surveillance. In general, the more critical or life-threatening the situation, the more frequently the parameters of interest should be monitored and evaluated.

Parameters of interest for an acute cardiac patient, such as B. S. in the case study, would be those that give direct indication of cardiovascular function. These would include blood pressure, urine output, neurological status, respiratory function, and laboratory values. These parameters would be monitored as frequently as necessary (every 5 to 15 minutes) in order to detect slight changes so that the appropriate measure might be initiated to prevent disaster or death (see Table 21–1 for an example of this tool).

Successful Surveillance used to prevent disaster or death in the critical care situation depends on the nurse's ability to diagnose the problem requiring the intervention of Surveillance and his or her ability to choose the appropriate parameters of interest for information gathering. Successful integration of the data, and predictions and action from this information, are the goals of Surveillance.

ASSOCIATED NURSING DIAGNOSES AND CLIENT GROUPS

The target population for the intervention of Surveillance is any client who is in a life-threatening situation in which death may be imminent. Types of client groups for whom Surveillance is an appropriate intervention include all patients who are in critical care situations, ranging from the emergency

Table 21–1. SURVEILLANCE TOOL

Parameters of Interest	Time Sequence (stated in seconds, minutes, or hours)									

area, where a patient may have been the victim of severe trauma, to the quiet area in the psychiatric ward, where a patient may be a potential victim of self-inflicted trauma. Other types of patients for whom Surveillance is indicated are those whose lives are "tube dependent," such as the person on a respiratory or cardiac assist device. All of these clients require close monitoring of certain parameters of interest in order to maintain their life status.

Of the 42 nursing diagnosis categories accepted at the Fourth National Conference for Classification of Nursing Diagnosis (Gordon, 1982), the following could use Surveillance as an appropriate intervention:

○ Ineffective Airway Clearance
○ Ineffective Breathing Patterns
○ Alterations in Cardiac Output
○ Impaired Gas Exchange
○ Potential for Injury
○ Potential for Violence

The degree to which the potential or actual problem is life-threatening will determine whether Surveillance, alone or in combination with some other intervention, is indicated in any given situation. To focus our discussion, the illustrations of Surveillance in this chapter will apply specifically to a patient with congestive cardiomyopathy who has a nursing diagnosis of Decreased Cardiac Output.

RECOMMENDATIONS FOR PRACTICE AND RESEARCH

Because our case study concerns a patient with severe alteration in cardiac output, the following discussion of implications for practice and research will apply to this client group.

Two related studies (Hubalik, 1981; Wessel, 1981) have demonstrated that Surveillance activities are legitimate and important in critical care situations involving patients with severe cardiomyopathy. In critical care situations such as these, nurses use both medical and nursing diagnoses to determine the parameters of interest for their surveillance activities. The acuteness of the situation generally determines the time sequence of monitoring. That is, the more acute or life-threatening the condition, the more frequently will the parameter of interest be monitored.

These studies describe the practice of medicine and nursing in Surveillance during treatment of patients with Decreased Cardiac Output as mostly collaborative. Both studies reported dependent, collaborative, and independent actions. Many of the independent and collaboration actions were surveillance activities, for example, taking vital signs, evaluating laboratory values and response to medications, monitoring ECG changes, and regulating fluid intake (Wessel, 1981).

In critical care situations, nurses are actively and independently monitoring numerous patient responses to illness and treatment. Some of the parameters of interest are identified through physician orders, whereas others are determined independently by the nurse. The responsibility for collecting all the information in an appropriate time sequence is the major responsibility of the nurse. Thus, Surveillance is a legitimate nursing intervention in the critical care situation.

The major research activity implied by this intervention is to test the two indices of the intervention tool (parameters of interest and time sequence) with different client groups who have different nursing diagnoses and who show differences in acuteness of condition.

Results of these research efforts could be used to verify the appropriateness of Surveillance as a nursing intervention for different client groups with different nursing diagnoses. Research findings could also be used to refine nursing diagnoses, with the etiological factors providing the parameters of interest used in the various Surveillance tools.

Systematic collection of data under a plan of Surveillance should help with the cognitive aspect of this intervention. That is, more valid and reliable data should lead to better evaluation, prediction, and action to maintain the life status of the patient in a life-threatening situation.

CASE STUDY

This case study concerns B. S., the 27 year old construction worker with severe congestive cardiomyopathy. B. S. was admitted to the hospital following a recent viral infection, for control of his congestive heart failure symptoms, for adjustment of his cardiac medications, and for relief of pedal edema. The major nursing diagnosis for B. S. was Decreased Cardiac Output, defined in this case study as a decrease in volume of blood ejected from the heart due to factors influencing stroke volume or heart rate, or both. The major antecedent condition leading to B. S.'s decreased cardiac output was a decreased ventricular contractibility resulting from the cardiomyopathy.

This episode of decreased cardiac output was not the first for B. S., but this time it was complicated by continued enlargement and dilation of the heart. Compensatory mechanisms, which normally aid in increasing cardiac output when a decrease in stroke volume has occurred, were ineffective in maintaining a steady state because the patient's cardiac reserve had been depleted. Because his cardiac output could not be maintained on the present medical regimen, and because the upper limits of medication administration had been reached, B. S. was being considered for a heart transplant as the only remaining medical treatment that could improve his condition.

After B. S. returned from the cardiac catheterization laboratory, where right and left heart catheterization was performed and an intra-aortic balloon pump (IABP) was inserted, he was reattached to all monitoring capabilities in the coronary care unit. Equipment utilized for monitoring included left femoral Swan-Ganz catheter, left femoral arterial line, right femoral IABP, two right femoral intravenous lines, urinary catheter, cardiac monitor, ventilator, nasogastric tube, and left subclavian intravenous line. At the time the primary nurse first came in contact with B. S., he was experiencing a further decrease in his cardiac output, indicating that cardiogenic shock and death were imminent if prompt intervention to reverse this trend was not instituted.

Goals

Factors leading to the selection of Surveillance as the intervention for B. S. included early detection of an impending cardiopulmonary disaster, early detection of complications, successful resolution of the decreased cardiac output, detection of minor changes in hemodynamic state, establishment of priorities of care so that important areas would not be overlooked, development of a plan to deal with future developments in care, and B. S.'s life. All these factors were found in the literature to be of primary importance for the critically ill cardiac patient.

Intervention

The nurse began the intervention of Surveillance immediately after the patient history and physical examination were completed. Instructions were given by the physician to the nurse, outlining the specific parameters of observation that medical personnel considered most notable for B. S. These are listed as the first 15 parameters on the Surveillance flow sheet, beginning with temperature and ending with heparin (see Table 21–2). All other observation parameters included on the flow sheet were determined to be important by the nurse (see Tables 21–2, 21–3, and 21–4). The time frame selected for the intervention was also determined by the nurse during this critical period, which would end either in recovery from the cardiogenic shock or in death. A vast amount of data were collected during the ensuing four day period, but the

Table 21–2. BASIC PARAMETERS OF INTEREST MONITORED DURING THE SURVEILLANCE OF B. S. (8 HOUR PERIOD)

Parameter	Time Sequence								
	1600	1700	1800	1900	2000	2100	2200	2300	2400
Temperature (celsius)	37.2		37.9		38.5		38.5		38.8
Apical Pulse	125	124	125	129	126	131	130	133	135
Respirations	12	12	12	12	12	12	12	12	12
Blood Pressure	104/33	105/41	104/33	115/21	104/22	86/36	80/33	81/32	84/32
Pulmonary Artery Systolic/Diastolic/Mean	42/35/39	37/28/30	35/24/30	48/30/42	48/33/37	36/20/29	32/18/26	32/20/28	35/18/24
Pulmonary Artery Wedge	30	28	30	34	32	25	19	20	24
Cardiac Output	5.25		2.86		2.74		3.78		3.07
Urine Output	7	17	55	13	12	18	15	38	22
Rhythm	RSR	RSR	RSR	RSR	RSR	RSR	RSR	RSR	RSR
Ventilator TV/FIO$_2$/Rate	800/40/12	800/40/12	800/40/12	800/40/12	800/40/12	800/40/12	800/40/12	800/40/12	800/40/12
Dopamine 1600 mg/500 cc	10	20	20	20	20	28	32	32	32
Dobutamine 1000 mg/500 cc	—	—	10	10	—	—	—	—	—
Nipride 200 mg/500 cc	—	—	—	14	10	18	18	18	14
IABP	1:2	1:2	1:2	1:2	1:2	1:2	1:2	1:2	1:2
Heparin units/hr	1000	1000	1000	—	1000	—	600	600	600
Lungs	clear R rales L	same	bibasilar rales	same	congestion	bibasilar rales	same	rales and ronchi	same

Heart	$S_1 = S_2$ 4/6 Systolic murmur	same murmur	4/6 Systolic murmur	same	$S_1 = S_2$ S_4	same	4/6 Systolic murmur	same	same
Pedal Pulses R/L	none	+/+	+/+	none	none	none	-/+	-/+	dop +/+
Skin Temperature/Color	cool/pale	same	dry/pale	same	cold/pale	same	same	same	same
Movement	paralysis	same	same	same	restless	paralysis	same	same	same
Pupils	PERL 2/2	same	same	same	same	same	same	same	same
JVD cm/hob	4/5 flat	same	same	6 flat	same	same	same	same	same
Secretions	—	oral	oral and nasal	—	ET suction oral	—	oral bloody	—	—
Abdomen	flat 0 sounds	same	same	same	same	same	same	same	same
Dressings	dry	dry	changed	dry	changed	dry	changed	dry	dry
Edema R ankle/L ankle	+3/ +2	+3/ +2	+3/ +2	+3/ +2	+3/ +2	+3/ +2	+3/ +2	+3/ +2	+3/ +2
Nose and Mouth Care	√/√	√/√	bloody √/√	bloody √/√	bloody √/√	√/√	√/√	√/√	√/√
Medications	MS 10 mg	Valium 5 mg	Maalox 30 cc	Lasix 80 mg	Heparin 10,000 Dilantin 300 mg	Pavulon 10 mg MS 10 mg	—	—	—

Table 21–3. ADDITIONAL PARAMETERS OF INTEREST MONITORED DURING THE SURVEILLANCE OF B. S. (24 HOUR PERIOD)—ENZYMES AND OTHER BLOOD TESTS

Parameter	Time Sequence				
	0300	0850	1320	1725	2235
Na		136			
K		4.9			
Cl		92			
BUN		62			
Cr		2.6			
PT	32		30	28	28
PTT	>150	118	57	53	77
LDH	>2000	4290			
AST	>3080	>3080			
CPK	2450	3420			
CPK-MM	100	100			
CPK-MB	0	0			
Hg/Hct	$\frac{13.1}{40}$	$\frac{11.6}{34.9}$			
WBC	21.9	18.7			

information presented here is limited to a brief period to illustrate implementation of the intervention.

Implemention of this intervention is summarized on the Surveillance flow sheet presented in Table 21–2. In this study, the behavioral aspect of Surveillance included inspecting, palpating, percussing, and auscultating B. S.'s body, equipment, and environment. This inspection encompassed vital signs, pulmonary artery pressures, cardiac output, urine output, oxygen status, medication titration, heart and lung assessment, peripheral circulation, skin color and temperature, secretions, hygienic care, intravenous titration, and laboratory values. The parameters identified as most important to monitor by the nurse were in agreement with those identified in the literature for acutely ill cardiac patients. In this case study, the physician was primarily interested in data concerning B. S.'s hemodynamic and medication status. These parameters were also of priority to the nurse. Although the physician was notified when significant changes occurred with B. S., he was not informed of the frequency of observations made, the titration of medication according to the observations, the administration of prn medications, or the results of laboratory tests.

The cognitive aspect of Surveillance for B. S. included looking, seeing, estimating, knowing, understanding, interpreting, analyzing, and evaluating all of the parameters identified. These cognitive aspects may not always be readily apparent to someone observing the nurse doing Surveillance, particularly if the nurse is merely standing at the patient's bedside and thinking. But, because the frequency of recording and reporting are common to the nurse in a critical care setting, this cognitive component is often reflected in the nurse's notes, which imply that a judgment was made. This cognitive component is also observable when the nurse notes an abnormality and either acts by reporting it to the physician, expecting collaboration and decision-making, or acts independently by titrating medications, changing the position of the patient, increasing the rate of intravenous fluids, giving emergency drugs, implementing protocols, drawing subsequent laboratory values, or making a conscious effort to continue to survey a particular parameter.

Table 21–4. ADDITIONAL PARAMETERS OF INTEREST MONITORED DURING THE SURVEILLANCE OF B. S. (24-HOUR PERIOD)—BLOOD GASES AND OTHER INDICES

Parameter	Time Sequence					
	0030	0430	0850	1225	1630	2030
pH	7.40	7.38	7.46	7.44	7.48	7.50
P_{CO_2}	40	40.7	42	40	40	34
P_{O_2}	77	72.4	88	86	77	94
HCO_3	24	23	29	26	28	25
O_2 delivery	40% ventilator					
Chest film	ET tube and Swan-Ganz in good placement; cardiac silhouette enlarged; pulmonary vascular congestion					
ECG 12—Lead II	Sinus tachycardia rate 120 across precardium; P.R. 20; notching of R waves; ischemia V_1–V_6; poor R wave progression across precordium					

In reviewing the Surveillance flow sheet for B. S., it is obvious that the nurse was busy manipulating cardiac monitor equipment, adjusting intravenous fluids and medications, and checking various other equipment. It is also demonstrated that changes in B. S.'s blood pressure, cardiac output, and pulmonary artery pressure were associated with changes in medication administration (at 1800 and 2100 hours); changes in laboratory values were associated with changes in medication (at 1900, 2100, and 2200); changes in arterial blood gases prompted positioning and suctioning (at 1600, 1800, and 2000); and neurological status changes were associated with medication administration (at 1700 and 2100). In noting these associations, the cognitive portion of Surveillance becomes observable, and the actions that followed careful and consistent watching become apparent.

To summarize, in this case study, Surveillance was implemented as a nursing intervention for the purpose of preventing cardiopulmonary disaster and death. In this instance, Surveillance was operationally defined as physically observing the parameters of temperature, pulse, respiration, blood pressure, pulmonary artery pressure, urine output, cardiac rhythm, ventilator settings, medications, IABP, lung and heart sounds, peripheral pulses, skin temperature and color, movement, pupil size and reaction, jugular venous distention, edema, secretions, abdomen, dressings, mucous membranes; surveying serum electrolytes, coagulation times, enzymes, blood counts, arterial blood gases, chest films, and electrocardiograms, interpreting the findings as normal or abnormal; and reporting significant findngs regarding B. S.'s life status in order to make early interventions and plan subsequent care.

Evaluation

The final step of this process involves an evaluation of the success of this intervention in reducing B. S.'s problem of decreased cardiac output. In this case study, it would be unrealistic to think that B. S.'s cardiomyopathy could be reduced by merely monitoring and watching important signs and symptoms. From the time that the nursing intervention was instituted, B. S. remained alive and in reasonably stable condition for four days. By close observation, assessment, and early intervention, it was hoped that the cardiogenic shock could be stabilized so that B.S. could be transferred for a heart transplant. Surveillance of hemodynamics, urine, laboratory values, and medications prevented major cardiopulmonary disasters and complications of decreased cardiac output until approximately 1 hour before his death. Surveillance prompted prioritizing needs, quick intervention, and detection of minor changes, and most likely it extended the life span of B. S. beyond what would be expected in such a situation if trained personnel had not been available. This intervention allowed time for family members to begin the grief process in coping with this crisis.

Although decreased cardiac output was not ultimately relieved by this intervention, B. S.'s condition was maintained and stabilized at a level that was compatible with life for a critical time period. For this nursing diagnosis of Decreased Cardiac Output, Surveillance provided the best overall results that could be expected. The general goal of increasing cardiac output was not met with this intervention because an overwhelming infection kept B. S. from receiving a heart transplant in time to save his life. Nevertheless, at points along the way, major decreases in cardiac output were prevented. Thus, we believe that Surveillance is an important nursing intervention in the care of the critically ill patient, in this case the patient with Decreased Cardiac Output.

EDITORS' COMMENTS AND QUESTIONS

The term "surveillance" has appeared in the public health literature, the maternal–child health literature, and the ANA's *Nursing: A Social Policy Statement* (1980). This chapter defines the concept as an intervention and delineates how it differs from assessment and observation. The conceptual framework for the concept was borrowed from the literature on spying, and the authors have developed it for the critical care nursing arena. Critical care nurses have expressed concern over being left out of the nursing diagnosis movement because of questions about the independent versus dependent aspects of their role. Surveillance clearly illustrates that critical care nurses develop advanced knowledge, skills, and decision-making abilities to work with their clients.

Questions for Discussion

1. *How can Surveillance be utilized in settings other than the acute care unit?*

2. *Is there a difference between medical and nursing Surveillance?*

3. *What distinguishes Surveillance from observation and assessment?*

References

Askin, F. Surveillance: The social science perspective. In Columbia Human Rights Law Review (Ed.), *Surveillance, data-veillance, and personal freedoms*. Fair Lawn, N.J.: R. E. Burdick, 1973.

Blum, R. H. *Surveillance and espionage in a free society*. New York: Praeger Publishers, 1972.

Carlson, J. H., Craft, C. A., and McGuire, A. D. *Nursing diagnosis*. Philadelphia: W. B. Saunders Company, 1982.

Carrieri, V., Stotts, N., Levinson, J., Murdaugh, C., and Holemer, W. L. The use of cardiopulmonary assessment skills in the clinical setting. *Western Journal of Nursing Research*, 1982, 4(1), 5–17.

Chalmers, H. Return to basics. 3. Look and see. *Nursing Mirror*, 1977, 145, i–iv.

Dulles, A. *The craft of intelligence*. New York: Harper & Row, 1963.

Gordon, M. *Nursing diagnosis: Process and application*. New York: McGraw-Hill Book Company, 1982.

Griffin, P. T. New cardiac surveillance unit combines functions of ICU and CCU. *Hospitals*, 1976, 50, 111–114.

Hayward, R. P. Emergency care of the cardiac patient. *Nursing Mirror*, 1977, 144, 45–49.

Hubalik, K. T. Nursing diagnosis associated with heart failure in critical care nursing (unpublished Master's thesis). Chicago: University of Illinois, 1981.

Karch, A. M. This assessment habit saves lives. *RN* 1976, 39, 42–44.

Owen, J. Patient observation: Caring for acute respiratory patients. *Nursing Mirror*, 1982, 154, vii–x.

Papenhausen, J. L. Data-based criteria for cardiovascular nursing intervention. *Critical Care Quarterly*, 1981, 4, 1–7

Pool, M. STAT! How would you manage this patient? *Journal of Emergency Nursing*, 1976, 25–27.

Ross, M. Learning to observe. *Nursing Papers*, 1979, 11(1–2), 46–54.

Sedlock, S. Cardiac output: Physiologic variables and therapeutic interventions. *Critical Care Nurse*, 1981, 1, 14–22.

Seth, R. *The art of spying*. New York: Philosophical Library, 1957.

Seth, R. *Anatomy of spying*. New York: E. P. Dutton and Company, 1963.

Weil, M. H., and Carlson, R. W. Priorities governing the care of the critically ill. *Hospital Practice*, 1976, 11, 67–76.

Wessel, S. L. Nursing functions related to the nursing diagnosis' decreased cardiac output (unpublished Master's thesis). Chicago: University of Illinois, 1981.

Winslow, E. H. Visual inspection of the patient with cardiopulmonary disease. *Nursing Digest*, 1976, 4, 20–23.

22

PRESENCE

DIANE L. GARDNER

DESCRIPTION AND DEFINITION OF PRESENCE

Just being there. From the image of the Lady with the Lamp, Florence Nightingale, to the modern-day hospital nurse, the presence of the nurse has symbolized professional nursing and has formed the core of the nurse-patient relationship. The effect, both physical and psychological, of the presence of the nurse is hard to capture. This is an elusive concept, which is challenging to measure in quantitative terms. Yet it is recognized by both nurses and their patients or clients. Zderad (1978) states that presence is an experience that is verified by the awareness of both the nurse and the patient. She cites an example from her group therapy work in which spontaneous feedback from a patient demonstrated that the nurse's presence was valued. In this instance, Presence is described in terms of a something-is-going-on-here perception and is validated by having made a difference that was observable by a change in the patient's affective behavior.

A concern for the health and welfare of people as one's purpose in life is the essence of nursing. Patients hold an expectation that nurses will enter into a relationship with them characterized by attitudes of warmth, caring, liking, interest, and respect: Rogers (1962) termed this a "helping relationship." A helping relationship needs to be based on a valid perception of the patient's experience and on an ability to understand the patient's feelings. Training and knowledge are required for the nurse to be therapeutically valuable to the patient (Altschul, 1979). Paterson and Zderad (1976) state that nursing, as a clinical art, is transactional: It involves being with and doing with the patient or client. The patient sees in the nurse the possibility of help, comfort, and support. Nursing phenomena can be experienced from the reference point of the nurturing process. Gagan (1983) also asserts that the nurse-patient relationship in the general hospital setting primarily focuses on elements of support and nurturance. The nature of the work of nursing continually exposes nurses to the miseries of others. Nurses see the suffering and share the concerns of their patients. Yet, as Colavecchio (1982) points out, one of the major rewards for nurses of direct patient care derives from human contact and from the significance of being present with another during critical times.

316

The presence of the nurse is the key that opens the door to the nurse-patient relationship. Nurses have recognized and remarked about this phenomenon. Vaillot (1962), in discussing the role of student nurses, noted that they can be a presence to patients. They become so when they become available to patients, as opposed to being aloof or being mere spectators in nursing situations. Zderad (1978) stated that she sees Presence as basic to the whole process of nursing. Paterson and Zderad (1976) describe presence as the gift of one's self in interhuman relating. This flows from the nurse's reason for being there: to nurture. There is an implicit expectation that a nurse will extend himself or herself in a helpful way if a patient needs assistance. The presence of the nurse involves openness and availability to what is and to what is not the patient's state of being, weighed against a standard of what ought to be, with the intention of doing something about the difference.

Despite the use of the term "presence" in the nursing literature and despite an awareness of its centrality to the nurse-patient relationship, little has been done to formally conceptualize and define this idea. Central to the development of the concept of Presence is the work of nursing theorists with a background in psychiatric and mental health nursing. Paterson and Zderad (1976; Zderad, 1978) can be identified as the major theorists for delineation of this concept. Paterson and Zderad (1976) defined presence as being available or open in a situation with a wholeness of one's unique individual being. Presence, then, is a gift of the self. Their schema is derived from an existential, phenomenological, humanistic philosophical base. Their thoughts on Presence reflect an emphasis on the psychological aspects of nursing presence: dialogue, empathy, and interactive transactions. In this sense, the nurse uses himself or herself as an intervention tool to create a therapeutic psychological milieu that meets the patient's needs for help, comfort, or support.

Presence, however, has also been viewed from the perspective of the therapeutic value of the nurse using himself or herself as an intervention tool by merely remaining physically present with the patient. The literature here is mostly anecdotal and related to the general acknowledgment of the comforting aspect of the presence of a supportive, concerned other person with the anticipation of help being required. Nurses have recognized the comforting and supportive aspects of their physical presence with a client who is grieving or who is in acute crisis. The intervention is to be physically present; the meaning for the client is the availability of a helpful other in anticipation of the need for professional assessment and intervention at a crucial moment.

The two aspects of Presence, the physical and the psychological presence of the nurse, are intricately interwoven in the reality of nursing care. The nurse's presence for the patient is manifested in three dimensions: in the cognitive domain by verbal communication of empathy or understanding of the patient's experiencing; in the affective domain by a generation of positive regard, trust, and genuineness, which are evidenced by interpersonal rapport; and in the behavioral domain by being physically available as a helper. Presence as a nursing intervention is operationally defined to include all three dimensions.

A holistic nursing *conceptual definition of Presence* is the *nurse's physical "being there" and the psychological "being with" a patient for the purpose of meeting the patient's health care needs.* In this sense, the nurse uses himself or herself as the intervention tool in the process of nursing care. It is a dynamic, conscious, and interactive process based upon knowledge and skill in the art and science of skilled caring for the health care needs of human beings. Presence is conceived of as a core element of nursing activity. It is the availability of the nurse as helper for the patient.

Presence, as a nursing intervention, then, is the *nurse's use of self through availability and attention to needs.* Brodish (1982) has conceptualized this nursing helping relationship in an interaction model. She defines nursing as the therapeutic use of self for the benefit of others after first acquiring both the knowledge and the skill necessary to identify needs. Established nursing theorists have also emphasized the conceptualization of nursing as a therapeutic interaction. Orlando (1961) theorized that what is unique to nursing is the process involved in interacting with a patient to meet an immediate need. Orem (1971) viewed nursing as an interpersonal process requiring the social encounter of the nurse with a patient and involving a transaction between them. King (1971) defined nursing as a basic interpersonal relationship process of action, reaction, interaction, and transaction.

The concept of Presence integrates the thoughts of various theorists and is derived from a combination of existential, humanistic, and phenomenological philosophies as applied to nursing. Stevens (1979) describes the advantage of joining existentialism with phenomenology in nursing as permitting a holistic conception of humans. Paterson (1978) describes humanistic nursing as a perspective of nursing as a happening between persons, an approach to nursing as existential presence and awareness. She states that as a nurse she is a presence to others whose health and survival are an issue. This is confirmed by the difference the nurse makes.

As a concept, Presence is related closely to other concepts, such as empathy and support, caring, and the therapeutic use of self. Elements such as caring, self-awareness, commitment to helping others, knowledge, and skill are antecedents to the nurse's use of Presence as a nursing intervention of being physically and psychologically available for patients. To enhance the effectiveness of the nursing intervention of Presence, the nurse uses such techniques as listening, attending, empathy, touch, hope, reassurance, comforting, being there, and communicating. The outcomes from the nursing intervention of Presence include support, comfort, sustained assistance, encouragement, and motivation.

LITERATURE RELATED TO PRESENCE

The idea of Presence as a nursing concept is most clearly derived from the work of Zderad (1978; Paterson and Zderad, 1976). She has labeled and defined the concept and expanded upon its relationship to humanistic nursing theory. Beyond Zderad's work, Presence has not been developed as a concept. Awareness of Presence as a concept is at the level of intuition: Nurses and other helpers have used Presence as an intervention without conceptualizing it.

Presence and empathy are a dynamic duo for patient care. Empathy enhances the quality of the nurse's Presence as an intervention. Egan (1982) describes being with, attending to, and listening to another person as potent reinforcers in certain situations. He discusses how, at more dramatic moments of life, simply being with another person is extremely important: just another's presence can make a difference in terms of being comforting, even if few words are spoken. Egan believes that helping and other deep interpersonal transactions demand a certain intensity of presence: Being fully there is more than physical presence; it is psychological or social-emotional presence also. He relates this to the concept of attending, which he considers to be a basic and important helping skill. Attending and listening skills contribute to effective empathy.

Empathy, or understanding, has been defined as the ability to perceive the meanings and feelings of others and to communicate that understanding to the other person (Gagan, 1983). It also includes being able to accurately predict and anticipate the behavioral responses of the other (Kramer and Schmalenberg, 1977). Empathy has been perceived as a concept integral to therapeutic nursing and is related to the role of the nurse as the one who creates a caring and helping atmosphere in which healing can be facilitated (Gagan, 1983; Stetler, 1977). Empathy has been a difficult concept to operationalize. Furthermore, there appears to be a wide range of differences between and among people in terms of their empathic ability (Kramer and Schmalenberg, 1977). Research on the empathic ability of nurses has produced mixed results (Gagan, 1983). Kramer and Schmalenberg (1977) note that a relationship exists between helping behavior and empathy: One study found that helping behavior was a function of empathic tendency (Mehrabian and Epstein, 1972).

The concept of support is also related to the concept of Presence. Support is similar to the provision of psychological comfort and has been defined as acceptance. Nursing support is an activity within the context of the nurse-patient relationship; it is one of the basic principles of practice and is thought to be an activity that should be performed by all nurses (Gardner and Wheeler, 1981). Gardner and Wheeler studied nurses' perceptions of the meaning of support in nursing. Factor analysis showed that the availability or presence of the nurse was an important aspect of support. Critical incident reports elicited behaviors such as sitting and spending time with a patient, which imply the availability of the nurse to the patient. As perceived by the nurses in this study, supportive nursing interventions utilize communication to mediate and alleviate emotional stress.

Physical closeness, nearness, and touching are aspects of Presence in nursing. Care-giving activities are predicated on proximity and bring the nurse into the patient's physical space. Physical closeness was a factor of support in Gardner and Wheeler's (1981) study. In Ricci's study of personal space invasion in the nurse-patient relationship, (1981), anxiety scores of the experimental group showed a definite downward trend, indicating that the intrusion of a nurse into a patient's space had a calming rather than arousing effect. Thus, the presence of the nurse is not generally perceived by patients to be anxiety provoking.

The concept of Presence, the availability of the nurse, is linked intimately with the concept of caring. Caring is based on an interest in or concern for another human being. Caring is defined as providing assistance to others in need (Leininger, 1980). The presence of the nurse as a helper is the embodiment of caring in nursing.

Finally, Presence is closely related to the concept of the therapeutic use of self. This concept can be traced from the work of Peplau (1952) and has been defined by Uys (1980) as the ability of nurses to scientifically and purposefully employ their entire person or unique individuality and identity as a tool to promote health and to limit disease. Uys sees the concept of the therapeutic use of self as central to nursing. Krikorian and Paulanka (1982) note that therapeutic use of self is frequently identified as the nurse's major tool in the nurse-patient relationship. Uys (1980) prefers a very broad view of the nurse as a total person in the service of patients. Her operational definition of the concept therapeutic use of self includes the four facets of mental, physical, psychosocial, and spiritual aspects. She lists use of physical presence to reassure, encourage, set limits, and motivate as an example of behaviors or skills associated wih the use of physical aspects of self.

RELATED RESEARCH

No specific nursing research literature describing Presence as an intervention is available. In general, the dimension of the feelings experienced by the patient during the interaction with the nurse has rarely been investigated (Ricci, 1981). Evidence for the effectiveness of the presence of the nurse for the patient must be deduced from related literature.

Lynch and co-workers (1977) and Thomas, Lynch, and Mills (1975) have studied the effects of different kinds of psychosocial interactions on the cardiac activity of CCU patients. Cardiac responses to social interaction were monitored in patients who had received the drug curare. They observed abrupt heart rate changes in these patients of up to 30 beats per minute when a nurse simply held the patient's hand and comforted him or her. In this case, Presence was combined with touch and verbal communication.

In the pediatric literature, a study by Triplett and Arneson (1979) demonstrated that tactile comfort was an effective means of alleviating distress and maintaining trust in young hospitalized children. Sixty-three children between the ages of 3 days and 44 months old who were distressed (crying) at the time of intervention were studied to compare intervention techniques. In the verbal only group, seven of the interventions were successful in quieting the children, compared with 53 successes in 60 interventions in the tactile-verbal group. Thus, their data showed a highly significant difference when tactile comfort measures were used. Clearly, messages of care and comfort are conveyed to children through touch.

As already noted, Ricci (1981) studied the responses of the patient that arise during the interaction with a nurse by studying the relationship between personal space invasion by a nurse and patient anxiety level. Her results demonstrated that the intrusion of the nurse had a calming rather than arousing effect. The implications were that the nurses were perceived as not threatening.

Two other research studies included more direct elements of the presence of the nurse. Gardner and Wheeler's study (1981) on nurses' perceptions of the meaning of support utilized a critical incident technique. Behaviors of availability or nursing Presence, such as sitting and spending time with the patient, were shown to be important in the concept of support. Odell (1981) described a study of loneliness in which she asked adult patients how nurses could help. Her findings indicate that nursing interventions that prevent loneliness include the offering of psychological support by initiating short, frequent visits with the patient as an interested and concerned individual. Brief encounters were indeed therapeutic, and included patient requests to "just stop by," "drop in," and "check on me." One respondent indicated "just be there when needed."

INTERVENTION TOOLS

Owing to the poor conceptualization of and the paucity of research on Presence, identifiable intervention tools are not available. Presence is conceived of as the nurse's use of himself or herself as a therapeutic intervention tool. The effectiveness of this intervention is acknowledged in the literature despite little empirical validation to substantiate the claim.

An *operational definition of Presence* in nursing includes the following: *Presence in the cognitive domain by verbal communication of empathy or understanding of the patient's experience; Presence in the affective domain by a generation of positive regard, trust, and genuineness, which is evidenced by interpersonal rapport; and Presence in the physical domain by being physically available as a helper.* Presence is a basic nursing intervention. As the nurse assesses the nursing situation, Presence may be combined with other interventions (Touching, Counseling, Teaching, and so forth) in the delivery of patient care within the dynamic nurse-patient situation. Or, in certain situations, such as social isolation or loneliness, the nurse may choose to utilize the basic intervention of Presence as the intervention of choice.

ASSOCIATED NURSING DIAGNOSES AND CLIENT GROUPS

Presence is a concept that is basic and broad enough to be widely applicable to divergent client groups and to be useful as an intervention for various nursing diagnoses. The nurse can therapeutically intervene with Presence for adult clients experiencing loneliness (Odell, 1981) and through touch for young children experiencing distress during hospitalization (Triplett and Arneson, 1979). Supportive Presence of a nurse has been indicated as making a difference for adult patients newly diagnosed as having inoperable cancer (Gardner and Wheeler, 1981), for outpatient male cardiac patients (Ricci, 1981), and for psychiatric patients through use of empathic communication (Mansfield, 1973). It is theorized that the nurse's Presence and availability demonstrate caring, assist coping by implying psychological support, and diminish the intensity of feelings such as fear, powerlessness, anxiety, isolation, and distress by providing a physical and psychological anchoring of the patient to the nurse as a helpful other.

In just being there for the patient within the framework of the nurse-patient relationship, the anxious patient's sense of control is augmented by the availability of the nurse. The nurse uses the self as an intervention. The nurse assists patients to cope more effectively by being available as a helper. A sense of support is conveyed by the nearness of a nurse for those clients experiencing fear, grief, powerlessness, isolation, or distress. In the nursing intervention of Presence, the nurse uses the self to transmit psychological support and comfort to the patient or client by utilizing techniques such as physical nearness (e.g., sitting with the patient) or cognitive-affective awareness of and attending to the patient's needs.

Specific nursing diagnoses for which Presence would be most appropriate would include the following:

- Anxiety
- Ineffective Coping
- Impaired Communication
- Fear
- Grieving
- Potential for Injury
- Social Isolation
- Spiritual Distress

RECOMMENDATIONS FOR PRACTICE AND RESEARCH

It is important that nurses empirically validate that they do make a difference for their patients by asking what, how, and why. In this way nursing practice becomes more precise, reliable, and effective. As nurses recognize that their use of themselves can be a potent therapeutic intervention for their patients, the art and science of nursing practice will become more polished. The rewards for nurses of direct patient care will be augmented when nurses view themselves as a powerful force in the implementation of health care. As the value of the direct care-giving nurse is increased, so is the value of the profession of nursing.

The demonstration of the value of the nurse for the patient is predicated upon systematic research investigations of the effect of the nurse's behavior on the patient and on the feelings experienced by the patient during the interaction with a nurse. Very little research has been done in this domain. The value perception that nurses do make a difference will not suffice alone to improve practice. An explicit development by means of research investigation is needed. For example, a critical incident technique could be used to survey nurses regarding case examples of times when they have used Presence as an intervention. After initial investigation is done, further research concerning the question of what quality of Presence is necessary to be effective with patient groups would be useful to guide nurses in their utilization of Presence as an intervention tool. Patient outcomes must be validated through systematic research. This raises nursing practice beyond the level of intuition.

CASE STUDIES

Two case study examples are presented that illustrate the clinical application of the concept of Presence. One example is from psychiatric nursing practice and one is from pediatric nursing practice.

Case Study 1

D. W. was a 37 year old male hospitalized psychiatric patient. His medical diagnosis was schizophrenia. He had been hospitalized on psychiatric units on numerous occasions. When not hospitalized, D. W. had a history of getting into trouble for strange behavior, especially for urinating on the floor of his room at a hotel where he lived. D. W. was very quiet on the hospital unit. Much of his time was spent lying on his bed in a large ward. He would occasionally pace the halls anxiously and mutter in an angry or fearful tone. He would stand in the hall and very carefully watch what people were doing. He admitted to having auditory hallucinations in the form of "voices." D. W. would sometimes tell the nursing staff that people were going to harm him. His affect was usually flat. His behavior on the unit included only minimal interaction with other people. Environmental stimuli, especially people, were perceived by D. W. as threatening.

The nurse assessed D. W.'s nonverbal communication and diagnosed Fear (retreat to bed) and Anxiety (pacing and muttering). Initial intervention was acceptance of these behaviors. The nurse then used Presence with D. W. When the nurse came on the unit he greeted D. W. by name. When he sat in the dayroom, the nurse would sit nearby and watch television or make brief comments about activities on the unit. The actual message was nonverbal: that the nurse was not a threat and that it was safe to be near him. The nonverbal interaction with D. W. consisted of being nearby in a nonthreatening position. In this way, trust can be developed. The nurse utilized his presence by sitting with D. W. in as nonthreatening a manner as possible. The goal of intervention with D. W. was for him to be able to choose a greater degree of contact with others and to increase his ability to relate comfortably to others. The nurse was present to D. W. without demanding interactional responses from the patient which he was unable to make at the time. At one point, the nurse was called by another patient who needed pain medication. When the nurse arose to go, D. W. said, "Where are you going? I need you to keep me together!" This verbalization of the meaning of the nurse's Presence indicated D. W.'s active willingness to accept the nurse's presence in his time of anxiety (Wilberding, 1981).

Case Study 2

Michael was a 6 year old white male who had ingested a caustic lye solution when he was a 16 month old toddler. He suffered severe damage to his esophagus and was not expected to survive the ingestion incident. He did survive, but he had to endure multiple hospitalizations and surgeries. The aftermath has been a chronic handicapping condition. Michael underwent a colonic interposition at age 4, which was an attempt at surgical correction. Esophageal dilations every 2 weeks were begun to maintain patency of the reconstructed esophagus. Michael is still unable to swallow. He has a tracheostomy and a feeding gastrostomy tube. The esophageal dilations continue. They are now done under general anesthesia owing to Michael's level of apprehension and distress.

The nurse assessed Michael's apprehension and distress regarding dilation and diagnosed Fear and Threat related to security and independence needs. Initial intervention included acceptance of his protest behaviors. The nurse then explored alternative coping behaviors with the child and the family. The nurse arranged to stay with the child prior to the procedure, during induction of anesthesia, and afterward. Michael expressed eagerness for the nurse to remain with him. The nurse accompanied Michael up the elevator to the operating room and remained with him in the operating room during the induction of anesthesia. The nurse remained physically close to Michael and held his hand. Verbal reassurances ("I'll be right here") were given repeatedly. The actual message was: There is someone present who is focused solely on your welfare. The goal of the intervention was for Michael to accept induction of anesthesia without intense fear and physical resistance. The nurse was present for Michael to reduce his fear of abandonment in a perceived hostile situation and thereby helped to decrease traumatic aftereffects. As soon as Michael was under the anesthesia, the anesthesiologist who had witnessed the nursing intervention remarked to the nurse about how unusual it was for someone to accompany a child for anesthesia induction. The nurse replied that special permission had been obtained. The anesthesiologist commented about the success of the intervention. He noted that children of Michael's age usually fight anesthesia, yet Michael had remained calm and had fallen asleep quietly. He was aware of this induction as being less traumatic for the child. The threat and fear of the procedure for the child was alleviated by the Presence of the nurse.

EDITORS' COMMENTS AND QUESTIONS

This chapter is a good example of concept development at the symbolic level. Nurses have used this intervention a great deal, yet it has not been either defined or studied. There is little or no research base to support this intervention. Gardner does provide good case study illustrations of application of the intervention. Presence would also fit into the next section of this book, on communication.

Questions for Discussion

1. *How can Presence be operationally defined?*

2. *What type of methodology and tools are needed to study this intervention?*

3. *How can the concept be further developed?*

4. *Is Presence the same as empathy, physical closeness, caring, reassurance, or support?*

References

Altschul, A. T. Commitment to nursing. *Journal of Advanced Nursing*, 1979, 4, 123–135.

Brodish, M. S. Nursing practice conceptualized: An interaction model. *Image*, 1982, 14, 5–7.

Colavecchio, R. Direct patient care: A viable career choice? *Journal of Nursing Administration*, 1982, 12, 17–22.

Egan, G. *The skilled helper: Model, skills, and methods for effective helping* (2nd ed.). Monterey, Calif.: Brooks/Cole Publishing Company, 1982.

Gagen, J. M. Methodological notes on empathy. *Advances in Nursing Science*, 1983, 5, 65–72.

Gardner, K., and Wheeler, E. C. Nurses' perceptions of the meaning of support in nursing. *Issues in Mental Health Nursing*, 1981, *3*, 13–28.

King, I. M. *Toward a theory of nursing: General concepts of human behavior*. New York: John Wiley & Sons, 1971.

Kramer, M., and Schmalenberg, C. The first job . . . a proving ground basis for empathy development. *Journal of Nursing Administration*, 1977, *7*, 3–20.

Krikorian, D. A., and Paulanka, B. J. Self-awareness—the key to successful nurse-patient relationship? *Journal of Psychosocial Nursing and Mental Health Services*, 1982, *20*, 19–21.

Leininger, M. Caring: A central focus of nursing and health care services. *Nursing and Health Care*, 1980, *1*, 135–143.

Lynch, J. J., Thomas, S. A., Paskewitz, D. A., Katcher, A. M., and Weir, L. O. Human contact and cardiac arrhythmia in a coronary care unit. *Psychosomatic Medicine*, 1977, *39*, 188–193.

Mansfield, E. Empathy: Concept and identified psychiatric nursing behavior. *Nursing Research*, 1973, *22*, 525–530.

Mehrabian, A., and Epstein, N. A measure of emotional empathy. *Journal of Personality*, 1972, *40*, 525–543.

Odell, S. H. Someone is lonely. *Issues in Mental Health Nursing*, 1981, *3*, 7–12.

Orem, D. E. *Nursing: Concepts of practice*. New York: McGraw-Hill Book Company, 1971.

Orlando, I. J. *The dynamic nurse-patient relationship*. New York: G. P. Putmam's Sons, 1961.

Paterson, J. G. The tortuous way toward nursing theory. In *Theory development: What, why, how*. New York: National League for Nursing, 1978, pp. 49–65 (Publ. No. 15–1708).

Paterson, J. G., and Zderad, L. T. *Humanistic nursing*. New York: John Wiley & Sons, 1976.

Peplau, H. E. *Interpersonal relations in nursing*. New York: G. P. Putnam, 1952.

Ramaekers, S. M. J. Communication blocks revisited. *American Journal of Nursing*, 1979, *79*, 1079–1081.

Ricci, M. S. An experiment with personal space invasion in the nurse-patient relationship and its effect on anxiety. *Issues in Mental Health Nursing*, 1981, *3*, 203–218.

Rogers, C. The characteristics of a helping relationship. *Canadian Mental Health*, Supplement 27, 1962.

Stetler, C. B. Relationship of perceived empathy to nurses' communication. *Nursing Research*, 1977, *26*, 432–438.

Stevens, B. J. *Nursing theory: Analysis, application, evaluation*. Boston: Little, Brown & Company, 1979.

Thomas, S. A., Lynch, J. J., and Mills, M. E. Psychosocial influences on heart rhythm in the coronary-care unit. *Heart and Lung*, 1975, *4*, 746–750.

Triplett, J. L., and Arneson, S. W. The use of verbal and tactile comfort to alleviate distress in young hospitalized children. *Research in Nursing and Health*, 1979, *2*, 17–23.

Uys, L. R. Towards the development of an operational definition of the concept "therapeutic use of self." *International Journal of Nursing Studies*, 1980, *17*, 175–180.

Vaillot, S. M. C. *Commitment to nursing: A philosophic investigation*. Philadelphia: J. B. Lippincott Company, 1962.

Wilberding, J. Z. *A. comparison of two theories of nursing* (96:201 Conceptual and Theoretical Foundations of Nursing) (unpublished manuscript). Iowa City: University of Iowa, 1981.

Zderad, L. T. From here-and-now to theory: Reflections on "how." In *Theory development: What, why, how?* New York: National League for Nursing, 1978, pp. 35–48 (Publ. No. 15–1708).

COMMUNICATION

Overview: Communicating with and for the Patient

GLORIA M. BULECHEK
JOANNE C. McCLOSKEY

Communication is essential for the effective delivery of nursing care. Nurses need communication skills for good interpersonal relations with other health care workers and for assessing patient problems and explaining treatments. Communication is a process that involves more than one person. Barriers to communication can occur anywhere in the process: in the sender, who must use appropriate behavior, be credible, speak and write well, have something to say, say it at a timely moment, and encourage feedback; in the message, which must be understandable, include sufficient details, and often be expressed in more than one way and at more than one time; and in the receiver, who must listen, attempt to understand, ask for clarification, and give feedback. As the professional in nurse-client relationships, the nurse is responsible for the quality of the communication. Although communication skills in the areas of patient assessment, relationships with co-workers, and carrying out doctor's orders (e.g., explaining to a patient what will happen during a medical procedure) are emphasized often throughout a nurse's education, relatively little emphasis has been placed on independent communication interventions. The chapters in this section include three interventions (Active Listening, Patient Advocacy, Discharge Planning) that have received some attention in nursing and two (Culture Brokerage and Truth Telling) that have received very little.

Listening is an important aspect of communication. In her chapter on Active Listening, titled such to emphasize the difference between the everyday type of listening that we all do and therapeutic listening, which occurs when a nurse makes a conscious effort to understand and empathize with a client,

Helms outlines the steps of the listening process. She discusses the use of listening both as a valuable aid to data collection and diagnosis and as a nursing intervention. No research exists on Active Listening as an intervention; in general, nursing textbooks and journals disregard the use of listening as an intervention. Building on the general literature, Helms identifies the reported benefits of listening and then connects these to identified characteristics and etiologies of identified nursing diagnoses. She concludes that Active Listening as an intervention could help patients with Fear, Anxiety, Social Isolation, and Body Image Disturbance. She outlines a research strategy to facilitate the study of Active Listening as an intervention. Leaders who are interested in this intervention will also want to read Gardner's chapter on Presence in the previous section.

Patient Advocacy is not new, as Donahue aptly illustrates in her historical review of the concept. However, in the past decade, with demands for professional accountability and consumer protection, nursing has renewed its interest in the idea. As Donahue puts it, the question is not whether nurses should be patient advocates but how they lost the role.

While a significant portion of nursing's literature of the past decade addresses patient advocacy, the concept, according to Donahue, is not well understood or accepted. She outlines three models of advocacy and points out that nothing has been published on the advocate role with incompetent patients and there are no reports of research on Advocacy. She says that Advocacy is probably not possible for a nurse working in a traditional role as an assistant to physicians dependent on hospital employment. Advocacy involves risk for the nurse; it calls for a nurse who "care and dares." If the profession wants nurses who are patient advocates the profession must sanction and encourage the role.

While the concept is included here as an intervention and Donahue believes it is one, she raises the interesting question of whether Advocacy may be, in the final analysis, the theory for nursing. Much work remains to be done on defining the process and strategies of Advocacy, but the concept holds exciting promise for the nurse-patient relationship and for the profession of nursing. Donahue outlines five recommendations to bring the promise closer to reality.

Culture Brokerage can be thought of as a type of advocacy. It requires the nurse to interpret the patient's culture and health beliefs to orthodox health care professionals. Sometimes it requires the nurse to teach new skills to patients so that they can cope with the dominant orthodox system. Culture Brokerage is an intervention in which the nurse is an intermediary between the patient and other health care providers. Although other health providers could do Culture Brokerage, the nurse, who generally has the closest relationship to the client and family, is in the best position.

Tripp-Reimer and Brink develop the intervention of Culture Brokerage from the discipline of anthropology. They identify numerous nursing diagnoses that could require Culture Brokerage, but the diagnosis most associated with Culture Brokerage is Noncompliance. The health beliefs of the unorthodox client often interfere with adherence to orthodox medical treatment.

In their chapter, Tripp-Reimer and Brink discuss the various techniques of Culture Brokerage, which include negotiation and the therapeutic use of time. Culture Brokerage takes time. It also requires that the nurse have knowledge of the subculture, knowledge of the disease and its orthodox treatment, and skill in interviewing, listening, and negotiation. The nurse must be flexible in attitude and not appear hurried. Although nursing textbooks of the past decades have emphasized cultural assessment of all clients, little has been written about Cultural Brokerage as an intervention. In their chapter, illustrated with five case studies, Tripp-Reimer and Brink provide nurses with a way to help the increasing numbers of clients from different cultures. As the authors point out, Culture Brokerage may be the key: that unlocks the door for other interventions.

Another intervention also related to advocacy is Truth Telling. With any communication there is the possibility for dishonesty, distortion, or omission. Nurses are often in the position in which they have to decide whether a painful truth should be told to a patient. The nurse's dilemma of truth versus deception is thoroughly discussed in the chapter by Livingston and Williamson. They define Truth Telling as "a process of responsible, caring, and honest communication based on ethical decision making." They propose a truth telling model that outlines five options for the nurse: whole truth, partial truth, silence, lying, and decision delay. A case study of a cardiac patient whose wife was killed in a car accident is woven throughout the text and illustrates the various options. In order to choose an option, a nurse may also have to use the intervention of Active Listening. If the whole truth is told and it is painful, the nurse may also choose to use the interventions of Presence and Crisis Intervention to support the patient through a difficult time. As the authors so well demonstrate in their chapter, Truth Telling is a complex intervention. It assumes good understanding of oneself, a sound knowledge base, excellent communication skills, rapport with the patient, and collaboration with other health professionals. Above all, it requires an accurate assessment of the risks, both to the patient who receives the truth and the nurse who tells the truth. More research is needed on the effects of Truth Telling, and the authority of nurses to use Truth Telling as an intervention needs to be acknowledged.

Discharge Planning is about communication between systems of care and among different health care professionals. The purpose of Discharge Planning is to achieve "continuity of care." In their chapter, Kelly and McClelland are very critical of past and present efforts at Discharge Planning. With their community health backgrounds they have a broad perspective of the discharge planning process and available resources. They offer a nursing process model for Discharge Planning with three key features: mutual problem identification and goal determination by patient or client and health professional; allowances for client withdrawal; and an ongoing evaluation of the process. Like the interventions of Preoperative Teaching and Advocacy, effective Discharge Planning requires administrative support. This chapter, about an intervention often implemented by hospital nurses, could have been placed in the previous section on acute care management. However, the key to successful implementation is cooperation and communication with other health care providers. The barriers to successful implementation are great, including the traditional medical model of health care that treats people chiefly in acute care settings. The potential benefits, improved delivery of care, reduced health care costs, and an expanded nursing role, are well worth the effort.

In conclusion, we concur with a statement made by Livingston and Williamson in their chapter, "As nursing assumes greater responsibility for making decisions about patient care, each nurse must accept responsibility for practicing honest communication." The chapters outlined in this section demonstrate the challenges, preparation necessary, and benefits of honest, open, and thoughtful communication interventions done by nurses.

23

ACTIVE LISTENING

JANET HELMS

The nurse's capacity to treat a client's problem depends to a large degree on his or her ability to recognize cues in the client's behavior that may indicate a problem. Lack of recognition may arise from a variety of factors, over which nurses can learn to develop some dimension of control by exploring their feeling toward the client and his or her problems. Obstacles to communication may also arise from situations that compel clients to express themselves in an acceptable manner, even at the expense of disguising their most critical needs. Other clients may be emotionally incapable of expressing their needs.

Listening has been credited with facilitating the nurse's recognition of a client's problem. When nurses listen to patients, they are consciously immersing themselves in the patient's frame of reference. Concentrating on the aural and sensory stimuli, all of which must be perceived and classified, is necessary for a response of interpretation and comprehension to be made. This dynamic process of attaching significance to what we hear is called listening (Hein, 1980).

Listening is more than just hearing (Lewis, 1973). To hear means specifically to become aware of sounds. It is passive, occurring automatically when sound waves stimulate the auditory nerves. Listening, however, requires a person to make an active, conscious effort to attend closely to the auditory stimuli.

Edwards and Brillhart (1981) point out that listening includes hearing, which occurs in the ears, as well as perceiving and interpreting the sounds, which take place primarily in the brain. While hearing acuity is important, listening depends more significantly on motivation, determination, and skills in empathizing and interpreting.

Listening is defined as a skill whereby a person consciously attends to the other's message. It is an active process that requires concentration and effort on the part of the listener. The desired outcome of the listening process is an inference about the speaker's message (Kron, 1972; O'Brien, 1974; Wilson, 1970).

Authors who have written about listening are in agreement that listening is a process. The major difference in the process of listening described by

328

authors is the classification and the depth of refinement. For example, Wilson (1970) recommended a seven-step process; Parsons and Sanford (1979) and Egan (1970) both described a four-step process; and Hein (1980) presented activities of listening. Wilson's seven-step process is described here.

Step One: Purpose. According to Wilson (1970), the first step in the listening process is to listen with purpose. Both participants in the listening interaction enter into a situation with conscious and unconscious purposes. These purposes are associated with individual goals and needs, as well as with the roles and functions of the participants. Hein (1980) indicates the major value of purpose is that it determines the extent to which a patient will share himself or herself with the nurse. Rankin (1966) purports that the initial behavior of the listener is to establish the purpose for the interaction.

Travelbee (1971) asserts that the interest displayed by nurses is crucial to the listening process. Failure to show interest in a client is often interpreted, and probably correctly so, as disinterest in the client altogether. Whether implicit or explicit, rejection by the listeners results in less disclosure by the client. Anticipation of rejection and viewing nurses as busy and overworked both influence the listening process. Several researchers have found similar attitudes—generally nurses are perceived as being too busy, disapproving, and likely to refuse requests (Gowan and Morris, 1964; Skipper et al., 1963).

Step Two: Emotion. The second step of listening, according to Wilson (1970), is to be aware of the emotional influences acting on the participants and to determine the meaning of the message intended by the sender. The meaning can be influenced by attitudes, past experiences, and the situation at the moment.

Step Three: Attention. Paying attention to the speaker requires focusing complete attention on the speaker as well as other aspects of the environment. To maintain total attention, the listener must put forth the necessary effort to suppress prejudice, bias, preoccupying personal concerns, and any other distracting factors (Wilson, 1970). The interest and attention conveyed by the listener set the tone of the verbal communication the patient will share with the nurse during this interaction as well as in subsequent interactions (Hein, 1980). Showing interest in the speaker and the message is essential for a productive interaction (Nichols, 1966). Concentrating on the message enhances this step (Barker, 1971).

Step Four: Verbal Reception. Attention is a prerequisite to verbal reception. While a participant is listening, the purpose, emotion, and attention will primarily determine which spoken words will be heard, when meaning will be attached, and which ideas will be formulated. The listener experiences an influx of words, but they must be familiar and organized into a sequence before comprehension takes place. The degree of experience and educational level of the listener will determine to some extent the accuracy of the verbal reception (Wilson, 1970). Using insight and accepting the speaker's statements as they are enhances this step (Rankin, 1966).

Step Five: Assessment. Assessment implies interpreting ideas expressed in verbal symbols. Implicit in this phase is listening between the lines for the unexpressed message. This impels the listener to be cognizant of the words the speaker chooses and how, when, and where in the message they are used. The words provide clues for the listener to arrive at the meaning of the message. The listener also needs to be aware of which words are avoided as well as the nonverbal message that accompanies the expressed words. In addition, the listener is aware of the tone, tempo, volume, pitch, and inflection of the voice. The listener attempts to listen for predominant themes. The effective listener derives relationship between the ideas expressed (Wilson, 1970). This step also includes appraising the value or significance of statements (Rankin, 1966). Bois (1966) points out that having an open mind enhances the interaction.

Step Six: Response. Response is the the listener's reaction to the message that has been received. The response may be communicated either verbally or nonverbally. The effective listener appropriately times his response so that it reflects understanding of the received message. The listener's response to the speaker's message is the only way to test how well the message was understood and if there is a need for more clarification or correction. At this point the message is complete. The feedback aspect of listening is essential to determine if the listener understood the message (Wilson, 1970). The listener should clarify the message through the use of feedback (Barker, 1971). In order to respond to the speaker appropriately, the listener critically analyzes the message, draws conclusions, and makes an inference about the message. The listener is then ready to provide feedback or reflect on the speaker's message (Duker, 1961; Rankin, 1966).

A speaker who has experienced having his message understood and has received an accepting response from a listener now reaches satisfaction. A reciprocal feeling of satisfaction is experienced by the listener. Satisfaction conveys the message that the speaker is worth listening to and gives him or her a sense of importance. The freedom to express oneself and having the opportunity to clearly sense what is going on leads to responsibility and cooperation. Mutual efforts toward the goal of understanding and movement directed toward other inherent goals leads to satisfaction.

Listening can be summarized into specific actions so that a nurse can implement them.

1. Determine the purpose of the message on both conscious and unconscious levels.
2. Display an awareness of and sensitivity to emotions.
3. Be attentive and convey interest.
4. Hear the words spoken.
5. Interpret the message. Draw conclusions. Make inferences.
6. Respond to the message. Seek feedback.
7. Demonstrate an understanding and acceptance of the message.

BENEFITS OF LISTENING

Listening has been found to be influential in clarifying meaning of statements, enabling persons to draw conclusions, and allowing them to make inferences about the message (Wagner, 1971). Other values of listening are cited as enabling one to comprehend and evaluate the message (Barker, 1971).

Psychosocial advantages of listening have been identified as reducing tension, improving a person's self-image and self-confidence, establishing a sense of identity, and assisting individuals in recognizing the cultural and ethnic influences on their behavior (Barker, 1971).

Additional gains from listening are clarifying values, enhancing ability to problem solve, defining problems, increasing ability to share self, and nourishing a sense of community in relationships (Koile, 1977). Resolving conflicts, satisfying the human need to communicate, and altering attitudes and behavior patterns are identified by Nichols and Stevens (1957).

NURSING LITERATURE ON LISTENING

Hein (1980) proposes that listening is assessment. As a sensory tool, listening helps the nurse attach meaning to a patient's behavior regardless of how it is communicated. Listening denotes discovery—identifying relationships between verbal and nonverbal behavior.

Many interactions using listening with the patient are necessary if the nurse is to discover the meaning of the behavior. A one-time interaction provides insight, but a series of exchanges unfolds the interconnected aspects of the patient's personality and ways in which a need is expressed (Hein, 1980).

In all patient's verbal communication there is a common core of beliefs, feelings, and ideas. It may be subtle or quite obvious, but it always exists. These common cores are labeled themes—unifying, repetitive thoughts that connect various forms of expression.

Listening is of major importance to the nurse in identifying the theme of the patient's behavior. While themes exist in a patient's behavior, their significance is frequently communicated through variations in a basic theme. Therefore, themes are not always distinguishable through overt behaviors. In fact, the greater the need, the more it is disguised. Until the patient reaches a feeling of interpersonal safety, varying his or her particular theme serves as a protective device. Many variations will be displayed until the patient is sure of the nurse's purpose and ability to help resolve the need.

Because of the infinite ways a theme may be expressed, nurses must exercise their skill in listening to secure an accurate recognition of the theme. Hein (1980) maintains that listening for themes is a major component of assessing the patient's needs. She presented six themes representing some of the areas nurses encounter with patients in hospitals, in families, and in the community.

If nurses listen, to whom do they listen and what do they do with the data received during a listening interaction? Wallston and Wallston (1975) initiated an investigation to answer these questions. The study was carried out in a laboratory setting which resembled a patient care unit. Conversations with four simulated patients with medical diagnoses of diabetes mellitus, alcoholism with bleeding ulcer, ulcerative colitis, and cancer of the large intestine were tape-recorded on 12 topics pertaining to their illnesses. Of the 12 topics, six were physiological problems and six dealt with psychological aspects. To test a nurse's willingness both to listen and to communicate data to the next nurse, the 48 tape-recorded segments of patient information were played for the 16 volunteer nurses. Nurses in this study had an option of listening to these patients or preparing medications for other patients. Overall, nurses chose to listen 60 per cent of the time, indicating nurses saw this as a more valuable task than preparing medications. Following this, they were then asked to tape-record a report on the patient for the nurse who would follow them. Nurses reported to the next shift more information for the patients with the medical diagnoses of alcoholism with bleeding ulcer and cancer. Although the results are not conclusive, there is evidence from this study that a patient's diagnosis significantly influences the nurse's decision to listen.

Another significant study was conducted by Elder (1965) to determine how clearly patients expressed their state of comfort or discomfort and their needs for nursing care in an initial interaction with the nurse. Elder, in the role of participant observer, collected data on 60 nurse contacts with 41 patients. During the contacts, the researcher noted verbal and nonverbal behavior of the patients and responded to them in accord with aspects of the thought, feeling, or question that the patient's behavior evoked in the researcher. The response to behavior was made in an exploratory and nonjudgmental manner to allow patients to confirm, deny, or elaborate upon the researcher's perception of the patient's behavior or situation. The goal of the interaction was to obtain a mutual understanding of the patient's present condition and areas of discomfort or distress. Thus, the data collected encompassed (1) verbal and nonverbal behavior; (2) the state of comfort, discomfort, concern or distress; and (3) the type of nursing assistance that patients required. The finding of this study indicate that patients did not adequately communicate their needs for assistance upon the initial interaction. In 47 contacts, patients expressed no aspect of their needs clearly in their presenting behavior.

A typical interaction of nurse-patient contact in this study is evidenced by the example of the patient who was labeled a "demander" within a few hours of admission. Upon passing this patient's room, the nurse researcher heard, "Nurse, will you put down this window? I'm in a draft." This female patient was described as being thin, middle-aged, and pale, with a birdlike face and restless and fluttering hands. Before the researcher had closed the window the patient asked if the nurse could tell her when her doctor could come to see her. Instead of going to find out when the physician could visit with the patient, the researcher asked the patient if she had a particular reason for desiring to see the doctor. Later it was discovered that the patient had asked several other nurses the same question. With encouragement, the patient talked of her hospitalization, the scheduled operation, and the fears and concerns of what was going to happen to her. The nurse showed interest and encouraged her to continue. Many of the patient's fears were related to misconceptions and misinformation about the hospitalization and recovery period. The nurse clarified with the patient the misconceptions and indicated what she might expect in the postoperative period. As the nurse and patient continued to converse, the nurse noticed the patient's facial expression had changed, the muscles around the mouth and eyes had relaxed, and her hands were resting quietly. The nurse researcher verified her impression with the patient. The patient confirmed the nurse's perception and stated how anxious she was initially during their conversation and how much better she felt now.

Major implications of the findings of this study are the inability of patients to express their needs adequately and the significance of the listening process in helping patients identify their needs. Listening allowed the nurse in this study to respond to the patient's verbal and nonverbal behavior before employing another intervention that was based on misinterpreted behavior.

Tarasuk, Rymes, and Leonard (1965) designed an experimental study to test the importance of communication skills for effective nursing. Results of the study indicate that administering pain medication automatically, without first finding out the nature of the patient's report of pain, is often useless and perhaps at times harmful. The design of the study allowed for all patients whose communications were interpreted as meaning "pain" to be included in the study. The research nurse arranged with the medication nurse to place every other patient complaining of pain in the experimental group, while the remaining patients were placed in the control group and taken care of by the staff medication nurse. The patients in the experimental group were seen by the nurse researcher, who determined the type of nursing action needed based on statements of pain. All patients in the control group who said they had pain were given pain medication. In contrast, only 31 per cent of the patients in the experimental group were treated with pain medication; the remaining patients were determined to have pain that would not be alleviated by medication.

The two groups were compared on their relief from the original complaint of pain. The experimental approach resulted in faster relief of the patient's complaint and in more complete relief. This was measured by cues such as facial expression, color, and posture as well as by the patient's response to the question: How is your pain now? The majority of patients in the experimental group had immediate relief, whereas only a few in the control group did. The degree of pain relief was noted in three categories: "marked relief," "some relief," or "nonrelief." Although all the control group patients were treated with pain medication, none ever reached "marked relief" and 20 per cent reported no relief at all. In contrast, the majority of experimental patients achieved "marked relief." Relief was more effective in patients receiving pain medication in the experimental approach than in patients receiving pain medication in the control group.

What accounts for the drastic differences in the reports of relief in the two groups? The nurse treating the patients in the experimental group approached patients through a deliberative process which assumed that in order to intervene in a patient's needs, the nurse must first identify what the needs are. The nurse used her perceptions and explored them with the patient, by identifying and responding to verbal and nonverbal messages. She continually sought feedback from the patient about the accuracy of the message and, when action was taken, checked with the patient to determine its effectiveness. On the other hand, the control approach made assumptions about the meaning of the patient's behavior without obtaining feedback. Judgments about the needs of patients were also made. Occasionally no communication between patient and nurse took place except the administration of the pain medication.

The behaviors utilized by the nurse in the experimental group are synonymous with the behaviors of listening. Listening significantly reduced patients' pain. This study supports the assessment value of listening and implies that listening in some cases was used as an intervention to treat the patient's needs.

IS LISTENING AN INTERVENTION?

Thus far, listening has been presented as a dynamic process which, when applied, is a significant tool that helps the nurse accurately assess a patient's problems. As nurses incorporate diagnosis in the nursing process, the assessment phase becomes paramount as a prerequisite for accurate diagnosis. In the essence, the use of listening during nurse-patient interaction provides the nurse with data to make a precise diagnosis.

Listening has also been reported as being an intervention. Robinson (1983), an author of a psychiatric textbook, identifies listening as a therapeutic intervention. Smith and Duell (1982), authors of a basic nursing textbook, describe listening with therapeutic communication interventions. These authors are unique in their approach to listening. The majority of nursing textbooks do not discuss listening at all. The few textbooks that do address listening present it as a skill that facilitates communication between the patient and the nurse (Sorensen and Luckmann, 1979).

Is Listening an intervention? Smith and Duell (1982) define an intervention as the action component of performing a skill. Since listening has been described by numerous authors as a skill, when the nurse initiates the actions of the skill it is then an intervention. Listening therefore is an intervention. It does have significance in treating patients' problems.

Nursing journals also provide minimal discussion of listening as an intervention. One of the few authors who views listening as an intervention is Burkhardt (1969), who states that listening is the appropriate approach to use with patients who have mild or moderate anxiety. Listening is also cited by Burkhardt as being appropriate with patients who have fear.

Goldin and Russell (1969) concur with this use of listening, and describe some of the benefits that listening has for patients. Listening, they say, is helpful because it brings patients' feelings out in the open, helps them redirect their energies, and promotes better health.

Listening is also reported to be a method that aids patients in making their own decisions, allowing them to come to their own conclusions. A component of listening is to summarize a patient's dialogue—a method of mirroring his thoughts back to him. Thus, the patient can see himself, his attitudes, and his opinions in a clearer light. By pinpointing his most salient remarks, the nurse clarifies meaning to the patient and herself, thereby enhancing the patient's capabilities of making his own decision.

Henrich and Bernheim (1981) report the value of Listening as allowing a patient to identify, express, and accept his own feelings, and providing emotional relief. Another benefit is paving the way for more effective coping. Their report implies that listening may be effective in resolving a patient's diagnosis.

No scientific support for Listening's effectiveness as an intervention was found. In addition, tools with which to measure Listening were not found in the literature search. This is not surprising, since minimal research has been undertaken on this concept. Of the few studies reported, Listening was measured primarily through the listener's behavior.

LISTENING AS AN INTERVENTION

The importance of Listening as an assessment tool has been well documented in the literature. Therefore, Listening is essential to the nurse as a diagnostician. As the nurse employs the diagnostic process, listening will enhance the nurse's ability in generating an accurate diagnosis. Thus, Listening can then be employed by the nurse when diagnosing any patient's problems. Since no research has been completed where Listening was used as an intervention with a specific nursing diagnosis, suggestions for the use of Listening with several nursing diagnoses will be made.

The author supports Burkhardt's (1969) and Goldin and Russell's (1969) suggestion of using Listening as an intervention with the nursing diagnosis of *Anxiety*. Some of the defining characteristics of mild to moderate anxiety are restlessness, increased muscle tension, pacing, expressed feelings of apprehension or concern, and increased questioning (Gordon, 1982a, pp. 156, 158). Since Listening has been reported to decrease tension, enhance an individual's ability to define a problem, and increase problem-solving ability, Listening may address these aspects, thus enhancing the nurse's ability to treat anxiety with Listening. As causes for this diagnosis are identified, the intervention may increase or decrease in its effectiveness. Or, perhaps Listening will be used in conjunction with another intervention to treat the condition diagnosed.

The diagnosis of *Fear*, with an etiology of perceived inability to control an event, may also be treated with Listening. Some of the defining characteristics of this diagnosis are restlessness, increased muscle tension, and increased questioning or information-seeking (Gordon, 1982a, p. 168). Listening has been reported as relieving tension and enhancing a person's ability to clarify and make inferences about the message. These benefits offer support that the defining characteristics of fear can be reduced or removed. The etiological factor could be reduced through the capacity of Listening to enhance the client's ability to solve problems.

Listening may also be used in the treatment of *Social Isolation*. Some of the defining characteristics that Listening may influence are apathy and verbalization of isolation from others (Gordon, 1982a, p. 190). Perhaps the major value of Listening with this diagnosis is that Listening has been identified as satisfying the human need to communicate and as increasing an individual's sense of identity.

The diagnosis of *Body Image Disturbance* has the defining characteristics of "refusal to verify actual change in body, preoccupation with change in body, verbalized fear of rejection or retractions by others, change in social involvement, not touching or looking at body part, verbalized negative feelings about body" (Gordon, 1982a, pp. 162–163). The majority of these characterstics are psychosocial in nature. Listening has been cited as helping to improve an individual's self-image and self-confidence, clarifying values, and resolving conflict. These benefits from Listening may reduce the defining characteristics.

All of the diagnoses and defining characteristics are presently being used and studied by nurses. As data about these diagnoses are obtained with research, the utilization of Listening as an intervention may be altered. Etiological factors identified in the diagnosis are the focus of intervention (Gordon, 1982b). In order for Listening to be effective, it should be aimed at removing the etiological factors. However, the development of Active Listening as an intervention is only in the beginning stage. Once Active Listening has been further developed, the relationship between the intervention and particular causes can then be established. At this time, Listening can only be used in a speculative sense at reducing or removing defining characteristics.

PRACTICE AND RESEARCH

All actions by the nurse should be based on the goal of maintaining or improving the client's state of health. How the nurse communicates with the client impacts significantly on this goal. As Hein (1980) wrote: "Of all the skills we practice in relating to our patients, Listening is the primary sensory skill we use to effect therapeutic communication" (p. 224).

It is therefore recommended that Listening be used by the nurse when interacting with patients. Listening should be employed as an assessment tool in identifying the client's problems as well as an intervention in treating nursing diagnoses. Listening may be used as the primary nursing intervention or in conjunction with another intervention.

While Listening has been suggested as an assessment tool, research is needed to support or refute this. An experimental study could be designed involving patients being admitted to the hospital. Listening would be employed by the nurse during the initial assessment for the experimental group, and the traditional approach to assessment would be used with the control group. An experimental approach using Listening during the assessment phase while admitting a patient to the hospital will facilitate the nurse's ability to diagnose a client's problem and would be generated as a hypothesis for this study.

Experimental data on Listening as an intervention are nonexistent. Therefore, an exploratory study is necessary to determine why the nurse listens. This type of study would validate patient behaviors that require Listening. Once these behaviors were identified, nurses could then study Listening as an intervention. Experimental studies could be designed to test Listening's effect on the patient's behaviors. Finally, Listening could be researched as an intervention in treating nursing diagnoses.

CASE STUDY

Listening was found to be influential in assessment of a client's behavior as well as in treatment of the particular behaviors displayed. The client was a middle-aged woman who had been hospitalized for 45 days with a medical diagnosis of pancreatitis.

As an assessment tool, Listening was believed to decrease the time it took for the nurse to identify the client's problems, as well as increase the accuracy of determining the client's problems. The behaviors the nurse identified in the client were validated by the client. The client exhibited a poor self-image, made statements about being lonely, verbalized feelings of hopelessness and powerlessness with regard to physical condition, stated she had little contact with close personal friends, expressed concerns about no one understanding or accepting her, stated that nurses and doctors compared her with other clients, questioned values, inquired frequently about her physical condition, and stated she was having difficulty making decisions.

The nurse interacted with this patient over a period of several weeks. She used the seven steps and actions identified in the process of listening. Once the client's problem had been validated (nursing diagnosis of Social Isolation), Listening was continued during the interactions. Gradually, the originally identified behaviors of the client disappeared. At termination of the nurse-client relationship the patient displayed only the original behavior of concern about physical condition; all other behaviors were no longer manifested.

In general, although the results of this case study are far from conclusive, there is evidence that Listening was significant in helping the nurse identify the client's problem with accuracy and in modifying the majority of behaviors the client expressed, since Listening was the only intervention used with this client.

EDITORS' COMMENTS AND QUESTIONS

Active Listening, like Presence in the previous section, is an example of an intervention nurses do all the time but have not systematically defined or studied. The literature to develop the intervention is borrowed from the fields of speech pathology and communication. Little nursing research has been conducted, but Helms gives a good example for generating research relating to the intervention.

Questions for Discussion

1. *How does the intervention of Active Listening differ from listening used in the nurse-patient communication process?*

2. *What are the similarities and differences between the interventions of Active Listening and Presence (see Chapter 22)?*

References

Barbara, D. A. On listening. *Today's Speech*, 1957, 5(1), 12–15.

Barker, L. L. *Listening behavior*. Englewood Cliffs, N.J.: Prentice-Hall, 1971.

Bois, S. J. The art of listening, in S. Duker (Ed.), *Listening: Readings* (Vol. 11. New York: Scarecrow Press, 1966.

Brammer, L. M. *The helping relationship*. Englewood Cliffs, N.J.: Prentice-Hall, 1973.

Burkhardt, M. Response to anxiety. *American Journal of Nursing*, 1969, 69(10), 2153–2154.

Duker, S. Goals of teaching listening skills in the elementary. *Elementary English*, 1961, 38:170–174.

Edwards, B. J., and Brillhart, J. K. *Communication in nursing practice*. St. Louis: C. V. Mosby Company, 1981.

Egan, G. *Encounter: Group processes for interpersonal growth*. Belmont, Calif.: Brooks/Cole Publishing Company, 1970.

Elder, R. G. What is the patient saying? in J. K. Skipper, Jr., and R. C. Leonard (Eds.), *Social interaction and patient care*. Philadelphia: J. B. Lippincott Company, 1965, pp. 102–110.

Goldin, P., and Russell, B. Therapeutic communication. *American Journal of Nursing*, 1969, 69(9), 1928–1930.

Gordon, M. *Manual of nursing diagnosis*. New York: McGraw-Hill Book Company, 1982a.

Gordon, M. *Nursing diagnosis process and application*. New York: McGraw-Hill Book Company, 1982b.

Gowan, N. G., and Morris, M. Nurses' response to expressed patient needs. *Nursing Research*, 1964, 13, 68–71.

Hein, E. C. *Communication in nursing practice* (2nd ed.). Boston: Little, Brown and Company, 1980.

Henrich, A. P., and Bernheim, K. F. Responding to patients' concerns. *Nursing Outlook*, 1981, 29(2), 161–170.

Koile, E. *Listening as a way of becoming*. Waco, Texas: Word Books Publishers, 1977.

Kron, T. *Communication in nursing*. Philadelphia: W. B. Saunders Company, 1972.

Lewis, G. K. *Nurse-patient communication*. Dubuque, Iowa: Wm. C. Brown Company, 1973.

Nichols, R. G. Listening instruction in the secondary school, in S. Duker (Ed.), *Listening: Readings* (Vol. 1). New York: Scarecrow Press, 1966.

Nichols, R. G., and Stevens, L. *Are you listening?* New York: McGraw-Hill Book Company, 1957.

O'Brien, M. J. *Communications and relationships in nursing*. St. Louis: C. V. Mosby Company, 1974.

Parsons, V., and Sanford, N. *Interpersonal interaction in nursing*. Menlo Park, Calif.: Addison-Wesley Publishing Company, 1979.

Rankin, P. T. Listening ability and its components, in S. Duker (Ed.), *Listening: Readings* (Vol. 1). New York: Scarecrow Press, 1966.

Robinson, L. *Psychiatric nursing as a human experience* (3rd ed.). Philadelphia: W. B. Saunders Company, 1983.

Skipper, J. K., Jr., Mauksch, H. O., and Tagliacozzo, D. Some barriers to communication between patients and hospital functionaries. *Nursing Forum*, 1963, 2(1), 14–23.

Smith, S., and Duell, D. *Nursing skills and evaluation*. Los Altos, Calif.: National Nursing Review, 1982.

Sorensen, K. C., and Luckmann, J. *Basic nursing: a psychophysiologic approach*. Philadelphia: W. B. Saunders Company, 1979.

Tarasuk, M. B., Rymes, J. P., and Leonard, R. C. An experimental test of the importance of communication skills for effective nursing, in J. K. Skipper, Jr., and R. C. Leonard (Eds.), *Social interaction and patient care*. Philadelphia: J. B. Lippincott Company, 1965, pp. 110–120.

Travelbee, J. *Interpersonal aspects of nursing* (2nd ed.). Philadelphia: F. A. Davis Company, 1971.

Wagner, G. Teaching listening, in S. Duker (Ed.), *Listening: Readings* (Vol. 2). New York: Scarecrow Press, 1971.

Wallston, K. A., and Wallston, B. S. Nurses' decision to listen to patients. *Nursing Research*, 1975, 24(1), 16–22.

Wilson, L. M. Listening, in C. E. Carlson (Ed.), *Behavioral concepts and nursing intervention* (2nd ed.). Philadelphia: J. B. Lippincott Company, 1970.

24

ADVOCACY

M. PATRICIA DONAHUE

> Turning points occur in the history of a profession when radical questioning
> and clarification of major tenets become essential for further growth. We
> recognize such a turning point now in nursing. The direction in which
> nursing develops will determine whether the profession draws closer to
> the medical model, with its commitment to science, technology, and cure;
> reverts to historical nursing models, with their essentially intuitive ap-
> proaches; or creates a philosophy that sets contemporary nursing distinc-
> tively apart from both traditional nursing and modern medicine.
>
> SALLY GADOW, 1980, p. 79

HISTORICAL PERSPECTIVE

Reasons currently abound supporting incorporation of the concept of advocacy
within the health care delivery system. Most are predicated on the fact that
crucial changes within society and, concomitantly, within health services and
medical science have mandated a means of protection for the consumer
requiring care. Inherent in this perspective, however, is the issue of ethics,
which is closely aligned to any discussion of advocacy. The question of ethical
health care practices has provided the driving force behind the outcry for
"patient advocates." Concern for and implementation of *quality* health care,
with emphasis on human worth, dignity, and rights, is thus becoming a
permanent feature of the working environment of health professionals.

Contrary to popular belief, the idea of advocacy is *not* new. Since the
turn of the century, it has been developed in conjunction with the consumer
protection and consumer rights movements. The consumer movement has
been destined to be a recurrent aspect of the American scene initiated by the
persisting problems of ill-considered application of new technology that results
in dangerous or unreliable products, changing conceptions of social responsibilities to be assumed by government, and the operation of a dishonest fringe
and occasional lapses of others in the business world (Hermann, 1978).

As consumer issues escalated, government regulations and legislation
were enacted in an attempt to benefit public welfare as well as eventually to
protect particular consumer groups (Nadel, 1971). This phenomenon ulti-

mately led to the development of a new—although at times a very controversial—figure, the consumer advocate. According to Nadel (1971), three basic types of consumer advocates emerged and are in evidence today: the *traditional advocate*, who works through political channels for the benefit of private or public interest groups; the *consumer crusader*, who plays a type of Ralph Nader activist role; and the *press*, who provide feedback and transmit information to the public. These actions, however, have only begun to deal with the ever-increasing consumer dissatisfaction and certainly have not provided totally acceptable solutions. Perhaps the inherent difficulty lies in Stone's argument that although legal rights of consumers may have been protected, their actual needs may not have been met (1979).

Consumer unrest is not confined to the economic, political, and social realms of society, but has eroded into the vital arena of health care services. Kelly (1976, p. 26) labels this movement "the social revolution of consumer action" which is "now being directed to the care given to *people*, not just to separate parts of their bodies." She proposes that this action will have a greater impact on health care than "any series of exotic scientific discoveries." She, as well as other writers, lends credence to the urgent need of a patient advocate role in the health care system (Annas and Healey, 1974; Chapman and Chapman, 1975; Christy, 1973; Curtin, 1979; Donahue, 1978; Gadow, 1980; Kosik, 1972).

The exact point at which advocacy became a real concern within health care is difficult to ascertain. Yet, it is an old term receiving new recognition. Kahn and associates (1972), after conducting a review of the aspect of advocacy, made the following statement:

> Historically, advocacy has existed as long as there have been powerless groups in need of a champion. The self-advocacy of suffragettes and the class advocacy of social reformers are as integral parts of American history as the more traditional form of legal advocacy. Recently consumer health and family advocacy programs have mushroomed. (p. 14)

Indeed, the concern for consumers of health care services has been inevitable and directly parallels the approach toward overall consumer protection exhibited in this country.

Several societal trends have occurred that have escalated interest in the advocacy movement. Each, however, is directly related to the twentieth century success of two distinct phenomena: democracy and technology (Thompson and Thompson, 1981). Democracy has focused on human rights and human responsibility, including self-government and education. Yet, as the focus on rights and obligations progressed, enormous changes in technology in most fields of human endeavor occurred, which added to the complexities of life and the delivery of health care.

In retrospect, two trends can be identified that have produced the greatest impact: an erosion of the professional knowledge monopoly and the decline of trust in professional decisions. Although not peculiar to health care, the significance of these issues to a concept of patient advocacy mandates an examination of their specific relationship to health care professionals.

Historically, it can be demonstrated that the command of knowledge has set the professional apart from the rest of society. The acquisition of special information was limited to the elite (professionals) who gained power by convincing the public that they had cornered their relevant knowledge market. These "professional claims of being the sole repositories of esoteric knowledge useful to society and the individual" are currently being "undermined by public education, computerization, and the sharing of expertise in new divisions of labor" (Haug, 1975, p. 206). According to Haug, the erosion of the knowledge monopoly has been the result of rising levels of public schooling and expanded public sophistication. This position is supported by Wilensky (1974, p. 158), who proposed the paradox that education not only could result in greater utilization of professional services but also could produce " greater sophistication about matters professional, more skepticism about the certainties of practice, some actual sharing in professional knowledge [the mysteries lose their enchantment]." Thus, the more educated general public are challenging professionals' exclusive command over health care.

A similar point can be made about the use of computers, which has given rise to knowledge availability and utilization. Potentially, the storage and retrieval systems will afford accessibility to professional knowledge to those who know how to get it. In addition, patients can now penetrate the mysteries of the health care system. Components of health education and regimens for various ailments, as well as other types of medical information, are constantly being disseminated to consumers through a variety of mechanisms, such as books, magazines, television programs, and so forth. Furthermore, new divisions of labor have emerged to create a wider spread of practice skills and information (Haug, 1975). No longer is the health care consumer ignorant of the complex machinery of the human mind and body. The demand for quality care and the protection of individual rights relative to that care are fast becoming a reality.

The age of consumerism has also produced a decline in trust in professional decisions, as evidenced by the rise of malpractice suits and limitations on medical experimentation. It is clear that there is a definite change in the public's view of appropriate behavior for themselves as patients and for health care workers as well. The demand for accountability and patient protection is apparent. The role of advocate has been proposed as a reliable means for achieving these goals.

NURSING AND ADVOCACY

The terms "advocate" and "patient advocate" seem to be popular in nursing circles today, although they did not appear in the *International Nursing Index* as a subject heading until 1976. It could be questioned whether this concept represents a fad or whether it indeed merits careful scrutiny and incorporation into the essence of nursing. Kohnke (1982) proposed that "advocacy" is an example of familiar buzz words that become popular every few years. The fact remains, however, that patients have become aware of themselves as something other than simply objects of care; their view has expanded to incorporate roles for themselves in scientific inquiry and as consumers of a valuable product.

It is difficult to delineate the progression of nursing in relation to the development of patient advocacy. Yet, if one considers advocacy in the context of "an act of loving and caring," there is no doubt that it has been a viable construct underlying the very foundation of nursing. In this sense, it has existed since the earliest origins of nursing, although it has received other types of labels. Certainly, the early nurse leaders were patient advocates; they "were nurses who were concerned about and committed to human rights, dignity, humanitarianism, and accountability" (Donahue, 1978, p. 146). Their definition of nursing included autonomy, advocacy, and independent practice, which focused on the prevention of illness as well as the maintenance of health. These ideas are consistent with current thought regarding advocacy and, more important, provide a holistic, humanistic approach to nursing care. Perhaps the question to be answered here is not whether the nurse should be a patient advocate but rather how nursing lost this role. It would seem that our present scope of practice has been severely limited compared with that of our illustrious predecessors. A concerted effort is now being made to reclaim a vital component present in early nursing.

A glimpse into nursing's history indeed can demonstrate the incorporation of the advocacy role. One need only to read about such individuals as Lavinia Dock and Lillian Wald to realize that nursing not only was concerned about patient advocacy but also practiced it. Delving even further into the roots of nursing, one cannot help but be impressed with the endeavors of Florence Nightingale, the founder of modern nursing. She was truly an independent practitioner who viewed herself as the patient's advocate. She thoroughly understood the importance of economics and the stratagems of power, and sought to establish a system whereby nurses themselves controlled nursing practice and nursing education. In her book, *Notes on Nursing: What It Is and What It Is Not* (1860), she set forth a clear concise charge to nurses for a broad definition of nursing: caring for and caring about, encompassing the care of the whole individual. It has taken the focus on consumer protection and human rights, however, for the emphasis on patient advocacy to resurface within nursing.

Only within the last 25 years has interest in the preservation of human rights become emphasized among health care professionals. Several documents are now in existence that affirm patient rights, including one issued as early as 1959 by the National League for Nursing, entitled "What People Can Expect of Modern Nursing Service." Since 1970 the Joint Commission of Accreditation of Hospitals has included a "Patient's Bill of Rights" in its list of standards for accreditation (Taubenhaus, 1976). The best known of these statements was issued in 1973 by the American Hospital Association (AHA) with the expectation that observance of these rights would contribute to more effective patient care. (No nurses were included in the committee membership to develop this statement!) "Since the issuance of the AHA statement, patient's rights have been explored separately, by such groups as hospital administrators, nurses, and lawyers" (Carnegie, 1974, p. 558). According to Kelly (1976), what is disheartening is the fact that the majority of the rights about which patients are concerned are theirs legally as well as morally.

The ideas expressed in the AHA Bill of Rights are not new to nurses. They have been delineated in a code of ethics (American Nurses' Association, 1976) which states that "the nurse provides services with respect for human dignity and the uniqueness of the client unrestricted by considerations of social or economic status, personal attributes, or the nature of health problems." This Code for Nurses, first developed in 1950, further states that "the nurse acts to safeguard the client and the public when health care and safety are affected by the incompetent, unethical, or illegal practices of any person." Nurses worldwide agreed on a similar code titled "Ethical Concepts Applied to Nursing," adopted in 1973 by the International Council of Nurses. This document maintains that "the nurse takes appropriate action to safeguard the individual when his care is endangered by a coworker or any other person." The nurse is obligated to actively ensure patients' rights and safety according to these codes. Although not *explicit*, the concept of advocacy is *implicit* in these statements. Unfortunately, these codes are not generally legally enforceable. However, they contain a certain moral power in terms of the respect for the rights of individuals.

At the present time, a significant portion of nursing literature addresses the issue of advocacy and, more specifically, patient advocacy. There has emerged a spectrum of ideas that either support or oppose the ultimate and legitimate role of the nurse as a patient advocate. It would seem that the value of such a concept in nursing is yet to be determined.

DESCRIPTIONS AND DEFINITIONS OF ADVOCACY

Currently, there is an abundance of nursing literature that attempts to define or describe advocacy, provide a rationale for the assumption of the advocacy role in nursing, or promote a specific model of patient advocacy. Yet the concept, although popular, does not seem to be totally understood or supported. It is evident that there is a wide diversity of opinion regarding an acceptable definition. Even more glaring is an obvious lack of descriptive empirical investigations that could provide the basis for putting advocacy into practice. In Wilberding's opinion (1984, p. 6) much of what has appeared in the literature "is philosophical reflection and opinion which provides a good intellectual basis for patient advocacy. There is little that examines how patient advocacy has been operationalized in practice aside from some anecdotal accounts."

An advocate has long been defined as one who pleads the cause of another; one who acts on behalf of another (Webster's New Collegiate Dictionary, 1973, p. 18). Transferring this definition to the situation involving a patient results in a simple definition of patient advocacy: one who pleads the cause of the patient; one who acts on behalf of the patient. Yet the majority of nurses who have contributed even minimally in the attempt to define advocacy do not seem to embrace the foregoing definition. The key element here seems to be a hesitancy over the word "act," which implies a variety of functions that may force the nurse into a more than passive role. They may even potentially force the nurse into situations that can be both risky and hazardous. This would naturally evolve, since the concepts of assertiveness, risk-taking, power, human rights and dignity, noncompliance, and involvement are entangled in advocacy and would require not only an understanding and support of these but also a commitment (Donahue, 1981). In essence, to be an advocate is easier said than done. Thus, it is difficult to accept such a definition and still more difficult to achieve it, since no clear-cut mechanism has been developed to accomplish such a formidable task.

An examination of the available nursing definitions of advocacy reveals a wide range of views, which progress from the very simple to the extremely complex. The major themes that emerge from these definitions include human rights, interpersonal relationships, support, information-giving, self-determination, and humanism. The primary factor that is emphasized—the patient—is consistent with a statement made by Goodnow (1921, p. 19) early in this century: "the patient is the main thing—the reason for it all—the unit—the one chief consideration, the one [to] whose welfare all else must be subordinated." It is, however, beyond the scope of this chapter to enumerate *all* current definitions. A selected list is provided in Table 24–1, which will give the reader an overview of existing ways to define advocacy.

It is apparent that an attempt must be made to unify the diverse descriptions of patient advocacy; this is imperative if its true value to nursing practice is ever to be determined. In addition, for the advocate role to become a reality for nursing, it must become a professionally sanctioned responsibility that will be internalized, taught, and utilized.

Table 24–1. NURSING DEFINITIONS OF ADVOCACY

Author(s)	Definitions and Related Statements
Chapman and Chapman (1975)	"Actions are taken in behalf of patients when it has been determined that *on their own* they or their representatives cannot bring the needed resources to bear on the situation" (p. 68) "Advocacy requires (1) the statement of a humane goal, or cause, (2) assertive action to accomplish the goal, and (3) an attitude of concern that the best be obtained for those for whom one advocates" (p. 60)
Kosik (1972)	"Patient advocacy is seeing that the patient knows what to expect and what is his right to have, and then displaying the willingness and courage to see that our system does not prevent his getting it" (p. 694) "Nurses must become actively involved not only in nurse-patient relationships but also in social-political relationships in order to be a patient advocate" (p. 698)
Nowakowski (1977)	"Client advocacy is aimed at helping the client move from passivity to action in his own behalf—assisting him to become actively responsible for his own health and decisions about it" (p. 299) "It is *not* fighting for what *advocates* think is best for the client but what the client believes is best or is willing to support" (p. 227)
Donahue (1978)	"Advocacy ... involves concern for and defined actions in behalf of another at both the individual and the system's organizational level" (p. 144) "It is the third element, knowledge, which is the key to nurses' attainment of the value of patient advocacy" (p. 150)
Donahue (1981)	"It simply means the acceptance that patients and family members have rights, as do nurses—the acceptance of the premise that man as a human being has the right to choose the manner in which he is to live or die" (p. 732)
Curtin (1979)	"The concept of adovacy implied here is not the concept of the patients' rights movement nor the legal concept of advocacy, but a far more fundamental advocacy founded upon the simplest and the most basic of premises" (p. 2) "This proposed ideal of advocacy is based upon our common humanity, our common needs, and our common human rights" (p. 3) "We must, as human advocates, assist patients to find meaning or purpose in their living or in their dying.... Whatever patients define as their goal, it is their meaning and not ours, their values and not ours, and their living or dying, not ours" (p. 7)
Thollaug (1980)	"Patient advocacy, then, is a kind of reform movement aimed at restructuring the relationship between providers and consumers according to the interests of the latter" (p. 37) "It is a profound challenge to each nurse that he/she conduct his/her own practice with the patient as the main focus and the first priority" (p. 58)
Kohnke (1980)	"The decision a client makes is his own, even if, in your own opinion, it is not the best decision for him. He has the right to make decisions freely and without pressure. This is advocacy in the finest sense of the word" (p. 2039) "I suppose the bottom line of the advocate role can be summarized in the term *knowledge* or *to know*.... The act of advocacy is, at its basic level, an act of loving and caring for others as you would love and care for yourself" (p. 2040)
Kohnke (1982)	"The role of the advocate is to *inform* the client and then to *support* him in whatever decisions he makes" (p. 2)
Gadow (1979)	"The concept of existential advocacy ... is based upon the principle that freedom of self-determination is the most fundamental and valuable human right" (p. 82)
Gadow (1980)	"We can summarize advocacy nursing as the participation with the patient in determining the *personal meaning* which the experience of illness, suffering, or dying is to have for that individual" (p. 97)

Table continued on next page

Table 24–1. NURSING DEFINITIONS OF ADVOCACY (*Continued*)

Author(s)	Definitions and Related Statements
Castledine (1981)	"The ideal which existential advocacy expresses is this: that individuals be *assisted* by nursing to *authentically* exercise their freedom of self-determination" "Advocacy is 'the act of informing, supporting, and protecting a person who is making, or has made, a decision regarding their own health care needs to increase their opportunities to get what they want.' If we do not start with this aim in mind then the nursing process will not be implemented for the good of the patient but for the sole benefit of nurses" (p. 14)

LITERATURE ON ADVOCACY

The era of advocacy is upon us and is being heralded in the literature. Yet advocacy still seems to be a myth rather than reality. In nursing it is in a stage of infancy and needs to be nurtured for growth and development to occur. More important, it must be made credible if it is ever to be incorporated in nursing as a valuable, necessary, and valid construct.

Although many nursing authors have been defining advocacy, others have been supporting the premise that the role of advocate is not only suitable for nurses but crucial for humanistic care. Christy (1973) viewed advocacy as the nursing challenge of thae 1970s that would involve nurses acting as patient sponsors, supporters, and counselors. This would be achieved through the acceptance of new responsibilities: the development of a deeper understanding of broader definitions of nursing, the acceptance of the components inherent in accountability, and the collective group becoming social activists. Knowledge would be essential (Donahue, 1978) and would be the key to attaining the role of patient advocate. Without it, nurses would be powerless to make independent judgments and decisions or unable to act on them.

The justification of the nurse's advocacy role is evident according to Fay (1978), who believes that it is implicit in the definition of nursing practice. Storch (1978) supports this position, since nurses have sustained contact with the patient and his family, have a large number of members in their ranks, and are distributed throughout the health care system. In addition, acting as the patient's advocate when he is unable to act on his own behalf is consistent with the nurse's traditional role. Anderson (1977) calls this simply "caring about" in her view of the nurse as a "lover of humanity."

The concept of patient advocacy has indeed received widespread endorsement in nursing literature. Yet Jenny (1979) questions why the need for another worker in the health care system has arisen. She cites reasons from the literature:

> (1) The advocate helps solve problems that may fall between the traditional job descriptions of other health professionals.
> (2) an adversary relationship exists between patient and therapist, and the advocate is needed to forge a redefinition of this relationship in favor of the patient.
> (3) Observance of patients' rights produces a conflict of interest between those of the patient and those of the providers of service or the institution. (p. 179)

These statements cast doubt about an advocacy role for the nurse. Jenny (1979) views them as potential barriers to the assumption of such a role, since they are concerned with the traditional nurse's role, adversary relationships, and potential conflict of interests. Consequently, shifts in nurses' self-concepts, allegiance, and repertoire of skills would have to occur before advocacy could be incorporated as a function of nursing.

Abrams (1978) also questions the appropriateness of nurses acting as patients' advocates on the basis of their dependence on employing agencies and their paternalistic relationship to the patient. She suggests that viewing patient advocacy as part of the nursing function may be fraught with difficulties since patients have the right to an *impartial* advocate in situations of conflict, when certain types of advocacy are most needed.

It is clear that there is still not total acceptance of this role for nurses. Although a large number of authors lend credence to the idea of the nurse as a patient advocate, a minority raise interesting points concerning the likelihood of the nurse's being effective in the advocate's role. Still other nurses have used case studies to demonstrate those situations in which they believed they functioned as advocates (Clark, 1978; Danielson et al., 1980; Nelson, 1977; Robb, Peterson, and Nagy, 1979; Smith, 1980; Vinyard, 1980).

Perhaps the most crucial information to come forth from the literature has been the description of models of patient advocacy that have been developed in all social arenas. A variety of models have been proposed and used, which tend to focus on a specific aspect of concern for either a consumer or a patient. These models include patients' rights advocate, ombudsman, legal advocate, sociopolitical advocate, and patient representative. However, it is difficult to determine how effective these particular models have been and whether they are indeed models of true advocacy or simply stop-gap measures to solve annoying and immediate problems. It would seem that an advocacy model for nursing would need to encompass the total individual (patient) rather than one aspect of concern, would need to consider long-term or projected outcomes, and would need to focus on helping the patient to ultimately become his own advocate when appropriate. In other words, a much broader concept of the advocate would be imperative.

Several nurses have proposed specific models in which nurses would assume the patient advocate role (Curtin, 1979; Gadow, 1980; Kohnke, 1980). The advocate in all of these models facilitates patient decision-making by giving or providing information. What is entailed in the information-giving process, however, varies with the particular model.

According to Kohnke (1982, p. 2), "the role of the advocate is to *inform* the client and then to *support* him in whatever decision he makes." Thus, advocacy is a twofold process of action that focuses on the patient's decision-making power. Consequently, the autonomy of the individual is upheld.

In this model, patients are informed of their rights in specific situations, patients receive all necessary information to make an informed decision, the nurse's opinions or biases are not revealed, and patient decisions based on rational ways of thinking are supported. The patient in this framework is free to make decisions without pressure, decisions that may be in conflict with the wishes and desires of family, friends, or health professionals. Kohnke (1980, p. 2039), therefore, cautions that the professional or advocate must not get into the position of rescuer (making decisions for others when they are capable of doing so themselves), as this role would rob the patient of responsibilities and rights. With this model, constraints will be placed on the advocate, who frequently will be in an adversary position.

Existential advocacy is the model proposed by Gadow (1980), who carefully and clearly distinguishes it from consumerism and paternalism. It, too, is concerned with decision-making and "is based upon the principle that freedom of self-determination is the most fundamental and valuable human right" (1980, p. 84). Gadow describes this type of advocacy in three ways:

1. The nurse's assistance to individuals in exercising their right to self-determination, through decisions which express the full and unique complexity of their values.
2. A mode of involvement with patients which necessarily engages the entire self of the nurse.
3. Assistance to patients in unifying the experience of the lived body and the object body at a level that incorporates and transcends both. (1980, p. 97)

Inherent in these descriptions are five conceptual themes that underlie this advocacy model—self-determination, the patient-practitioner relationship, the patient's values, the practitioner's values, and individuality (Gadow, 1981, p. 138). All of these are integral components of the self-determined decision-making process.

The need for relevant information is also vital in Gadow's model. However, the existential advocate does not merely supply the patient with information that is to be presented (Gadow, 1981). Thus, the patient decides how much information he needs; the nurse advocate enables and assists his decision.

Although it is beyond the scope of this chapter to completely analyze this model, existential advocacy can be summarized as "the participation with the patient in determining the *personal meaning* which the experience of illness, suffering, or dying is to have for the individual" (Gadow, 1980, p. 97).

A third model was developed by Curtin (1979), who distinguished it from patient rights advocacy and legal advocacy. She proposes that the nurse as advocate is a philosophical foundation for nursing as "it involves the basic nature and purpose of the nurse-patient relationship" (1979, p. 3). This model, entitled human advocacy, "is based upon our common humanity, our common needs and our common rights" (1979, p. 3).

The nurse-patient relationship in this model is similar to that in existential advocacy. Here, the emphasis is on the uniqueness of the patient, which parallels Gadow's concept of individuality. This theme of uniqueness extends into the information process since the patient must receive enough information to choose among options. However, patient readiness and ability to assimilate information must be the principles behind how, when, and how much patients are told (see Chapter 26 for an expanded discussion of this topic). In addition, human advocacy will lead to illumination of the meaning and purpose of an individual's living or dying. In essence, "the concept of human advocacy is as natural as living and dying" (Curtin, 1979, p. 9).

The fact that much has been written about advocacy is beyond dispute. Yet, two areas related to the topic remain virtually untouched—the advocate role with incompetent patients and reports of conducted research. Circuitous comments are infrequently found regarding the difficulty of functioning as an advocate for an incompetent patient. In these instances, Kohnke (1980, p. 2039) suggests that the advocate must become the rescuer "when the client may be too young or in a coma, and thus is unable to make the decision." Indeed, decision making does become more complex when the individual, because of age or disease state, cannot choose for himself and must be protected. In addition, controversy and at times conflict surface, since a decision is being made for someone else. Unfortunately, there is no universal agreement as to who has the right to make such a decision. Consequently, the question of ethics may be particularly evident in these situations.

Published reports of research specific to nurse advocacy are nearly impossible to find. In fact, only one study was found by this author, which was an attempt to measure nurses' attitudes regarding nursing autonomy and advocacy, patients' rights, and rejection of traditional role limitations. Pankratz and Pankratz (1974) reported that positive attitudes toward these factors were highly correlated with advanced education, leadership, academic setting, and nontraditional social climate. However, how these attitudes are reflected in the nurses' behavior remains unanswered. It is painfully clear that additional studies are needed, both descriptive and experimental.

An initial step in the process of developing a conceptual description of advocacy was begun by Kraus (1981), who found that the nursing concept of patient advocacy comprised three basic elements:

> These include a guiding perspective of the nurse-client relationship that respects the patient's right to autonomy, a caring professional nurse who embodies certain qualities that are necessary for advocacy to be effective, and the facilitation of patient autonomy through the implementation of specific advocacy actions. (p. 53)

Kraus investigated the role of the nurse as a patient advocate through an analysis of current articles addressing advocacy as a nursing function, personal interviews with registered nurses with an expressed interest in patient advocacy, and presentations at workshops incorporating content on patient advocacy. In the author's words, "advocacy is expert professional care that is tailored to the specific needs of the patient and his family as the advocate coordinates and humanizes what would otherwise be fragmented, impersonal interventions" (p. 53).

A second descriptive study currently in the data collection phase promises additional information. Wilberding (1984) is conducting an investigation of nurses' concepts of patient advocacy and how they use these in practice. This study should give an empirically based account of the state of the art of patient advocacy as a nursing role—i.e., whether patient advocacy as a nursing role has found its way into the *real world*.

Although the latter two studies are at present unpublished, they provide beginning information relative to the nurse in the advocate role. It is hoped that they will be the catalysts for increased research in this area.

ADVOCACY—AN INTERVENTION?

Unlike other strategies of nursing intervention, advocacy currently has no formal tools or instruments. As previously described, the concept itself in nursing is still in its infancy. Yet, patient advocacy is relevant for and applicable to any patient or group of patients in any setting in which nursing is practiced. Questions remain, however, as to whether advocacy is appropriate for nursing and, more important, what it really is. Even more fundamental is the question of whether advocacy is an intervention. In the opinion of this author, advocacy, in the *narrowest* sense, can be and is an intervention if intervention is defined as an independent nursing action designed to treat a specific diagnosed problem or situation. In this sense, advocacy is not simply an intervention but *the* intervention underlying every action a nurse takes. In other words, advocacy is the basis or foundation upon which any nursing intervention rests. The level of the action will be determined by the assessed situation. For example, an intervention may involve patient education, in which case the nurse will inform and teach. If, on the other hand, a patient does not wish to accept a prescribed medical treatment, the nurse may not only inform and teach, but also support, protect, defend, and potentially be placed in an adversarial position (nurse and patient against the health care system). In either case, the nurse performs in a specific manner for the ultimate benefit of the patient.

As an intervention, advocacy would relate to all of the nursing diagnoses approved by the Fourth National Conference on the Classification of Nursing Diagnosis (1980) from Activity Intolerance to Potential for Violence. The breadth and depth of nurse involvement, however, would be determined by all aspects of the particular situation. For example, Knowledge Deficit would of necessity have to be approached in a very different manner from Alteration in Tissue Perfusion or Rape-Trauma Syndrome. The major themes that emerge from the definitions of advocacy (human rights, interpersonal relationships, support, information-giving, self-determination, and humanism) would thus have to be considered to a greater or lesser degree with each specific nursing diagnosis. The two nursing diagnoses that seem of particular relevance are Powerlessness and Impaired Communication.

To consider advocacy, however, as simply an intervention would be a grave injustice. Advocacy must be considered and utilized in a much broader context—as a dynamic process which underlies the entire care philosophy of nursing and which provides the very structure basic to the nurse-patient relationship. As Thollaug (1980) stated:

> From the foundation of a strong nurse/patient relationship, we can help patients identify their alternatives, cope with their limitations within their own framework of values, and support them in defending their rights and prerogatives. Finally, we must represent patients' own wishes when they are unable to do so. This kind of relationship could be the tie that binds a person to the health care system: one of trust, and one directed by the interests, philosophy, and concerns of the patient. (p. 37)

The end or purpose of this process is the welfare of other human beings. Thollaug (1980, p. 58) carries this one step further and suggests making patient advocacy the conceptual framework for nursing. As such, nurses would need to be courageous and open and to conduct their practice with the patient as the main focus and the first priority.

Advocacy, in the final analysis, may possibly be the theory for nursing. It is interesting to note that it closely parallels the theory of goal attainment postulated by King (1981) and mirrors her process of human interaction, as seen in Table 24–2.

It is, however, beyond the scope of this chapter to adequately discuss and analyze the similarities between the concept of advocacy and the theory of goal attainment. Suffice it to say that both encompass a humanistic viewpoint, with a major emphasis on interpersonal relationships. The role of the nurse advocate could very well be what King (1981) defines as the nurse's role:

> an interaction between one or more individuals who come to a nursing situation in which nurses perform functions of professional nursing based on knowledge, skills, and values to identify goals in each situation and to help individuals achieve goals. (p. 93)

Role in this instance is not just a function of the individual but is interactional. "When two individuals come together for a purpose, such as in a nursing situation, they are each perceiving the other person and the situation, making judgments, taking mental action, or making a decision to act" (King, 1981, p. 145).

According to Kosik (1972), patient advocacy is nursing's hope for the future. It appeals to nurses at the present time for a variety of reasons: it is a way to flee from traditional bondage; it becomes a vehicle to achieve greater

Table 24–2. A PROCESS OF HUMAN INTERACTIONS

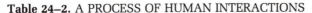
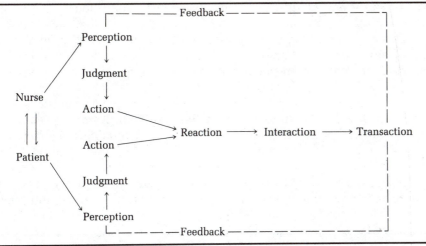

*Reprinted with permission from I. M. King, *Toward a Theory for Nursing.* New York: John Wiley & Sons, 1971, p. 92.

power and accountability; it represents a commitment to human ideals; and it can provide a sense of independence never before felt in nursing. Whether advocacy becomes a viable model for nursing, however, depends on the determination and commitment to overcome the barriers that stand between the movement from ideal to real. "Advocacy is no task for the uncommitted. It requires initiative, innovation and action" (Robb et al., 1979, p. 1737). In addition, other changes in the health care system will have to occur. As Jenny (1979) states:

> Patients will have to develop different expectations of nurses, physicians will have to begin to trust nursing autonomy, and employers will need to be more discriminating in personnel selection and role descriptions if advocacy is to become more than another cliché in nursing. (p. 181)

Advocacy can become a reality in nursing. The method whereby it can be accomplished rests with each and every nurse. A statement by Kelly (1976, p. 32) encapsulates the process in a most effective manner: "the situation calls for a nurse who cares and dares, multiplied by a million and a quarter."

While much has been done to define the word advocacy itself, much work remains in order that this concept may be applied to actual nursing practice and may become internalized as a vital construct of nursing. With this thought in mind, the following recommendations are made:

1. Further refinement and redefinition of advocacy as a concept related to nursing is necessary. In addition, numerous studies are needed to determine exactly what advocacy is: an intervention, an interactional process, a conceptual framework, a theory?

2. The characteristics of a nurse advocate must be identified as well as the process a person follows to become an advocate. Strategies for learning to be an advocate need to be identified and empirically tested. At the current time, no formal process or program exists, although certain criteria have been hinted at in the literature: adequate knowledge base, formal and informal coursework, and a belief in and commitment to patient advocacy.

3. Planned curriculum offerings dealing with advocacy should be developed and made available at both the undergraduate and graduate levels.

Advocacy content could be integrated into current course offerings without much difficulty and could thus be evaluated for application in the clinical area.

4. The question of the nursing community's commitment to the incorporation of advocacy into nursing practice must be resolved. The role of the nurse as advocate must become professionally sanctioned since advocacy functions can be decidedly at odds with the traditional role of the nurse.

5. Strategies of advocacy in nursing practice must be identified, tested, and evaluated. Advocacy must be more than an ideal. It must be applicable in the real world of nursing, applicable to clinical nursing practice. Unless advocacy can become operationalized, it will remain forever a philosophical ideal.

Advocacy is a concept that has been discussed for about 10 years in the literature. It is now time to *put advocacy into action* or let it rest in peace!

EDITORS' COMMENTS AND QUESTIONS
This chapter is a theoretical presentation of Patient Advocacy. Several definitions of advocacy are presented. Donahue points out that Patient Advocacy is a popular term but one that is not well understood. There are no reports of nursing research on advocacy. Because of the length of the theoretical presentation no case study was included.

Questions for Discussion
    1. *Which definition of Patient Advocacy do you prefer for your practice?*
    2. *Is Patient Advocacy a nursing intervention, nursing theory, or philosophy of nursing?*
    3. *Do nurses have enough power to be advocates?*
    4. *Describe a situation in which you have been a patient advocate. What was the outcome?*
    5. *How can Advocacy be taught to nursing students?*

References

Abrams, N. A contrary view of the nurse as patient advocate. Nursing Forum 1978, 17(3), 258–267.

American Hospital Association. A patient's bill of rights. Chicago, American Hospital Association, 1972.

American Nurses' Association. Code for nurses with interpretive statements. Kansas City, Mo.: American Nurses' Association, 1976.

Anderson, N. The nurse as a lover of humanity. Imprint, 1977, 24(4), 36–37. 55–57.

Annas, G. J., and Healey, J. The patient rights advocate: Redefining the doctor-patient relationship in the hospital context. Vanderbilt Law Review, 1974, 27, 243–269.

Carnegie, M. E. The patient's bill of rights and the nurse. Nursing Clinics of North America, 1974, 9(3), 557–562.

Castledine, G. The patient's advocate. Nursing Mirror, April 30, 1981, p. 14.

Chapman, J. E., and Chapman, H. H. Behavior and health care: A humanistic helping process. St. Louis: C. V. Mosby Company, 1975.

Christy, T. E. New privileges . . . new challenges . . . new responsibilities, Nursing '73 1973, 3(11), 8–11.

Clark, S. M. Midwives: Advocates or adversaries? Midwives Chronicle and Nursing Notes, 1978, 91, 257.

Curtin, L. L. The nurse as advocate: A philosophical foundation for nursing. Advances in Nursing Science, 1979, 1(3), 1–10.

Danielson, C., et al. Patient fact sheets: Nurses demonstrate patient advocacy. *Journal of the New York State Nurses' Association,* 1980, *11*(2), 5–8.

Donahue, M. P. The nurse: A patient advocate? *Nursing Forum,* 1978, *17*(2), 143–151.

Donahue, M. P., Euthanasia: An ethical uncertainty, in J. McCloskey and H. Grace (Eds.), *Current issues in nursing.* Boston: Blackwell Scientific Publications, 1981, pp. 726–734.

Fay, P. In support of patient advocacy as a nursing role. *Nursing Outlook,* 1978, *26,* 252–253.

Gadow, S. Advocacy nursing and new meanings of aging. *Nursing Clinics of North America,* 1979, *14*(1), 81–91.

Gadow, S. Existential advocacy: Philosophical foundation of nursing, in S. F. Spicker and S. Gadow (Eds.), *Nursing: Images and ideals.* New York: Springer Publishing Company, 1980, pp. 79–101.

Gadow, S. Advocacy: An ethical model for assisting patients with treatment decisions, in C. B. Wong and J. Swazey (Eds.), *Dilemmas of dying.* Boston: G. K., Hall Medical Publishers, 1981.

Goodnow, M. *First-year nursing* (3rd ed.), Philadelphia: W. B. Saunders Company, 1921.

Haug, M. R. The deprofessionalization of everyone? *Sociological Focus,* 1975, *8*(3), 197–213.

Hermann, R. O. The consumer movement in historical perspective, in D. A. Aker and G. S. Day (Eds.), *Consumerism.* New York: Free Press, 1978.

International Council of Nurses. Code of nurses—ethical concepts applied to nursing. *International Nursing Review,* 1973 20(166).

Jenny, J. Patient advocacy—another role for nursing? *International Nursing Review,* 1979, *26*(6), 176–181.

Kahn, A. J., et al. *Child advocacy report on a national baseline study.* New York: Columbia University School of Social Work, 1972.

Kelly, L. Y. The patient's right to know. *Nursing Outlook,* 1976, *24*(1), 26–32.

King, I. M. *Toward a theory for nursing.* New York: John Wiley & Sons, 1971.

King, I. M. *A theory for nursing: Systems, Concepts, Process.* New York: John Wiley & Sons, 1981.

Kohnke, M. F. The nurse as advocate. *American Journal of Nursing,* 1980, *80*(11), 2038–2040.

Kohnke, M. F. The nurse's responsibility to the consumer. *American Journal of Nursing,* 1978, *78*(3), 440–442.

Kohnke, M. F. The nurse as advocate. *American Journal of Nursing,* 1980, *80*(11), 2038–2040.

Kohnke, M. F. *Advocacy: Risk and reality.* St. Louis: C. V. Mosby Company, 1982.

Kosik, S. H. Patient advocacy or fighting the system. *American Journal of Nursing,* 1972a, *72*(4), 694–698.

Kosik, S. H. The nursing profession as health care advocates. *Maine Nurse,* 1972b, *3*(4), 12–17.

Kraus, K. J. Patient advocacy as a nursing role (unpublished thesis). Iowa City, University of Iowa, 1981.

Nadel, M. V. *The politics of consumer protection.* Indianapolis: Bobbs-Merrill Company, 1971.

National League for Nursing. *What people can expect of modern nursing service.* New York, National League for Nursing, 1959.

Nelson, L. J. The nurse as advocate: for whom? *American Journal of Nursing,* 1977, *77,* 851.

Nightingale, F. *Notes on Nursing: What It Is and What It is Not.* New York: D. Appleton and Co., 1860. (Reprinted by Dover Publications, New York, 1969.)

Nowakowski, L. A new look at client advocacy, in J. E. Hall and B. R. Wearcer (Eds.), *Distributive nursing practice: A systems approach to community health.* Philadelphia: J. B. Lippincott Company, 1977, pp. 227–238.

Pankratz, L., and Pankratz, D. Nursing autonomy and patients' rights: Development of a nursing attitude scale. *Journal of Health and Social Behavior,* 1974, *15*(3), 211–216.

Robb, S. S., Peterson, M., and Nagy, J. W. Advocacy for the aged. *American Journal of Nursing,* 1979, *79*(10), 1737–1738.

Smith, C. S. Outrageous or outraged: A nurse advocate story. *Nursing Outlook,* 1980, *28,* 624–625.

Stone, A. A. The myth of advocacy. *Hospital and Community Psychiatry,* 1979, *30*(12,), 819–822.

Storch, J. L. Nurse as consumer advocate, *AARN Newsletter,* 1978, *34*(6), 12–15.

Taubenhaus, M. The rights of patients. Public Affairs Pamphlet No. 535, 1976.

Thollaug, S. C. The nurse as patient advocate. *Imprint,* 1980, *27*(5), 37, 58.

Thompson, J. B., and Thompson, H. O. *Ethics in nursing.* New York: Macmillan Publishing Company, 1981.

Vinyard, N. D. Whose advocate are you? *Surgical Rounds,* 1980, *3*(9), 15.

Webster's new collegiate dictionary. Springfield Ill. G & C Merriam Company 1973.

Wilensky, H. The professionalization of everyone? *American Journal of Sociology,* 1974, *70,* 137–158.

Wilberding, J. Patient advocacy as a role for staff nurses: a descriptive study (unpublished thesis). Iowa City, University of Iowa, 1984.

25

CULTURE BROKERAGE

TONI TRIPP-REIMER
PAMELA J. BRINK

DEFINITION OF INTERVENTION

Culture Brokerage is essentially an act of translation in which messages, instructions, and belief systems are manipulated and processed from one group to another. As a nursing intervention, Culture Brokerage involves the nurse's acting as a mediator between clients and members of the orthodox health professions. Culture Brokerage may be used whenever there are separate culture groups and a need to establish links between them. As a nursing intervention, Cultural Brokerage occurs most obviously between minority clients and orthodox health professionals. Brokerage, however, is sometimes necessary between the popular culture of the lay client and the scientific culture of the health professional. Culture Brokerage may be thought of as *bridging, negotiating, or linking the orthodox health care systems with clients of different cultures.*

Brokers are individuals who occupy linkage roles between sectors of a society. Sussex and Weidman (1975) identified nursing personnel as the bearers and transmitters of a professional health culture in which patients and staff are interlocked in processes of learning, supporting, and changing behavior in mutually beneficial ways. Culture Brokerage is a nursing intervention more than an intervention for other health professionals because nursing education emphasizes the social as well as the biological sciences, and nurses generally have the closest relationships with the client's family and significant others.

Weidman (1982) states, "In the context of clinical activities, culture brokerage encourages behavior by health professionals which theoretically should lead to greater success for the clinician and a better outcome for the patient. In order for the health practitioner to negotiate between divergent health beliefs and practices, it is necessary to determine the nature of the beliefs and concerns that guide the patient's behavior. Only then can areas of difference or incompatibility be determined. And only after these are identified can mediation be attempted" (p. 211).

If used properly, the intervention of Culture Brokerage can result in the following benefits in clinical situations:

1. A more comprehensive understanding of the client and a more realistic treatment plan.

2. More congruence between the patient's perception of illness and the practitioner's perception of the patient's pathology.

3. Increased compatibility between the client's notions of desired treatments and the scientific therapeutic regimen.

4. Increased client satisfaction and adherence and decreased practitioner frustration.

Culture Brokerage has a broader scope than that in most nursing interventions, which are directed primarily toward altering aspects of the client's system. Culture Brokerage may focus on the client, on the health professional, or on mediation between both. Thus, Culture Brokerage may take three basic forms:

1. Culture Brokerage may focus on the client and help the client to handle the implications of the illness. This presumes the nurse broker understands what is important to the client and how the illness is interpreted. Culture groups differ in role expectations, family lifestyles, childrearing activities, patterns of authority, occupational patterns, religious requirements, educational achievements, political affiliation, and dietary practices. Nurses who understand the client's specific orientation in these areas can anticipate illness-oriented problems that derive from the particular culture base.

2. Culture Brokerage may focus on the practitioner by assisting the orthodox practitioner to adapt scientific methods, communications, or intervention strategies into culturally appropriate ones.

3. Culture Brokerage may focus on both the client and the orthodox health practitioner, as when the client and the practitioner have different views about the cause, meaning, or treatment of an illness. In this case, each person's perspective needs to be translated to the other.

Basic to Culture Brokerage is an understanding of the distinction between the concepts of disease and illness (Eisenberg, 1977; Kleinman, Eisenberg and Good, 1978; Tripp-Reimer, 1984b). Diseases are abnormalities in the structure and function of body organs and systems; they are problems of biological malfunctioning. Illness, on the other hand, encompasses the subjective experiences of the individual who is sick, and includes the way in which this sickness is perceived and experienced by the individual and social group. The client is predominantly concerned with illness. Medicine is primarily concerned with disease: its etiology, pathology, and treatment. Nursing uses both the model of illness and the model of disease and mediates beween the two.

In order to use Culture Brokerage successfully, the nurse needs knowledge of the client's culture and its influence on health beliefs and behaviors. The nurse also must have insight into the culture of scientific health professionals to ascertain which elements are crucial to clinical effectiveness and which are superfluous. Finally, the nurse needs skills in communication and negotiation for mediating the two systems.

RELATED LITERATURE

The concept of the culture broker emerged from the discipline of anthropology. The earliest work on culture brokers by Wolf (1956) and Geertz (1960) looked at individuals who served as middlemen between groups at local and national levels. These local men usually lived in small villages and served as the economic or political intermediaries between their own group at the local level and a group at the national level. Brokers tend to emerge in situations involving culture change or culture conflict. Consequently, the broker role has been apparent particularly in Latin America (Adams, 1970; Press, 1969; Salovesh, 1978; Wolf, 1956) Southeast Asia (Geertz, 1960), and sometimes Africa (Silver, 1979), the Arctic (Paine, 1971), or the United States (Hannerz, 1974).

In anthropological literature, the term "culture broker" has been applied to a variety of roles that link various sections of society: teachers; religious and political leaders; artists; public health physicians, and agricultural extension agents. For example, Adams (1970) notes that in Guatemala, as in many other Latin American countries, the male schoolteacher is a cultural representative of the national system working in a culture different from that which he is used to operating. Although the teacher may serve to make national traits available to members of the local community, he usually has no power of his own. Adams also notes that the same may be said for the public health physician and the agricultural extension agent. Adams defines the culture broker as an individual from one level who lives or operates among individuals of another level. Whatever influence he or she may have on the other level depends basically not on the power that the broker can wield but on personal skill and personal influence. Culture brokers are usually sponsored through upper level decisions and act at lower levels. Their tasks are seldom of high priority, however, since the failure in performance of their duties is not a threat to the position of the individuals sponsoring them at the national level.

Essential to the functioning of the broker is the broker's marginal status (Press, 1969). From his study of a Yucatan peasant community, Press suggests that role ambiguity serves as a crucial mechanism in the genesis of the broker role. During the development of the innovative role, ambiguity allows novel behavior while retarding negative sanction. In this study, Press described the manner in which culture brokers arise, receive permission to innovate, and create a role in which innovative behavior becomes an expectation.

As cited by Whitten and Wolfe (1973), Boissevian conceptualized brokers as dealing through interpersonal linkages by transforming and using interpersonal relations for some perceived advantage. In the process, they affect social relationships. These brokers transmit, direct, filter, receive, code, decode, and interpret messages. Such strategically placed persons may turn their skills as brokers into personal power, manipulating networks to their own advantage.

Similarly, Wolf (1956), Press (1969), Salovesh (1978), and Silver (1979) all discuss the notion that it is to the benefit of a person in a permanent culture broker role to deliberately leave tensions unresolved or perhaps even increase them in order to ensure his or her continuing need as a buffering agent. Wolf (1956) contends that the position of these brokers is an exposed one since, Janus-like, they face two directions at once. They must serve some of the interests of the groups operating on both the community and the national levels, and they must cope with the conflicts raised by the collision of these interests. Permanent brokers, however, cannot afford to totally resolve conflicts, since by doing so they would abolish their usefulness to others.

Weidman (1973, 1982) and Sussex and Weidman (1975) developed the concept of culture broker in the health care delivery system. The culture broker role, according to Weidman (1973), is that of an intermediary, and this could be applied whenever there is a need to recognize the existence of separate cultural or subcultural traditions and to acknowledge an individual's role in establishing meaningful linkages between them. As Weidman conceived the role, however, the culture broker was an anthropologist who was placed in a health care setting and would be emulated by health care professionals. She views the culture broker as having the responsibility of linking, negotiating, and meshing aspects of two health cultural systems that confront each other the moment the physician and patient meet.

There is an important distinction between Culture Brokerage as a full time role and as an intervention. As a full time role, the concept had its origins in political anthropology. There the broker needed to maintain distance, barriers, and tensions between groups. Otherwise, the broker's role would end; that is, if brokerage is too successful, the broker is out of a job. On the other hand, when Cultural Brokerage is used as a nursing intervention, it is only one possible intervention among many. As such the nurse is not bound to maintain barriers between groups. Other interventions can proceed once Culture Brokerage is successful. In other words, the success of Brokerage is an advantage; the nurse can move on to new and more health oriented interventions after the broker role has been fulfilled.

ASSOCIATED NURSING DIAGNOSES

Because culture pervades all domains of life, there are no nursing diagnoses that specifically indicate the intervention of Culture Brokerage. That is, virtually any behavioral category of nursing diagnosis may have a culturally based etiology and need Culture Brokerage. For example, language differences may result in a diagnosis of Impaired Verbal Communication; the consequent Brokerage intervention would be to find methods or individuals for translating information between practitioner and client. Similarly, the client's home treatments for a health problem may result in a diagnosis of Noncompliance with prescribed scientific therapy. In this case, the Brokerage intervention would be to mediate between the folk and biomedical models of therapy. Other nursing diagnoses that may call for this intervention are the following: Anxiety, Ineffective Coping, Fear, Alteration in Health Maintenance, Knowledge Deficit, Alterations in Nutrition, Alterations in Parenting, Powerlessness, Disturbance in Self Concept, Social Isolation, and Spiritual Distress.

Frequently, it is the diagnosis of Noncompliance that triggers the identification of the need for culture brokerage because it may be only when the patient is noncompliant that health professionals become aware that there is a problem that cannot be solved in the usual way. Culture Brokerage is a time-consuming intervention and is not usually chosen when there is little time to spare. Only when there is a disruption of the routines of the health professionals and their work becomes impaired or inefficient does the need for further assessment and different intervention strategies become apparent. At this time, the intervention of Culture Brokerage may be the most appropriate.

INTERVENTION TECHNIQUES

Within nursing, Culture Brokerage has been described in almost every case example involving nurse-client interactions when the nurse is from one culture or ethnic group and the client is from another; none of the descriptions, however, have labeled the intervention as Culture Brokerage. For the most part, the nursing textbooks that deal with cross-ethnic or transcultural issues have devoted considerable space to the content necessary in a cultural assessment, and have provided suggestions on how to work with persons of culture groups different from that of the nurse (Bauwens, 1978; Branch and Paxton, 1976; Brink, 1976; Clark, 1978; Henderson and Primeaux, 1981; Leininger, 1970, 1978; Orque and Block, 1983; Spector, 1979). Each textbook also devoted chapters to particular ethnic groups. Again, the emphasis has been on what Leininger (1978, pp. 85–106) calls a "culturalogical assessment." Each textbook has also emphasized the *content* of a culturalogical assessment rather than the *process*, on the assumption that nurses know *how* to assess patients but do not know *what* to assess when the patient comes from a different culture.

In contrast, Brosnan (1976) and Winn (1976) emphasized the *process* of arriving at a nursing diagnosis and an appropriate nursing intervention using culturalogical assessment techniques. In each case the nurse used Culture Brokerage as an intervention but was not identified as doing so. These two papers were unusual in that their point was to plan a specific intervention based upon knowledge of the client group. The process of planning the intervention was the single theme of the papers. A plan for a nursing intervention was systematically created, however, based upon available literature. Whether or not the intervention will work waits for the implementation and evaluation of the plan. More nursing papers of this nature are necessary in order to analyze the nurse's actions relevant to Culture Brokerage.

One book, *Community, culture and care: A cross cultural guide for health workers* (Brownlee, 1978), is devoted to the process of practical assessments in situations demanding Cultural Brokerage. Brownlee states that she wrote the book to "provide a readily accessible and practically oriented guide for health workers and students on what they need to learn about their own culture and organization and the culture around them, why the information is important and how to go about gathering it" (p. vi). Each chapter deals with three aspects of assessment: (1) what to find out, (2) why it is important, and (3) how to do it. The sheer practicality of the volume, its simplicity of language, and its almost outline format is the best description of Culture Brokerage that nursing has to offer.

Although nursing does not, to date, have a specific intervention strategy for Culture Brokerage, the intervention of Patient Advocacy comes close to it. Anthropology, on the other hand, does offer several useful techniques that might be immediately adaptable to the nursing situation.

The intervention technique of "negotiation" is described by Katon and Kleinman (1981) for clinical interviews between the health professional and the patient. Katon and Kleinman define negotiation as a "bilateral arrangement in which the two principal parties attempt to work out a solution. . . . The goal is to reduce conflict in a way that promotes cooperation" (pp. 262, 276). Negotiation, as an intervention strategy for Culture Brokerage, is used when the diagnosis is reached that a conceptual difference exists between the patient and the health worker. In other words, the patient and health professional (1) may be using the same words but actually mean different things; (2) may apply the term to the same phenomenon but have different notions of its causation; or (3) may have different memories or emotional associations with the term and its use. When conflicts do arise between clients and health professionals, the following model of negotiation is offered:

> 1. The initial questioning is for the health professional to find out how the patient explains the illness or health problem.
> 2. The health professional then clearly and fully presents (in lay terms) an explanation of the disorder, including the recommended treatment, and invites questions from patient and family, to which full explanations are

given. The point here is to work within the patient's frame of reference and level of understanding.

3. A working alliance is possible when the patient's personal explanation of the illness either agree with or shifts to the health professional's model, or if the health professional shifts recommendations more toward the patient's expectations of treatment.

4. At times, discrepancies remain. When this occurs the health professional can openly acknowledge and clarify conflict. The health professionals are ethically entitled to provide references and data to argue their position, but should also allow the patients (or patient's family) to provide references and data to argue their position. The health professional continues to elicit the patient's explanatory model until understanding is reached.

5. At this juncture, either the professional or patient will change sides to arrive at a mutually desired treatment.

6. When a conflict cannot be resolved, the health professional should attempt to arrive at an acceptable compromise of treatment based upon biomedical knowledge, knowledge of the patient's point of view, and ethical standards.

7. When all else fails, health professionals need to recognize that their role is to provide expert advice and rationale for the treatment recommendations, but that it is the patient (or patient's family) who is the final decision maker in this situation. If a complete stalemate is reached, the health professional is responsible for offering a referral to another person. Finally, the patient may seek advice from another health provider without fear of reprisal by the system.

8. Throughout this process, each negotiation involves an ongoing monitoring of the agreement and of each party's participation in the agreement (Katon and Kleinman, 1981, pp. 270–276).

The concept of negotiation in Culture Brokerage is based upon the idea that health professionals and patients should meet and interact with each other as equals in an attempt to achieve an outcome satisfactory to both parties in the interaction. In order to achieve this goal, power must be taken from the clinician and given to the patient or patient's family. Only by doing this first step can Culture Brokerage be successful.

A second strategy of the Culture Brokerage intervention is the therapeutic use of time (Zola, 1981). Clients and their families need time to absorb information. Time, therefore, needs to be set aside, specifically, for the processing of information between the history, the physical examination, and the diagnosis; between the diagnosis and the treatment alternatives; and between the treatment alternatives and the decision by the patient or family to accept or reject the information provided. Instant decisions in health-illness situations deprive clients of the right to work through decision making at their own pace. Concomitant with the client's decision making is the encouragement and presence of significant others during all phases of the health encounter. "What patients are responding to when they do not cooperate is not the medical treatment but how they are treated, not how they regard their medical regimen but how they themselves are regarded" (Zola, 1981, p. 250).

Health professionals need to be aware that interactions with clients of different cultures or ethnic groups will take more time and that an important skill of the professional is to appear relaxed and unhurried. Longer appointment periods can be scheduled to allow for the time it will take for translation, for discussion and clarification of concepts, for explanation of diagnosis, for negotiation of treatment regimen, and for socialization to the health care delivery system (Harwood, 1981). Culture Brokerage takes time. Even when the client is of the same culture as the health professional, the same process of negotiation needs to take place and time must be given to the process. Many times health professionals forget that they represent the "health culture"

culture" with its jargon and belief systems, whereas the client represents the "lay culture" with its particular belief systems. Just because two people speak English and grew up in the United States does not automatically translate into clear communication.

The client expects the health professional to be knowledgeable about the illness, its symptoms, and its cure, and to care for the patient as a person, not as a case. These characteristics are demonstrated by the practitioner's ability to use nontechnical language, to explain the symptoms of the illness that the patient is experiencing rather than the biomedical causes (or the pathology), and to explain the relationship between the symptoms, the diagnosis, and the treatment plan with the prediction of the outcome. This is, of course, done in the "professional manner," which is projected by careful listening, politeness, warmth, and an unhurried manner (Harwood, 1981).

The third strategy of Culture Brokerage is to treat cultural assessment as a process rather than simply a content area. Culture Brokerage requires a clinically appropriate cultural assessment of the patient (whether individual or group) that elicits several basic data sets by using the patient as a cultural informant who is more knowledgeable about the culture than is the health professional. The health professional, therefore, uses the patient as the resource for cultural data. The nurse enters into the clinical interview with an eye toward gaining an increased understanding of the culture from which the patient comes, in addition to learning the patient's health history and eliciting a description of symptoms.

In the first level of cultural assessment, the nurse needs to discover with which ethnic group the patient identifies. The patient's cultural affiliation should not be assumed simply because of skin color or accent. Since culture is a system of shared beliefs and values, nurses need to ask patients what health and illness beliefs are common to their group. These shared rules and values need to be discovered in order to place the individual patient's beliefs and values in context. Here the nurse tries to establish a "belief variability ratio" in which the patient's degree of adherence to the group's belief system is established. What the nurse is looking for is the shared meaning with a group of people and the degree of distance the individual sees between self and culture group.

In order to understand the client's specific reaction to an illness situation, the health professional needs to know if this reaction is idiosyncratic (held only by the individual) or if it is a commonly held belief or value (idiosyncratic variability).

In summary, clinically relevant cultural assessments are based upon interviewing skills that attempt to elicit the shared beliefs and values about a health problem and its treatment outcome that may assist or interfere with the planned medical treatment regimen or nursing intevention. In health care delivery, it is not enough to diagnose a health problem; something needs to be done about it, so that the cultural assessment is valuable in yielding data that assist the health professional to predict the possible outcome of the intervention.

Another strategy of Culture Brokerage, frequently described in the literature, involves the nurse's calling in a translator for the client who has difficulty with English. In this case, either the translator or the nurse serves as broker and creates the link between the two parties. Although the translator may assist in translating from one language to another, the nurse is still responsible for determining the meaning of the words and their emotional impact upon the situation. Again, taking time, appearing to be unhurried, and selecting a place that is comfortable to the client are all Brokerage techniques.

One goal of Culture Brokerage may be adherence, which means that the client is expected to follow the prescribed treatment regimen correctly. Adherence can be enhanced by enlisting the family or significant others to reinforce the treatment regimen; by including the most influential member of the family in the treatment plan; discontinuing the treatment when the symptoms have gone or explaining why treatment should continue; using the client's preferred methods of treatment when they are not directly contradictory to the treatment needed; and placing treatment in the setting where it is most wanted—home or hospital.

Harwood (1981) has a series of suggestions for methods health professionals can use to promote adherence:

> 1. For most lay persons (non-health professionals), relief of pain or a decrease or cessation of specific symptoms generally indicates the person is cured. Discuss with patient whether treatment is necessary beyond relief of symptoms and if so, explain why.
> 2. Discuss in depth those symptoms that appear to be most anxiety provoking for the client or the client's family, especially with regard to cause, severity, and ways in which treatment will affect them.
> 3. Determine which forms of medical treatment are most anxiety provoking for the patient and family.
> 4. Discuss with the patient and family alternative ways of fulfilling the sick person's responsibilities while the individual is sick.
> 5. Discuss any limitations on valued activities due to medical treatment and help patients devise ways of coping with them (Harwood, 1981, pp. 492–495).

As we noted earlier, Culture Brokerage does not involve simply a one-way interaction in which the health professional learns to adapt and translate the patient's needs and meanings; Culture Brokerage may be directed toward health professionals as well. There are times when the nurse will "broker" between patients and other health professionals. At these times the same strategies apply to the health professional as they do to the patient. One key to assisting the health professional to work with a patient of another culture is for the nurse to translate what the patient means in terminology readily understood by the health professional. Whereas patients may need lay terms to understand, the health professional sometimes needs professional language in order to make sense of an interaction. Physicians, for example, take justifiable pride in arriving at sound "diagnosis" on the basis of a thorough "review of systems" (Nurge, 1978, pp. 388–400). Yet patients rarely offer personal histories that readily fit within the system-review format. Some Italians may provide "florid descriptions," whereas a Puerto Rican may provide a "long symptoms list" yet neither may be a "hypochondriac." The Haitian may provide a very "truncated description of symptoms" and need to be drawn out (Harwood, 1981, pp. 498–499). For this reason, Nurge (1978) sensitized medical students into cultural awareness by placing cultural content within the medical student's frame of reference. She provided an easy to read, rapid checklist format on two axes—horizontal and vertical. On the vertical axis she organized medical information according to (1) infectious diseases, (2) nutritional deficiencies, (3) diseases by organ system, and (4) "other diseases," such as alcoholism or drug addiction. On the horizontal axis the columns were headed by the following items: (1) disease; (2) agent; (3) mode of transmission; (4) environmental factors; and (5) familial and social factors (which were further subdivided into (a) biological and social arrangements in the family and (b) the beliefs and behaviors relating to a state of well-being, illness, and therapy). In this way Nurge was able to incorporate a logical system for including social and cultural content in a "systems review" of the patient's problem list. Nurge was acting as a culture broker between patients and medical students with the intervention focused upon the medical student. She was "translating" the patients' symptoms into a frame of reference the medical student could understand.

One example of a Brokerage tool used in clinical nursing education was developed by the School of Medicine at the University of Miami in an in-service training program (Scott, 1983). A chart composed of two axes is given to the students. On the vertical axis are five categories of data: (1) symptoms that identify the disease; (2) causes of the disease; (3) labels for the disease; (4) perception of bodily function when the disease is present; and (5) ways of preventing, curing, and treating the disease. On the horizontal axis, there are two categories: the traditional folk beliefs of the patient or client group and the orthodox or Western biomedical beliefs about the disease. The chart is used in a group work session in which a group of students is assigned a particular disease, such as diabetes, and is then asked to fill in all areas of the chart. The chart easily identifies the patient's idea of illness and contrasts it with the professional's concept. In this way, areas of cultural conflict are immediately apparent. The same sort of Cultural Brokerage tool could be developed for graduate programs in nursing, particularly in nurse practitioner programs, in order to "translate" culture content into the frame of reference of the student.

Whether the client is a foreigner or an American, the hospital is seen as a foreign environment which the patient must learn, and part of the role of the nurse is to teach the patient to behave appropriately in this new environment (Brink and Saunders, 1976). In this way the nurse acts as a culture broker between the patient and the system. When the nurse functions as the link between patient and system, the role may be one of Brokerage or Patient Advocacy and meets all the criteria for clinical intervention (as described by Harwood, 1981) or clinical negotiation (as described by Katon and Kleinman, 1981).

There are three options in Culture Brokerage that the health professional can plan with the patient or patient's family: (1) do nothing, (2) translate one culture to the other to provide the knowledge base for understanding, and (3) teach or learn new skills to cope with the new cultural environment. Culture Brokerage demands much of the nurse in relation to flexibility of approach to nursing problems and in relation to searching out new knowledge with which to adequately nurse the patient. Culture Brokerage requires interviewing skills very similar to those necessary for research. Painstaking, in-depth interviews are required to learn the patient's knowledge base and system of beliefs about the presenting problem and its treatment outcomes.

CASE STUDIES

The following are examples of Culture Brokerage as an intervention and reflect the three major options for the nurse: (1) do nothing, (2) translate one culture to the other, and (3) teach new skills.

Case Study 1

One of the authors was called in for a consultation on an inpatient acute care unit. The nursing staff stated that too many visitors were in the room at one time and that this was against the hospital policy. In assessing the situation, the culture broker established the environmental parameters of the situation by determining whether or not there was any contraindication to nursing care by having a large number of people in the room at one time. The social environment was also assessed in relation to whether or not the patient had a roommate and whether this was causing a problem. On establishing that the large number of visitors was not bothering anyone but was simply violating a hospital rule, the nurse consultant suggested that the patient be allowed to have the visitors no matter how unusual the situation was. The culture broker recommended the option of "do nothing." Although the patient and patient's family were not adhering to a hospital rule the nonadherence was not a true problem, but simply an infraction of a nonfunctional rule. The culture broker translated to the nursing staff the social needs of the patient (who was Amish) during hospitalization to show that these needs took precedence over a general rule that did not apply to the particular situation. In this case, the nurse consultant was a culture broker to the staff and not to the patient.

Case Study 2
A patient was placed on bed rest but was constantly found out of bed. The nursing staff diagnosed the problem as Noncompliance. On further assessment, the nurse-consultant found that the patient was a Muslim and was trying to face east in order to pray. The solution, similar to that described by MacGregor (1976), was to place the patient's bed near the window facing east. The patient subsequently remained in bed. In this situation, the culture broker established that the patient's cultural identity included his Muslim religion, which provided the clue to asking further questions about his religious beliefs. (The nurse was not a Muslim and did not understand the religious requirements of this group.) Finding that the patient's religious practices were not excused during illness, it became a simple matter of attempting to find ways of supporting the patient's religious beliefs while hospitalized. The patient's beliefs were translated to staff, who were then able to decide how best to meet the patient's cultural needs while ill.

Case Study 3
A Native American woman had a below-the-knee amputation due to gangrene of the leg secondary to diabetes, but refused to follow a diabetic diet. The staff were unable to accept the patient's decision. She was labeled by the nursing staff as uncommunicative, hostile, and uncooperative. The nursing diagnosis was Noncompliance. The nurse-consultant, however, found her to be quite communicative. She was completely aware of the danger of nonadherence but simply did not wish to diet as prescribed by the staff. The work of the consultant, as a culture broker, was with the staff in relation to having them accept the patient's decision. The solution was to allow the patient to eat as she wished. The nursing action, again, was "do nothing" in relation to the client but to focus on the staff and decrease their frustration.

Case Study 4
An infant was brought into the county hospital with severe burns on the top of the head. The nursing staff called the police to report what they perceived to be a case of child abuse. One of the nursing staff, familiar with Hispanic customs, interviewed the parents and discovered that the family had diagnosed the baby as having "fallen fontanel," which required the treatment of holding the infant upside down over a pot of boiling water to "pull the fontanel out." Although the police took the parents to court, the nurse went along to explain to the judge about the custom. The judge gave the parents a suspended sentence but asked the nurse to teach the parents other methods of treating "fallen fontanel," which would be in keeping with their custom but less damaging to the child. In this situation the nursing diagnosis was Maladaptive Parenting in a new culture and the nursing action was to teach the parents new skills more appropriate to their new environment. In addition, the newly immigrated parents were introduced to the neighborhood health worker, who was asked to refer the parents to a curandera (Hispanic folk healer) more familiar with American laws regarding folk treatments.

Case Study 5
A nurse in a large western city was doing a home visit to find out why a child was not attending school. The child was in the special education program for the mentally

retarded. The mother was a Native American and was a new arrival from a reservation. During the interview the nurse discovered that the child had refused to return to school and the mother had not insisted. The nurse understood that many Native Americans have the right to make their own decisions about and for themselves. It was up to the nurse to explain the school system, the beliefs about truancy, and the benefits of the special education program. Once the mother was convinced, then the nurse enticed the child back to school. The original nursing diagnosis that triggered the "clinical negotiation" strategy of the Cultural Brokerage intervention was, again, Noncompliance. The action was to translate the new urban environmental requirements to the mother and to counsel her on survival strategies. The second aspect of the intervention was for the nurse to change her beliefs and behavior about how much responsibility a child should have and to talk to the child in the child's terms and at the child's level of understanding. Once the nurse accepted the fact that the child had the final decision-making power about going to school, the nurse was able to adapt her clinical strategies to those of a different belief system.

Frequently, it is the nursing diagnosis of Noncompliance that triggers Culture Brokerage. The nurse then moves into an unhurried time strategy and assumes that flexibility of beliefs and values will be needed as differences will probaby exist in these areas. The nurse may find that the patient needs to be allowed to retain a belief rather than abandon it. At other times, just listening is enough. Finally, there are times when the staff must be taught to accept the patient's position and allow the patient to dictate a style of health care more in keeping with that of the patient's beliefs and values.

EDITORS' COMMENTS AND QUESTIONS

This intervention has been adapted from the field of anthropology. As cultural minority groups are recognized in our society, nurses have become more conscious of working with these groups. No nursing research has been done on the intervention. The authors provide five case studies to illustrate this unique intervention.

Questions for Discussion

1. *What are the differences and similarities between Culture Brokerage and Patient Advocacy?*

2. *What research methods would be useful to test this intervention?*

3. *Can all nurses do Culture Brokerage?*

4. *Can other health providers do Culture Brokage?*

References

Adams, R. Brokers and career mobility systems in the structure of complex societies. *Southwestern Journal of Anthropology*, 1970, 26:315–327.

Aron, W. S., Alger, N., and Gonzales, R. T. Chicanoizing drug abuse programs, in M. H. Logan and E. E. Hunt, Jr. (Eds.), *Health and the human condition: Perspectives in medical anthropology*. North Scituate, Mass.: Duxbury Press, 1978, pp. 340–344.

Bauwens, E. (Ed.). *The anthropology of health*. St. Louis: C. V. Mosby Company, 1978.

Branch, M., and Paxton, P. P. *Providing safe nursing care for ethnic people of color*. New York: Appleton-Century-Crofts, 1976.

Brink, P. J., and Saunders, J. Culture shock: theoretical and applied, in Brink, P. (ed.), *Transcultural nursing: A book of readings*. Englewood Cliffs, N.J.: Prentice-Hall, Inc., 1976.

Brosnan, J. A proposed diabetic educational program for Puerto Ricans in New York City, in P. J.

Brink (Ed.), *Transcultural nursing: A book of readings.* Englewood Cliffs, N.J. Prentice-Hall Inc., 1976, pp. 263–275.

Brownlee, A. T. *Community, culture, and care: A cross cultural guide for health workers.* St. Louis: C. V. Mosby Company, 1978.

Bullough, B., and Bullough, V. L. *Poverty, ethnic identity, and health care.* New York: Appleton-Century-Crofts, 1972.

Clark, A. *Culture, health professionals and childbearing.* Philadelphia: F. A. Davis, 1978.

Eisenberg, L. Disease and illness: Distinction between professional and popular ideas of sickness. *Culture, Medicine and Psychiatry,* 1977, *1,* 9–23.

Geertz, C. The Javanese Kijaji: The changing role of a culture broker. *Comparative Studies in Society and History: An International Quarterly,* 1960, *2,* 228–249.

Good, B., and Good, M. The meaning of symptoms: A cultural hermeneutic model for clinical practice, in L. Eisenberg and A. Kleinman (Eds.), *The relevance of social science for medicine.* Boson: Reidel Publishing Company, 1981, pp. 275–295.

Hannerz, U. Ethnicity and opportunity in urban America, in A. Cohen (Ed.), *Urban ethnicity.* New York: Tavistock, 1974, pp. 37–76.

Harwood, A. Guidelines for culturally appropriate health care, in A. Harwood (Ed.), *Ethnicity and medical care.* Cambridge: Harvard University Press, 1981, pp. 482–507.

Henderson, G., and Primeaux, M. (Eds.). *Transcultural health care.* Menlo Park, Calif.: Addison-Wesley Publishing Company, 1981.

Hessler, R. M., Nolan, M. F., Ogbru, B., and Kong-Ming New, P. Intraethnic diversity: Health care of the Chinese Americans, in M. H. Logan and E. E. Hunt, Jr. (Eds.), *Health and the human condition: Perspectives in medical anthropology.* North Scituate, Mass.: Duxbury Press, 1978.

Hopkins, N., Ekpo, M., Heileman, J., Michtom, M., Osterweil, A., Seiber, R., and Smith, G. Brokers and symbols in American urban life. *Anthropological Quarterly,* 1977, *50,* 65–75.

Katon, W., and Kleinman, A. Doctor-patient negotiation and other social science strategies in patient care, in L. Eisenberg and A. Kleinman (Eds.), *The relevance of social science for medicine.* Boston: D. Reidel Publishing Company, 1981, pp. 253–279.

Kleinman, A., Eisenberg, M., and Good, B. Culture, illness, and care. *Annals of Internal Medicine,* 1978, *88,* 251–258.

Leeds, A. Brazilian careers and social structure: An evolutionary model and case history. *American Anthropologist,* 1964, *66,* 1321–1347.

Leininger, M. Culturalogical assessment domains for nursing practice, in M. Leininger (Ed.), *Transcultural nursing: Comcepts, theories, and practice.* New York: John Wiley & Sons, 1978, pp. 85–106.

Leininger, M. *Nursing and anthropology: Two worlds to blend.* New York: John Wiley & Sons, 1970.

Leininger, M. (Ed.). *Transcultural nursing: Concepts, theories, and practices.* New York: John Wiley & Sons, 1978.

Leininger, M. Culturalogical assessment domains for nursing practice, in M. Leininger (Ed.), *Transcultural nursing: Concepts, theories, and practice.* New York: John Wiley & Sons, 1978, pp. 85–106.

Logan, M. H. Humoral medicine in Guatemala and peasant acceptance of modern medicine, in M. H. Logan and E. J. Hunt, Jr. (Eds.), *Health and the human condition: Perspectives in medical anthropology.* North Scituate, Mass.: Duxbury Press, 1978, pp. 363–375.

MacGregor, F. C. Uncooperative patients: Some cultural interpretations, in P. J. Brink (Ed.), *Transcultural nursing: A book of readings.* Englewood Cliffs, N.J.: Prentice-Hall, 1976, pp. 36–43.

Nurge, E. Anthropological perspective for medical students, in M. H. Logan and E. J. Hunt, Jr. (Eds.), *Health and the human condition: Perspectives in medical anthropology.* North Scituate, Mass.: Duxbury Press, 1978, pp. 388–400.

Orque, M. S., Bloch, B., and Monrray, L. S. *Ethnic nursing care: A multicultural approach.* St. Louis: C. V. Mosby Company, 1983.

Paine, R. A theory of patronage and brokerage, in *Patrons and brokers in the east arctic.* Newfoundland Social and Economic Papers #2. Institute of Social and Economic Research. Memorial University of Newfoundland, 1971.

Pfifferling, J. H. Cultural prescription for medicocentrism, in L. Eisenberg and A. Kleinman (Eds.): *The relevance of social science for medicine.* Boston: D. Reidel Publishing Company, 1981, pp. 197–222.

Polgar, S., and Marshall, J. F. The search for culturally acceptable fertility regulating methods, in M. H. Logan and E. E. Hunt, Jr. (Eds.), *Health and the human condition: Perspectives in medical anthropology.* North Scituate, Mass.: Duxbury Press, 1978, pp. 328–339.

Press, I. Ambiguity and innovation: Implications for the genesis of the culture broker. *American Anthropologist,* 1969, *71,* 205–217.

Salovesh, M. When brokers go broke: Implications of role failure and culture brokerage, in R. Holloman and S. Arutiunov (Eds.), *Perspective on ethnicity.* The Hague, Netherlands: Mouton, 1978, pp. 351–371.

Scott, C. S. Competing health care systems in an inner city area, in M. H. Logan and E. E. Hunt, Jr. (Eds.), *Health and the human condition: Perspectives in medical anthropology.* North Scituate, Mass.: Duxbury Press, 1978, pp. 345–347.

Scott, C. S. A technique for teaching transculturally oriented health care. *Medical Anthropology Quarterly*, 1983, *14*(3), 7, 1983.

Silver, H. Beauty and the "I" of the beholder: Identity, aesthetics, and social change among the Ashanti. *Journal of Anthropological Research*, 1979, *35*, 191–207.

Silverman, S. Patronage and community-nation relationships in central Italy. *Ethnology*, 1965, *4*, 172–189.

Spector, R. E. *Cultural diversity in health and illness.* New York: Appleton-Century-Crofts, 1979.

Sussex, J., and Weidman, H. Toward responsiveness in mental health care. *Psychiatric Annals*, 1975, *5*, 306–311.

Tripp-Reimer, T. Cultural assessment, In J. Bellack and P. Bamford (Eds.) *Nursing assessment.* Belmont, Calif.: Wadsworth Health Sciences, 1984a, 226–246.

Tripp-Reimer, T. Reconceptualizing the construct of health: Integrating the emic and etic perspectives. In *Research in Nursing and Health*, 1984b, *7*, 101–109.

Vincent, J. Political anthropology: Manipulative strategies. *Annual Review of Anthropology*, 1978, *7*, 175–194.

Weidman, H. Implications of the culture broker concept for the delivery of health care. Paper presented at the annual meeting of the Southern Anthropological Society, 1973.

Weidman, H. Concepts as strategies for change. *Psychiatric Annals*, 1975, *5*, 312–314.

Weidman, H. Research strategies, structural alterations and clinically applied anthropology, in N. Chrisman and T. Maretzki (Eds.), *Clinically applied anthropology: Anthropologists in health science settings.* Boston: D. Reidel Publishers, 1982, pp. 201–241.

Whitten, N., and Wolfe, A. Network analysis, in J. Honigman (Ed.), *Handbook of social and cultural anthropology.* Chicago: Rand McNally & Company, 1973, pp. 717–746.

Winn, M. C. A proposed tuberculosis treatment program for Papago Indians, in P. J. Brink (Ed.), *Transcultural nursing: A book of readings.* Englewood Cliffs, N.J.: Prentice-Hall, 1976, pp. 276–289.

Wolf, E. Aspects of group relations in a complex society; Mexico. *American Anthropologist*, 1956, *58*, 1065–1078.

Wolf, E. Closed corporate peasant communities in Mesoamerica and central Java. *Southwestern Journal of Anthropology*, 1957, *13*, 1–18.

Zola, I. K. Structural constraints in the doctor-patient relationship: The case of non-compliance, in L. Eisenberg and A. Kleinman (Eds.), *The relevance of social science for medicine.* Boston: D. Reidel Publishing Company, 1981, pp. 241–252.

26

TRUTH TELLING

DEBRA LIVINGSTON
CASSANDRA WILLIAMSON

Truthfulness is an ethical consideration in virtually all aspects of nursing. Since nursing is primarily an interaction process, there is constant potential for honesty or dishonesty, distoration, or omission. Furthermore, the question of truthfulness often awakens ambivalence about rights and values.

Nurses are often in the vulnerable position of having inconsistent obligations in the context of Truth Telling and the nurse-patient relationship. Since nurses provide most of the care and have the most extended contact with the patient and his or her loved ones, they receive the most requests for information. Nurses are caught in the middle between the patient and others in providing knowledge and the concern for the patient's best interest. Ethical challenges occur with confidentiality, Truth Telling, informed consent, and the right to read the medical record. There are few written guidelines to help in the decision of when to tell, how much of the truth to tell, and to whom to give the truth. Despite the widely held belief that Truth Telling is for the most part beneficial, it is an issue for all of those engaged in the patient-health professional relationship.

There is an emerging assertiveness by nurses to prove their independent, decision-making ability that is sound in judgment and knowledge. This is echoed in the nurse's role as patient advocate. Patients in turn are becoming increasingly aware of their rights in the health care system. Some are desiring to be treated as partners in health care. Nurses are taught health promotion and to actively involve patients in goal-directed activities that increase patients' responsibility for their own actions, thoughts, and feelings. The move away from an illness model in which patients are "cared for and done to" is timely, in that it will cause old myths about nurses being passive care givers, carrying out orders of others, to be relinquished. A wellness model emphasizes patient rights, but it also requires nurses to be more assertive about their coequal rights in providing health care. The increased involvement in health care generates the need for nurses to become responsible, accountable, and authentic. In order to achieve this goal, truthfulness is essential.

The focus of this chapter will be on truth as a concept and on Truth

Telling as a nursing intervention. A model for Truth Telling is presented to guide the nurse in delivering truthfulness. This model is based on the patient's right to determine his or her own destiny and the nurse's ability to use the intervention. The intervention is dynamic and complex. Truth Telling has great potential for enhancing relationships. The nurse has the authority, power, and responsibility to give quality care. Truthfulness is an intervention that belongs in the domain of nursing.

THE CONCEPT OF TRUTH

Although Webster's Dictionary defines truth as "that which is true. . . which accords with fact," Salzman claims truth is "more a matter of definition and varies according to the framework in which it is established . . . whether scientifically, as in natural laws, or morally, as determined by man or by God. . . . There are many definitions of truth; all of them are true, yet none of them are entirely true, and this is precisely the limitation of the concept of truth, unless we believe in absolute truth. To say that something is absolutely true is immediately to tell a lie, for truth is entirely dependent upon our frame of reference" (Salzman, 1973).

Truth can be seen as forming a continuum from truth to deception. The difficulty with being truthful is that there is rarely an absolute truth. For example, in medicine no one really knows the truth of prognosis. Anderson (1935) maintains, "It is meaningless to speak of telling the truth and nothing but the truth to the patient. It is meaningless because it is impossible" (p. 822). It is not possible to tell what you can't foresee. Bok (1978) suggests that truth and truthfulness are not identical. While the truth of any statement may be difficult to establish, truthfulness in communication is determined by one's intent. The nurse must ask, is the intent of the interaction to mislead or deceive?

What is the difference between a white lie and deception? Bok (1978) defines a lie as "an intentional deceptive message that is stated verbally or in writing" (p. 13). Deceit is a wider-ranging phenomenon that includes the indirect intent to mislead others and the omission of necessary information. The nurse could be deceptive in situations by purposely omitting information, giving false reassurances, administering placebos, coercing patients to receive treatments, and being dishonest with peers about substandard care. Deception can occur with patients, families, or physicians when needed information is withheld or misrepresented.

Truthfulness is delivering any statement that is as accurate as is humanly possible. We believe honesty and truthfulness are synonymous. Salzman (1973) states, "Honesty is a dynamic concept that is based on an an individual's sincere and objective attempt to appraise a total situation and that is limited by his inability to be totally unbiased" (pp. 1281–1282).

Truthfulness is affected by our sociocultural environment and our life experiences. Individuals come to the meaning of truth through their values, heritage, and educational influences. Therefore, each person carries some truisms, which are feelings, beliefs, attitudes, and values about a given situation. Lack of awareness, fear of rejection, and concern about the consequences of honesty may cause individuals to conceal information.

When we recognize the value of truthfulness and the importance of the nurse-client relationship, Truth Telling becomes an all-encompassing nursing intervention. We define Truth Telling as *a process of responsible, caring, and honest communication based on ethical decison making*. This process utilizes the nurse's own values, the application of ethical principles, the assessment of the patient, and collaboration with others. The nurse's intent in this interaction is to promote the patient's self-determination and enhance well-being.

THE VALUE OF TRUTHFULNESS

Curtin (1983) defines a value simply as "something so important to a person that he chooses (consciously or unconsciously) to live by it. Professional values, then, are those matters so important that nurses choose to practice by them" (p. 7).

Truth Telling is an intervention only when the value of truth is reflected in nursing care. If the nurse and the patient value truthfulness, the truth can be used as a means of facilitating the patient's well being. Values are developed throughout a person's life by the process of socialization, which occurs personally and professionally. However, a personal value may not be congruent with a professional value. A nurse may proclaim a belief about honesty but at the same time deliver care and communication that are inconsistent with the value of truthfulness.

Uustal (1978) focuses on this issue. "Values form your philosophy and the basis for your actions. If you do not take the time to examine and articulate your values you will not be fully effective with your patients." She further states, "The price paid for unexamined values and arising conflicts over values is confusion, indecision, and inconsistency" (p. 2058). The nurse may say, "The patient should be told the truth because he has the right to know the truth." Yet in an actual situation, when the patient asks for specific information about his or her progress, the nurse replies, "You're doing just fine," and quickly leaves. The nurse has no intention of exploring this issue with the patient.

Steele (1981) maintains that "values determine the selection made between competing alternatives, and therefore, they hold a key position in any decision making process" (p. 5). By clarifying values, nurses determine whether they prize honesty as a value. If the value of truthfulness is a priority, it will be reflected consistently in nursing care. The nurse will choose the option of truth, and communicate this honesty to the patient.

In contrast, Hartman (1976) proposes that a "necessary lie" in a patient–health professional relationship may ward off potential harm. Although we have heard many express a deep concern about the stress, anxiety, and harm Truth Telling can cause patients, our counterclaim comes in the form of a question. Who is to say that the patient's stress level won't be made even greater by the unknown? Certainly many patients sense the avoidance of honesty when the truth is withheld. The patient may then create a "truth" that is much worse than what he would be told by the health professional.

CONFLICTS WITH TRUTH TELLING

The dilemma of Truth Telling arises with the conflict of information sharing versus withholding information, or deceiving the patient. Kant (1963) states that without truth social intercourse and conversation become valueless. "The duty of being truthful ... is unconditional. To be truthful in all declarations ... is a sacred and absolutely commanding decree of reason, limited by no expediency" (pp. 147–154).

How can the nurse resolve the dilemma of truth versus deception? There are several alternatives. The nurse can rely on the traditional position of simply following the physician's orders, react impulsively on the basis of emotion or intuition, or be a detached problem solver. The nurse can emerge, however, as a compassionate risk taker who has developed and applied a critical thinking process.

Paternalism versus Self-Determination

Historically medicine has promoted the principle of paternalism, which is reflected in the codes of medical ethics. Dworkin (1972) states that paternalism "is that which is justified by reason of the welfare, happiness, needs, interests, or values of the person being constrained" (p. 65). The decision to shed the truth or use a "benevolent lie" is based on the principle of paternalism.

Paternalism seeks beneficence but denies the patient control of information. Beneficence requires the health professional to produce or provide good in greater amounts than harm. The autonomy principle strives for beneficence, but maintains the patient's right to self-determination. We view autonomy and self-determination as the same. These terms are used interchangeably in the literature on ethics. What is best should be decided by the patient, not by the professional, if upon his request the patient has been adequately informed. Professionals have the legal responsibility to provide informed consent. Informed consent includes an explanation of the condition, an explanation of procedures to be used and the consequences, description of possible benefits, alternative treatments, and an answering of the patient's inquiries. There is also an understanding that the patient is not to be coerced and may withdraw from treatment (Kelly, 1976). If Truth Telling is based on paternalism, the decision to tell or withhold information rests with the professional. With autonomy the decision rests with the patient; however, truth may still be waived. The patient may directly state a desire not to know. The decision about the amount and type of information (the truth) to be shared often belongs to the patient.

The philosophy of autonomy maintains the patient's basic human rights, treats the patient with respect and dignity, and limits coercion, as much as possible, within the institutional environment. The nurse who accepts this philosophy of autonomy is morally aligned with the patient, not with other professionals or the institution.

The patient's right to self-determination in relation to Truth Telling involves the patient's being fully informed about his health status, alternative treatment modes, procedures, and outcome. When adhering to the right of self-determination, the patient shall have the freedom to choose to participate at any point. The difficult task for the nurse involves assessment of whether or not the patient wants information. The nurse must assess what information the patient has already received, his perception of the information, and the impact of this on the patient. The nurse must also forecast how the truth will affect the patient's behavior, and how his behavior affects others.

AUTHORITY AND TRUTHFULNESS

Some types of medical information are best delivered by the physician. It is the physician's duty to explain medical diagnosis and medical treatment. The nurse is then responsible for clarifying or reiterating this information with the patient. At times nurses experience interferences by physicians who prefer little or no explanation given about medical diagnosis or treatment. The nurse's duty rests with the patient. In providing nursing care, the nurse has the responsibility and authority to explain procedures and nursing treatments. If a physician chooses to withhold medical information which the nurse assesses as important for the patient to know, the nurse has the responsibility to collaborate with others. Based on the patient's right to self-determination, nurses extend their authority by requesting collaboration with health care members. From this collaboration, it will be decided whether or not the patient will receive the information, and who will provide it.

If more credit were given to each professional's knowledge base and authority with a shared notion of respect and interdependence, there would be less conflict between nursing and medicine about who tells the patient what. No professional, be it the nurse or the physician, has the legitimate power to dictate what is best in an ethical dilemma.

The nurse has the duty to protect the patient's right to be informed. The nurse is granted the authority to give this information by the 1976 American Nurses' Association *Code for Nurses with Interpretative Statements* and each state's Nurse Practice Act. These are minimum standards for practice and, in combination with their own values and critical analysis of each situation can be used by nurses to help clarify issues.

The 1976 ANA *Code for Nurses with Interpretative Statements* strengthens the nurse's position of fostering the patient's right to self-determination. As stated in Section 1.1, Self-Determination of Clients, "Each client has the moral right to determine what will be done with his/her person; to be given the information necessary for making informed judgments, to be told the possible effects of care, and to accept, refuse, or terminate treatment" (p. 4). It later states, "The nurse must also recognize those situations in which individual rights to self-determination in health care may temporarily be altered for the common good" (p. 4). While there is no specific reference to Truth Telling in the Code, we believe the first sentence supports the use of Truth Telling as a nursing intervention after assessing the patient's request for truth. The second statement from Section 1.1, although it may seem contradictory, allows the nurse to use professional discretion in either withholding the truth, telling the truth, or delaying a decision.

To further illustrate this, consider a cardiac patient in an intensive care unit who is asking for the truth concerning his wife's condition after a car accident. The nurse is aware that the wife was fatally injured and the patient has a history of stress-related myocardial infarctions. In this situation the nurse acknowledges the patient's right to know and his value system. The nurse has made a critical assessment of the data base and of her communication skills, and has collaborated with others. At this time the nurse temporarily chooses to withhold the truth, based on the long-term well-being of the patient and others.

Compare the ANA Code with the American Hospital Association's (AHA) Patient's Bill of Rights:

> The patient has the right to obtain from his physician complete current information concerning his diagnosis, treatment, and prognosis in terms the patient can be reasonably expected to understand. When it is not medically advisable to give such information to the patient, the information should be made available to an appropriate person in his behalf.
>
> Within the AHA's Bill of Rights there is a startling omission. The only relationship mentioned is the physician-patient relationship. Nothing is said about the duties the nurse or other health professionals have to the patient. Institutions and physicians within these institutions may assert that the physician is the appropriate person to decide upon and then deliver

diagnostic and treatment information to the patient. Yet Section 6.3 of the ANA Code states that with discretion, based on educational preparation, experience, legal guidelines, and professional policies, the nurse may intervene in diagnostic and therapeutic matters. Although the ANA suggests this is not always recognized as "established nursing practice," this direction in nursing is strengthened by the nurse's role as advocate. The nurse's primary commitment is to the patient and to safeguarding his "best interests."

The ANA Code stresses the importance of consultation and collaboration with others. It speaks to interdisciplinary efforts, sharing responsibilities, and promoting collaboration as ingredients that ensure quality care for patients and families. While the Code offers direction, it has not been updated and thus does not reflect the rapidly expanding role of the nurse.

Considering together the patient's right to self-determination, the nurse's power of discretion, his or her role as advocate, and the responsibility to foster collaboration, we believe that nurses are supported by the profession in making Truth Telling a nursing intervention.

THE ETHICS OF TRUTH TELLING

The nursing profession is emphasizing its individuality. As nursing gains recognition as an autonomous group of professionals, nursing is compelled to promote an understanding of ethical theory and ethical practice. The process of learning ethics includes an understanding that morals and ethics are not synonymous. Brody (Gilbert, 1982) holds that ethics is "the study of rational processes for determining the best course of action in the face of conflicting choices" (p. 50). Morals relates to "action in accordance to rules of 'right' conduct." Morality would teach one "how to behave," while ethics would teach one "how to think" when faced with a moral conflict. We are not telling nurses what is right and thus what they should do.

In every ethical dilemma the nurse confronts his or her personal value system and the obligation to carry out what is "sound" nursing practice. We believe that ethical nursing is a blending of critical thinking and is based on ethical theory and self-scrutiny.

According to Curtin (1978), nurses need to be able to identify, clarify, and organize their thinking about ethics and nursing. She states, "Nursing is vitally concerned with ethics because nursing is essentially a moral act! That is, its primary moral conviction shapes its fundamental nature. Its basic moral concern is with the welfare of other humans and its technical skills are developed and designed to that moral end" (p. 12). Nursing is concerned for human beings, their wholeness, and their integrity. This is reflected in Levine's statement, "The willingness to enter with the patient that predicament which he cannot face alone is an expression of moral responsibility: the quality of the moral commitment is a measure of the nurse's excellence" (Levine, 1977, p. 845).

Nurses often determine a sense of what is right and wrong about patient care. Beginning practitioners determine what is right by the direct feedback they receive from important others. These beginning nurses are limited in approach to ethical decision making. When confronted with an ethical dilemma new nurses are uncomfortable because they are bound by conformity and the need to please others. As nurses mature they are more able to apply a critical thinking process, assessing their own values and the patient's about truthfulness. This process involves the nurse delineating the various options for Truth Telling and finally acting on what is most likely to benefit the patient and create stability in the system.

With higher level moral development, nurses relinquish the need for paternalistic control. Nurses assume responsibility for making choices that reflect not what they feel is good for the patient but what the patient feels is good for himself. The patient's right to self-determination is protected by the nurse until it interferes with the higher good for all, in which case it may produce harm for another. At this point the nurse must forgo the good for one and strive for the good for all.

It is important that the nurse identify his or her own ethical framework and assess the ethical frameworks of the institution, the physician, the patient, and the family. By knowing all these pieces of information the nurse can use a critical thinking process and make the best choice when faced with opposing ethical principles.

We believe that a nurse's ethical decision is based on Kantian or Rawlsian deontological theory. Deontological theory supports the belief that there are parts of any act that make it right or wrong. Within this framework, being ethical means doing what is right; doing your duty. Deontologists consider autonomy, nonmalificence, beneficence, and justice as their most important principles.

Each principle in deontological theory can stand alone and be the ethical support for a decision made in an ethical dilemma. One deontological principle can conflict with another. Davis (1981) shows that being honest with a patient about his terminal condition would be justified by the bioethical principle of autonomy. Yet she states that in some instances the decision to tell would conflict with the principle of nonmalificence. To tell a patient the truth, says Davis, might add to the already extensive stress the patient is experiencing.

In rare circumstances autonomy could limit justice, and vice versa. What a patient deserves may be modified by the nurse's choice of the justice principle. Let us return to the cardiac patient who has requested information about the status of his wife who was killed in the motor vehicle accident. Knowing that this patient has had stress-related myocardial infarctions, and that he has three young children under the age of 10 years, does the nurse honor the patient's right to autonomy? He or she certainly could, under closely monitored cicumstances. But the nurse may, however, decide not to risk creating more stress at the moment. The nurse would delay the truth, choosing what is "just" or fair to the children over the patient's right to autonomy.

Most often, being honest will not in itself precipitate a life- or- death situation. Nor will it allow one person to receive care that another then would not have or would have to wait to receive. On the other hand, Truth Telling can put the nurse in a position of double jeopardy. The nurse must be willing to take a risk when favoring the patient's rights and what is best for the other parties involved in the truth dilemma.

As the nurse encounters a plethora of day-to-day experiences, he or she recognizes the ethical dilemmas that are a part of so many decisions. The nurse carries a moral obligation to confront each dilemma as such and not run away. With experience the nurse more easily identifies ethical issues and analyzes them.

The nurse must choose one theory and one principle per situation as a guide in decision making. To do this each nurse should list according to priority which principles are of greatest importance to him or her. The nurse is not being asked to negate his or her affective response. Gilbert (1982) states that ethics provide individuals with the means to recognize and legitimize their emotional reactions in the face of a dilemma and come forth with a caring and logical response.

Ethical Decision-Making Models

Nursing has only recently addressed ethical practices. Therefore, the literature contains few ethical decision-making models. In an interdisciplinary search for such models, we found several common components: gathering relevant data, identification of the ethical dilemma, understanding ethical theory, identifying one's values, selecting a course of action, and reflecting on one's reasoning and that of one's peers. All models emphasize a humanistic concern for the patient. "The client is placed in a position of prime importance and must be considered in the decision making process" (Steele and Harmon, 1981).

Brody (1981) a biomedical expert, propose an individual ethical decision-making model. This model involves a process of problem perception, listing alternatives, making a choice, framing an ethical statement listing immediate and long-range consequences, and then for each consequence comparing values. A short test he proposes for each consequence is "Would I be satisfied to have this action taken upon me?" Brody's model emphasizes the importance of making values explicit in order to judge acts by their consequences. If the value is consistent with the ethical statement, it is a reasonable choice.

TRUTH-TELLING MODEL

Our model involving Truth Telling as a nursing intervention utilizes the necessary components found in ethical decision-making models. The Truth Telling model provides the nurse with a practical approach for directing values and knowledge into a compassionate and logically reasoned response. It represents our definition and illustrates the nurse-patient interaction and the factors influencing the Truth Telling dilemma while using the decision-making process (Table 26–1).

The foundation of the truth-telling model is the nurse-patient relationship. The basis of nursing is in humanistic, holistic, and patient-centered practice. Nursing is also deeply concerned with providing competent care based on sound knowledge as well as communication skills necessary to deliver this knowledge. Nursing as a profession is involved in the current revolution against the illness model in which paternalism has control. We are joining together with individual patients to promote a wellness model. The effects of this are the patient's increasing demand for information and the acceptance of alternative treatments not prescribed by traditional medicine. It is to be hoped that the impact will be society's valuing of health promotion and a wellness model. Because the nurse has the most frequent contact with the patient, he or she has a unique, intimate connection. While this reflects quantity of care, quality is also included. The nurse-patient relationship enhances decision making about health care, and it puts the nurse in the front-line position of delivering truthfulness.

The intent of Truth Telling is (1) to promote greater coping for the individual; (2) to provide increased information for decision making; (3) to enhance trust in the relationship, and in care; and (4) to give patients what is rightfully theirs.

There are a myriad of factors that influence the nurse-patient relationship. Watson (1977) states, "The quality of one's relationship with another person is the most significant element in determining helping effectiveness" (p. 23).

Table 26–1. TRUTH-TELLING MODEL

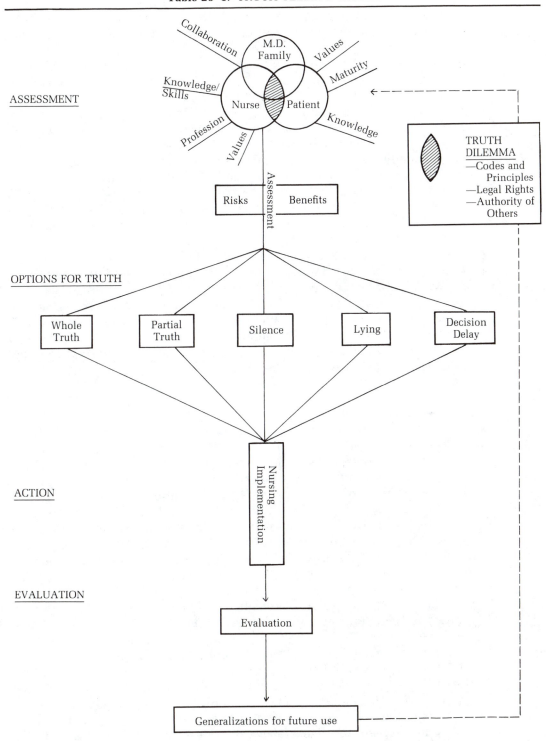

This is enacted by the communication process that promotes honesty, caring, respect, and growth in patient determined directions. Yarling (1978) maintains that "trust has traditionally been considered an essential ingredient in a therapeutically sound relationship" (p. 29, Part II). It is essential to have honesty if trust is to develop. Truth is the atmosphere in which trust thrives. Underlying the patient's request for information about his care, his condition, or probable outcome is a core of concern, often unspoken. The patient may indirectly ask, "Will you treat me fairly, have my best interests at heart?" Will you protect me from harm?" Bok (1978) states, "If there is no confidence in the truthfulness of others, is there any way to assess their fairness, their intentions to help, or to harm?" (p. 31). Once lying or deception has occurred, trust is eroded. This has far-reaching consequences. From this point on, any care or information given by health professional may be suspect by the patient and the family. It is impossible for the patient to enter into a mutual problem-solving process if he does not trust the health care professional or has not received the information necessary for sound decision making.

The consequences of mistrust and deception extend beyond the patient–health provider relationship. Bok (1978) discusses the dire consequences of lying. She states, " It [deception] can give rise to practice very damaging to human communities. Trust is a social good to be protected just as much as the air we breathe, or the water we drink. When it is damaged, the community as a whole suffers; and when it is destroyed, societies falter and collapse" (p. 26). We feel that health care institutions and professionals are morally responsible for protecting the patient's right to information and must adhere to the value of truthfulness. The authority of nurses to use truthfulness as an intervention, to protect patient rights, and to maintain competent care and good service must be acknowledged.

Nursing Diagnoses

Truth Telling encompasses genuine communication and can be a useful strategy for any nursing diagnosis. In particular, Anxiety, Fear, Ineffective Coping, and Powerlessness could be reduced by the nurse using one of the five options for truthfulness. The nurse, being morally aligned with the patient, is in the position of increasing his identity control and his right to self-determination by using Truth Telling as an intervention.

Being honest with patients with such nursing diagnoses as Decreased Cardiac Output, Impaired Physical Mobility, or Anticipatory Grieving might involve delivering the awesome truth or clarifying information about the illness. It is difficult for any health care provider to deliver information that may cause hardship to the receiver.

With a diagnosis such as Potential for Violence or Spiritual Distress, honesty in communication, providing relevant information, and giving feedback are essential. With an agitated patient, truthfulness shows respect. By providing information and feedback, the nurse may help the patient decrease anxiety and maintain self-control. The terminally ill patient who has suffered from loss of function and pain may be more anxious when he has not been given the truth about his condition. If truth is delivered and honesty conveyed, the patient often experiences a change in attitude about the meaning of life and what tasks must be completed before death is imminent. Cases in the literature, especially writings by Kubler-Ross (1969), indicate that terminal patients can handle the "awesome truth" when it is delivered with sensitivity, warmth, and directness. To let someone approach death, unaware that death may be near, is denying the patient and family the right to death with dignity and resolution. Family members appreciate this grim knowledge so that they may gather support and prepare themselves for the loss of a significant other. When a nurse chooses truth or partial truth he or she must provide the ingredients needed in delivering truthfulness: rapport, knowledge of the client and the disease, collaboration with others, communication skills, and timing. While much has been said about rapport, most patients tend to seek information from the person they trust the most. The nurse must decide if he or she is the best person to handle this matter and whether or not he or she has the ability and time to deal with the consequences of Truth Telling. The question of whether to tell the truth has been decided when the nurse chooses an option in our model.

Assessment

The first phase of the truthfulness model is assessment. This assessment differs from the assessment phase of the nursing process because the nurse is gathering information that will lead to the analysis of the risks and benefits of Truth Telling. Good fact gathering is essential. While this phase uncovers vitally important information about the patient, it allows the nurses to build a trusting relationship, so essential for the helping effectiveness. The information gathered will help the nurse and the patient make the optimal choice regarding truthfulness. It is necessary to consider factors influencing the patient's ability to choose, e.g., his age or maturity, level of consciousness, mental capacity, and knowledge base.

Based on the philosophy of autonomy, the nurse must ask, "What is important to the patient?" This helps the nurse determine the patient's values regarding health care, information he needs, his involvement in decision making, and his long-term goals. The patient's right to self-determination, which could include his quest for truth, is waived when the patient is a youth or has been found mentally incompetent by law. When the right to self-determination is denied, albeit temporarily, the nurse would make the decisions about care based on the deontological principle of beneficence, which is associated with paternalism. The nurse assumes the responsibility for protecting the patient from harm. This is justified when the patient's rational reflection is significantly impaired. We believe the nurse may waiver the patient's request for no truth when his refusal of relevant information may cause harm to others. Consider a patient recently given a prescription for a drug that frequently produces drowsiness. He impatiently disregards teaching about medication. It is the nurse's ethical responsibility to inform him of the potential dangers of driving or using heavy machinery. By doing this the nurse adheres to the principles of justice and the greatest good for the most.

Once the nurse has gathered information about the patient, he or she must consider ethical codes and principles, the patient's rights, and the authority of others. Dealing with these external factors, the nurse is forced to confront the truth dilemma. The truth dilemma is illustrated at the point where relationships intersect. In most states hospitals have incorporated the patient's Bill of Rights, but these rights are not upheld by law. Health care practitioners do have the legal obligation to provide information required for informed consent. Only a few states have laws giving the patient or his attorney the legal right to inspect hospital records. The nurse must reflect on his or her knowledge of ethical principles and incorporate nursing's ethical codes when choosing options for truthfulness.

A network of relationships intersect with that of the patient and the nurse, compounding the truth dilemma. These need to be assessed. Each person involved brings his or her own values regarding truthfulness. Before choosing any option, the nurse collaborates with the physician, other nurses, and the family. This collaboration may uncover more information about the patient, including his values, coping ability, and knowledge base. It allows the nurse to present his or her knowledge about the patient. This collaboration reveals each individual's position concerning truthfulness.

Decision Making

According to our model, the nurse considers the position of others and the patient's position, and yet makes the final decision about truthfulness as an intervention. Our model requires the nurse to honestly assess his or her own values, philosophy, knowledge base, and communication skills. Based on the assessment of these, the nurse may decide he or she is not prepared to tell the patient the truth. Since he or she honors the patient's right to self-determination, the nurse seeks to find another who has the rapport, knowledge, and skill to deliver the truth. The nurse takes a risk when he or she decides in favor of truthfulness with the patient, against the wishes of the physician, family, or institution. In the decision-making phase, the nurse considers the various options for truthfulness. These are *whole truth, partial truth, silence, lying,* and *decision delay.* Although the emphasis of this paper has been on the importance of truthfulness, this phase allows the nurse to rationally choose one option.

To offer guidance in selecting the best option, we will put forth hypothetical situations, and discuss benefits and risks.

Whole Truth

The option for whole truth may be easily selected when the patient, family, nurse, physician, and institution all value truthfulness. The patient has specifically requested that he be kept informed, saying, "Just give me the straight facts." Delivering the truth involves the nurse sharing an interpretation of the facts. The patient is alert and shows no mental impairments. The risks of Truth Telling in this example are minimal, although the patient may experience temporary anxiety symptoms. It can be anticipated that the immediate consequence of Truth Telling (about bad news) will be discomfort. The intensity and duration of this discomfort must be evaluated. At this time the patient needs support and reassurance that the nurse will not abandon him. The neophyte professional, eager to deliver truthfulness, needs to understand the complexity of truth telling as an intervention. "Compulsive candor" or "truth dumping," just for the sake of honesty, falls short of the intent, which is caring communication to enhance the well-being of the patient.

There are other times when the decision for truthfulness is more difficult. A terminal cancer patient repeatedly asks you about his pain and prognosis. The nurse is aware the family and the physician wish to protect the patient from the bad news, fearing that the patient will lose the will to live. The nurse assesses the patient's capacity for the truth and his values, and addresses the Truth-Telling dilemma. He or she justifies Truth Telling based on the deontological principle of autonomy. The nurse respects the authority of others and recognizes his or her own position of authority. At this point the nurse collaborates with the others involved. Even if collaboration does not yield consensus concerning Truth Telling, he or she has informed others of the choice to tell the truth.

Assuming the nurse has a sound knowledge base and good communication skills and rapport with the patient, he or she may then deliver truthfulness (Yarling, 1978). It is the nurse's duty to stand by the patient to provide clarity and ongoing support. The risk this nurse may encounter is disapproval, direct and indirect. The consequences of this disapproval may range from a simple reprimand to rejection by peers or the threat of losing one's job.

Partial Truth

The second option in the decision-making phase is partial truth. The nurse must carefully discern the risks and benefits of this option. "The harms of Truth Telling are not to be underestimated," states Gadow (1981, p. 858). She summarizes the three main risks of Truth Telling. The patient may relapse when the truth is delivered. He may experience overwhelming anxiety or depression or become suicidal upon learning his poor prognosis. Gadow recognizes the second risk as being confusion, and states that "the truth is of no benefit to some patients who cannot understand it" (p. 858). When given abruptly and explained in language unfamiliar to the patient, confusion and increased hopelessness can occur. Gadow's last risk is noncompliance with the recommended treatment. Too liberal disclosure fosters ambivalence in persons who might otherwise agree to treatment. An example would be an oncology nurse explaining chemotherapy to a patient. If truthfulness involves telling all the possible risks and side effects, the cancer patient may refuse treatment for fear of impending discomfort. He may not foresee the potential long-term benefits of controlling the cancer. The nurse must also be careful in using partial truth that is one-sided and would lead the patient to choose the health professional's preferred option for treatment, not the patient's. Partial truth would then be coercion. These risks mentioned by Gadow should be considered in each situation involving truthfulness. By themselves, they may not constitute reasons for withholding the truth. The risks must be weighed with specific information gathered during the assessment phase.

Partial truth allows the nurse to respond with sensitivity to the patient's request for information. What information is the patient requesting right now? What need is the patient expressing? Any patient who is hospitalized, away from his secure environment, and dealing with an illness is vulnerable. To immediately blast the patient with "the truth, the whole truth, and nothing but the truth" is insensitive. McCorkle (1981) states, "Telling is rarely an urgent question . . . the actual conveying of messages to a person about his diagnosis and future needs to be an ongoing process" (p. 408).

Unlike the patient in the whole truth option who asks directly for complete information, another patient may be more hesitant about wanting the facts. Before using partial truth the nurse assesses what the patient already knows. A more difficult task is to listen carefully to what is being asked, both directly and indirectly. The intent of partial truth is veracity, not to purposely deceive. This option allows the nurse to give ongoing information without the need to repair or disentangle misinformation. Partial truth is often used with children and individuals with altered levels of awareness.

Partial truth may be used in response to a surgical patient who has recently returned from the recovery room. Mr. Jones, who had an exploratory laporatomy for possible cancer, asks, "Am I going to be all right?" The nurse can reply, "You've come through surgery, and your condition is stable." He or she needs to assess whether this satisfies the request for information. If the patient continues to ask for further information—for example, "What did the surgeon find?"—the nurse has the responsibility to answer. The next response may be that the doctor found an inoperable tumor. At this point, the nurse determines if the patient is content with the amount now given. If the nurse is uncertain, based on the patient's verbal and nonverbal responses, he or she must continue to ask, "Would it be helpful to know more?" Partial truth involves delivering only the relevant information that answers the patient's questions and unspoken concerns.

Silence

Silence is the third option. Historically it has been used to protect the patient from harm. Part of this protection has only been possible by deception. Silence is reflected in the statement "I can't answer that for you. You'll have to ask your doctor." In our model, however, there are rare circumstances when silence is appropriate. When the risk of truthfulness appears to be overwhelmingly destructive, truth is withheld. Consider again the cardiac patient asking about his fatally injured wife. The nurse choosing silence might respond, "Right now we aren't addressing any concerns other than getting you in stable condition." There is no intent to mislead or deceive. The nurse remains open to giving the patient information about his wife later. This is a temporary choice until the patient is more stable and can be given partial truth or whole truth. If the cardiac patient continues to ask while in an unstable condition, what happened to his wife, the nurse may be forced to use decision delay, saying "I'll try to find out," or to lie, saying, "I don't know." Collaboration with others is often required and is frequently supportive for the nurse in such rare circumstances.

The greatest risk of silence is that the patient may feel anxious about the unknown. The patient may be aware that things are amiss because the care givers and family members are poor actors. Feelings of mistrust build if silence is interpreted as deception. Silence, when used by the nurse, may be interpreted by the patient as avoidance, indifference, or lack of knowledge. The benefits of this option would be protection from induced anxiety or despondency. Silence should be employed for a brief time only, and limited to the initial phase of the crisis. It may also be used when the patient requests no truth and this silence is not harmful to another. In this situation, the nurse is simply adhering to the patient's right to self-determination.

Silence in Truth Telling is not to be confused with the therapeutic use of silence. In Truth Telling, silence involves the temporary withholding of information "in the patient's best interest." The therapeutic use of silence denotes a presence, a supportive "being there," which is unencumbered by words. Each of these forms of silence may be used alone or may occur in the same interaction with one patient. If the decision has been made to withhold information, the nurse's presence may be one means of communicating caring, authenticity, and support.

Lying

There are rare circumstances when lying is necessary. Lying may be used when truth endangers the immediate health and well-being of the patient and silence or decision delay is ineffective. A young woman is about to be delivered of a stillborn fetus. She is highly anxious and repeatedly asks, "Is my baby going to be all right? How can I deliver a baby that is dead?" The nurse knows, but replies, "The baby is O.K. and we will get you through this."

The nurse needs to consider the perspective of the liar and the deceived. Is the liar affected by his or her own lies? As a health professional the ethics of the situation must be carefully weighed. The nurse's decision to lie may have consequences that affect her belief about herself, her integrity, and her credibility. From the perspective of the deceived there may initially be greater comfort but this turns to mistrust, disillusionment, increased anxiety, anger, and depression when deception is revealed.

There are many forms of lying in a health care setting. These range from concealment to exaggeration. Lying for whatever reason usually requires the nurse to produce an excuse. The energy of maintaining a lie, even for benevolent reasons, carries a future burden of protecting the liar's credibility.

Decision Delay

Decision delay is the last option. It can be used when there is missing information, lack of knowledge, or lack of rapport. The nurse uses decision delay when he or she has not assessed the patient's values, knowledge base, or mental status, and when he or she does not have the time to deliver information and offer the necessary support to the patient. Fear of being an incompetent communicator may also cause the nurse to choose this option. Such factors may lead the nurse to say, "I'll find someone who can give you the information." Decision delay gives the nurse time to responsibly plan the intervention for truthfulness, and it can be carried out by such a statement as, "I appreciate your concern. Let me find out for you. I'll get back to you this afternoon."

Whether the nurse uses whole truth, partial truth, silence, lying, or decision delay, he or she has the responsibility to evaluate the patient's responses to the interaction. If the nurse assesses that it is best for another person—possibly the physician, primary nurse, or family member—to provide the truth, he or she remains responsible for helping plan who, when, and what is said. Later the nurse determines if the intervention was carried out and what the outcome was. This allows for continuity of care.

Implementation

In the implementation phase of the Truth Telling model the nurse will carry out a planned strategy, having chosen the best option for Truth Telling. According to our definition, the intent of the intervention is to promote the patient's self-determination and enhance his well-being.

As stated previously, the essence of the nurse-patient relationship is communication. It is with trust that truth flourishes. There are important communication skills that the nurse must use effectively if he or she is to be successful in Truth Telling. Active listening, empathy, congruence, confrontation, nonpossessive warmth, immediacy, and self-disclosure may be utilized in all phases of our model. The beauty of each nurse combining these skills constitutes the art of nursing and the therapeutic use of self. Active listening and empathy involve attending to verbal and nonverbal cues during the communication process, and strategically validating the feeling tone of the patient's message. Immediacy and self-disclosure involve the nurse's participating in the relationship by being authentic and expressing beliefs and values, as well as perceptions of the relationship. "I hear you saying honesty is important to you, and you value being informed about your care. . . . Honesty is important to me also. Our being open, together, about what we want and value has been helpful to me and has strengthened our relationship. How has it been for you?"

Congruence is being truly genuine and without "professional armor." The nurse's verbal and nonverbal cues are congruent when both reflect the same message. If the nurse is showing interest and concern, he or she is expressing it verbally as well. She is not saying "I'm interested in what you have to say" while her nonverbal message is distraction and impatience. Confrontation is a higher level communication skill that is effective if trust and truthfulness have been established. Confrontation in Truth Telling involves the nurse's pointing out discrepancies between the patient's beliefs and behaviors. For instance, the nurse confronting a noncompliant patient might say, "On one hand you value getting better and going home. On the other hand, you are refusing to cooperate with the treatment plan. Can we sit down and honestly discuss our beliefs and expectations, so that we can work together toward your goal?"

The concept of integrity does not refer only to the patient; it is also important to the nurse in a patient-centered relationship. To be true to ourselves, and maintain our own integrity, is being authentic. Authenticity also denotes truthfulness, individuality, and becoming a risk taker about values or beliefs concerning health care and nursing practice that may depart from the existing norms. Nelson (1982) states, "Our authenticity lies in keeping in touch with ourselves as persons, in adhering to a personal value system, and having the courage to resist peer pressure for mediocre practice should this pressure exist" (p. 3). Some nurses struggle with the fear of losing "group acceptance" when being an innovator of change. A nurse who is a risk taker does not forsake the sense of this acceptance but preserves personal identity, accountability, and responsibility. Part of being treated as a confident, reasonable professional who can collaborate and cooperate is presenting oneself in an assertive manner. This requires leadership skill and honesty and maintains one's authenticity. It does not, however, deny the importance of promoting team efforts and group decision making.

Evaluation

Evaluation of the intervention is the next phase in the model. Documentation of the various stages and the patient's response to the intervention is vital for the interdisciplinary team to understand the process and to evaluate its outcome in order to make generalizations about truth telling for the future.

Truth Telling is part of the communication process, which may be ongoing. After evaluating the patient's response to a specific option for truth, the nurse may move toward or away from the whole truth. To do this the nurse must reenter the assessment phase and move through the Truth-Telling intervention. Our final conversation with the cardiac patient will illustrate this. As the patient's condition stabilized within 24 hours, he was physically and emotionally able to discuss the accident and the loss of his wife. The nurse previously used decision delay or silence and would progress to either partial truth or whole truth. The nurse, or person designated to provide the truth, might say, "You've asked so often about your wife. We have been concerned about your own well-being and have not discussed this with you. We regret to say that your wife was killed during the accident. We will address your concerns and do anything to support you through this crisis." To evaluate the Truth Telling intervention the nurse should reflect on the following:

Process Evaluation

1. Were the nurse's personal and professional values incorporated?

2. Did the nurse apply ethical principles in the decision-making process?

3. Did the process involve the careful assessment of the client and his situation?

4. Did collaboration occur with the primary care givers and the family if needed; in the data collection, assessment, and implementation phase?

Outcome Evaluation

5. Was the intent of the interaction to increase caring, respect, and self-determination of the patient? Was the nurse successful in communicating this? How was it received?

6. Has Truth Telling enhanced the well-being of the patient? What behaviors indicate this? Consider alterations in pain, decreased restlessness, increased involvement in care, synthesizing new information, ability to plan short and long term goals, increased socialization.

7. What were the patient's behavioral and emotional changes observed after the intervention? Consider decreased anxiety, mood change, increased ability to verbalize feelings, and reported satisfaction with health care.

8. What has the nurse learned about himself or herself? How will this affect his or her nursing practice?

RESEARCH

The professional nurse must balance scientific knowledge with humanistic caring. In nursing research the investigator is responsible for sound scientific inquiry and is obligated to protect the patient from harm, as well as safeguard the patient's rights. Honesty is essential during informed consent, scientific investigation, and the reporting of research findings. Patients must be given the freedom to refuse participation or to withdraw at any point in the study.

Other health professionals have examined Truth Telling from two main perspectives: whether the truth should be told, and the risk associated with telling. Although research in these areas is scant, most studies support the notion that patients prefer being informed of their diagnosis and treatment. Oken's (1961) research on what to tell cancer patients revealed that over 80 per cent of patients surveyed favored knowing their diagnosis. A 1981 study done by Faden and associates studied the detailed disclosure of side effects of phenytoin (Dilantin) medication to seizure disorder patients. It was found that physicians chose to be selective regarding the amount of information shared with the patient, disclosing only the most likely risks, and minimizing the alternatives to medication treatment. The majority of patients and families surveyed preferred detailed and extensive disclosures, particularly regarding risks and alternative therapy.

The biggest concern for telling the truth is the impact it will have on the patient. According to Mappes and Zembaty (1981) the damages associated with Truth Telling are less than one would believe. The benefits are substantial. Pain is tolerated more, recovery from surgery is quickened, and cooperation with therapy is improved. Schwarz (1978) studied compliance in a large psychiatric population and found that informed patients complied more fully with prescribed treatment than did uninformed patients.

Nursing research needs to examine professional values with regard to patient rights, informed consent, and Truth Telling. Research must verify that Truth Telling as a nursing intervention enhances the well-being and the self-determination of the patient. At this time, it is not known whether truthfulness is a consistent value for nurses. Generating new knowledge about nurses using truthfulness, using informed consent, and maintaining patient rights would increase nurses' power and authority to make decisions regarding care. This would protect nurses who are involved in the decision-making process of patient care, not merely implementing care. Research in these areas could strengthen patients' and nurses' rights.

Although our model for Truth Telling has not been tested, there are parts that have been strengthened by empirical research. Ketefian (1981) investigated the relationship between critical thinking, educational preparation, and levels of moral reasoning. Ketefian's data analysis supports the positive relationship between critical thinking and moral reasoning. Her findings suggest that a positive correlation exists between higher education and higher level moral reasoning. This reiterates the importance of ethics in nursing education and the practice of critical thinking in ethical decision making.

Nurses are in the unique position of having the most contact with the patient, which allows easy collection of data concerning what the patient values about nursing care and health care. Specifically, nurses might explore what value Truth Telling has for the patient and his family as it relates to length of hospital stay, acceptance of illness, and compliance with treatment. Investigating truthfulness could also dispel myths concerning the damages of being truthful.

CONCLUSION

The Truth Telling model has application for the nurse far beyond the day-to-day encounters with patients. Nurses can apply this same problem-solving process when examining the consequences of being honest with a peer, a nursing administrator, a physician, or any health care professional. As nursing assumes greater responsibility for making decisions about patient care, each nurse must accept responsibility for practicing honest communication. Nurses need to work at being honest by giving constructive feedback to others about the quality of care given. The ability to be honest varies from situation to situation. How honest anyone will be in an interaction depends upon the value placed on truthfulness and the person's commitment to the cause for which he or she proclaims the truth. The commitment to honesty is weighed against the perceived threat in the interaction. If a young nurse is to deal with a head nurse or supervisor about poor staffing, which caused unsafe care, he or she must ask, "What are the consequences for me? If I am honest and criticize, and make suggestions for change, will I have to work more weekends? Will I put my promotion in jeopardy? Will she turn others against me?" Using the Truth Telling model, the nurse can carefully assess the benefits and the risks of honesty, which are influenced by what he or she believes to be true about the superior. Drawing together this information helps the nurse choose the best option and plan the Truth Telling strategy.

The authentic nurse using honesty and Truth Telling as a nursing intervention, in a caring and assertive manner, serves as an excellent role model for any nurse entering into practice. In delivering the truth, it is not so much the correctness of the words we choose as the intention of our message and our commitment to stand by and support the patient that are important. Truth then becomes a garment that we wear. For some it is worn with comfort and ease. We convey honesty through our words, the unspoken language of our bodies, and the energy of our beings.

EDITORS' COMMENTS AND QUESTIONS

Nurses are constantly faced with complex ethical situations. The model presented in this chapter helps define the truth-telling dilemma and provides guidance to the nurse in decision making. The authors consulted literature in ethics, philosophy, law, and religion to develop this complex intervention.

Questions for Discussion

1. *How much of the truth would you tell in the following situations?*

   a. A telephone call to relatives of a client who was dead upon arrival in the emergency room.

   b. First contact with a client who has a recent medical diagnosis of a terminal illness. The purpose of the contact is to do a nursing assessment.

   c. Face-to-face discussion with relatives in the waiting room of an intensive care unit to which a client has just been admitted in serious condition.

   d. Direct questioning about recurrence of a malignancy by a long-term cancer patient for whom you cared during previous hospitalizations.

2. *Must the nurse have the physician's permission to tell the truth? What if the nurse and physician disagree?*

References

American Hospital Association. A patient's bill of rights. Chicago, American Hospital Association, 1973.

American Nurses' Association. Code for nurses with interpretive statements. Kansas City, Mo.: American Nurses' Association, 1976.

Anderson, L. Physician and patient and social system. *New England Journal of Medicine*, 1935, *212*, 819–823.

Aroskar, M. Anatomy of an ethical dilemma: The practice. *American Journal of Nursing*, 1980, 4, 658–661.

Bok, S. *Lying: Moral choice in public and private life.* New York: Random House, 1978.

Brody, Howard, *Ethical Decisions in Medicine.* Boston: Little, Brown and Company, 1981.

Curtin, L. A proposed model for critical ethical analysis. *Nursing Forum*, 1978, *17*(1), 12–17.

Curtin, L. Editorial opinion. *Nursing Management*, 1983, *14*(1), 7–8.

Davis, A. J. Dilemmas in practice: To tell or not. *American Journal of Nursing*, 1981, 1, 156–158.

Dworkin, G. Paternalism. *Monist*, 1972, *56*, 64–84.

Faden, R., Becker, C., Lewis, C., et al. Disclosure of information to patients in medical care. *Medical Care*, 1981, *19*(7), 718–733.

Gadow, S. Truth: Treatment of choice, scarce resource, or patient's right? *Journal of Family Practice*, 1981, *13*(6), 857–860.

Gilbert, C. The what and how of ethics education. *Topics in Clinical Nursing*, 1982, *4*(1), 49–56.

Hartman, N. From Truthfulness and uprightness, in S. Gorovitz and R. Maklin (Eds.), *Moral problems in medicine.* Englewood Cliffs, N.J.: Prentice-Hall, 1976.

Kant, I. *Lectures on ethics* (translated by L. Infield). New York: Harper and Row, 1963, pp. 147–154.

Kelly, L. Y. The patient's right to know. *Nursing Outlook*, 1976, *24*, 1.

Ketefian, S. Critical thinking, educational preparation, and development of moral judgement among selected groups of practicing nurses. *Nursing Research*, 1981, *30*(2), 98–103.

Kubler-Ross, Elizabeth. *On Death and Dying.* New York: McMillan, 1969.

Levine, M. Nursing ethics and the ethical nurse. *American Journal of Nursing*, 1977, *77*, 845–849.

Mappes, T., and Zembaty, J. *Biomedical ethics.* New York: McGraw-Hill book Company, 1981.

McCorkle, R. Communication approaches to effective cancer nursing care, in L. Marino (Ed.), *Cancer Nursing.* St. Louis, C. V. Mosby Company, 1981.

Nelson, M. J. Authenticity: Fabric of ethical nursing practice. *Topics in Cancer Nursing*, 1982, 4(1), 1–6.

Oken, D. What to tell cancer patients: A study of medical attitudes. *Journal of the American Medical Association*, 1961, *175*, 1120–1128.

Salzman, L. Truth, honesty, and the therapeutic process. *American Journal of Psychiatry*, 1973, *130*, 1281–1282.

Schwarz, E. Use of a checklist in obtaining informed consent for treatment with medication. *Hospital and Community Psychiatry*, 1978, *92*, 97.

Steele, S. M., and Harmon, V. M. *Values clarification in nursing*. New York: Appleton-Century-Crofts, 1981, p. 5.

Uustal, D. Values clarification in nursing: Application to practice. *American Journal of Nursing*, 1978, *78*, 12, 2058–2063.

Veatch, R. Nursing ethics, physician ethics, and medical ethics. *Law, Medicine, and Health Care*, 1981, 9(5), 19.

Watson, J. Nursing: *The philosophy and science of caring*. Boston: Little, Brown and Company, 1977.

Yarling, R. R. Ethical analysis of a nursing problem: The scope of nursing practice in disclosing the truth to terminal patients. Parts I and II. *Supervisor Nurse*, 1978, May-June, 40–50, 28–34.

27

DISCHARGE PLANNING

KATHLEEN KELLY
ELEANOR McCLELLAND

The Discharge Planning literature within the last decade has focused on the functional aspects involving staff and discharge planners. This chapter is designed first to synthesize salient issues in providing continuity of care that have been identified in the literature during the last 25 years and to create a bridge between current Discharge Planning strategies and these conceptual issues.

Discharge Planning has been defined frequently and with varied emphasis in the recent literature. Some definitions seem to isolate one aspect of Discharge Planning while others equate discharge planning activities with referral to another care source. We believe that Discharge Planning is a process, not merely an event formalized and culminated by referral.

Therefore, a more eclectic definition is offered. *Discharge Planning consists of a series of events that occur soon after a person is admitted to a given health care setting in order to facilitate continuity of care; is based on an assessment of individuals' health care needs; maximizes client independence; and gives consideration to comfort, compassion, and economical methods of delivering health care services.*

The goal of Discharge Planning is to enable the client to regain or maintain as normal and productive a role in life as possible. Effective Discharge Planning brings the client and the needed human and nonhuman resources together. The client is given the available options and is allowed some leeway in choosing among them. Discharge Planning should involve community-wide multiprofessional team planning on a regular basis. All staff professionals must appreciate the need for coordination among the client care providers in all settings if effective, individualized care is to be delivered.

STATE OF THE ART

Ideally, ensuring continuity between levels of care should be automatic. When health problems require resources beyond those of the client, a referral should be the next step. The current health care system in the United States does not always demonstrate an organized effort to plan and deliver a level of care that matches the needs and maximizes the potential of the individual. A 1980 study of home health utilization prepared by the Iowa Health Systems Agency (IHSA) described the state of Discharge Planning as follows:

> In determining potential barriers to increasing the utilization of home health services, the accessibility to these services must be examined. Patients may enter the home health care sector through a variety of courses, the most common of which is referral upon discharge from acute and long-term care facilities. Some of these facilities already have established very workable and comprehensive discharge planning programs. In many other facilities, however, discharge planning is uncoordinated and haphazard, and in some cases nonexistent. This results in many patients being discharged without an adequate treatment plan to guide them through the levels of care which best suit their medical and social needs. Poor discharge planning results in inappropriate placements and underutilization of home health services. (IHSA, 1980, p. 1)

A major weakness in the current system is that care is planned in terms of what an individual provider knows to be available and not necessarily in response to client care needs. The outcome of effective Discharge Planning (i.e., continuity of care) requires that there be open communication among health care personnel at all levels. The United States system isolates acute, long-term, outpatient, and community or home care delivery providers from each other, which often impedes communication. Agencies attempting to provide a continuum of services are often hampered by the limited scope of health problems served by a particular institution or policies regarding payment for services.

Discharge Planning initially involves defining the "at risk" population in order to determine priorities for health professionals. The internal resources of individuals within the at risk population should always be considered if planning is to be effective. When an at risk population is defined in writing within a particular care setting, it is possible to disregard the needs of other individuals outside the defined group who may also require continued health care. Therefore, effective Discharge Planning must evolve from the application of basic principles and guidelines as they are applied by the primary care provider interacting with the client and his or her significant others.

Giving legitimacy to Discharge Planning as an expectation in any health care setting or situation are statements from professional and governmental sources. For example, the American Nurses' Association has published the following:

> Health care occurs on a continuum which exists even though an individual's need and/or desire for care varies, and even when health care is given by numerous providers.
> To achieve continuity of care, it is necessary: (1) that the health care structure or system provides for and identifies linkages among the health care providers; (2) that each provider within this structure or system be identified as a contributor to a general health care plan for the individual; and (3) that there be planning, coordinating, communicating, referral and follow-up to achieve the mutually agreed-upon goals.
> Continuity of care is an ideal. An individual health care provider contributes to this ideal by: (1) developing and strengthening the linkage with other providers who give care to the patient/client prior to, together with, or following that provider's involvement; (2) relating the specific contribution to the general plan of health care for the individual; and (3) initiating and participating in coordinated planning.
> Continuity of care planning in an organized health care system estab-

lishes a process designed to meet the needs of the patient or client during every phase of care. The process involves admission planning, discharge planning, referral, and follow-up. (ANA, 1975, p. 2)

Skilled Nursing Facility Medicare and Medicaid rules (revised) published in the *Federal Register*, May 1974, have provided more detailed guidelines on Discharge Planning than previously included in the original work, "Condition of Participation, Utilization Review":

> (h) Standard: Discharge Planning. The facility maintains a centralized coordinated program to ensure that each patient has a planned program of continuing care and/or follow-up which meets his/her post-discharge needs. (1) The facility has in operation an organized discharge planning program. . . . (DHEW, 1974a, p. 15232)

In 1974, the Department of Health, Education, and Welfare issued guidelines for the Professional Standards Review Organization (PSRO), which include a section on Discharge Planning located under the Continued Stay Review (CSR), Section 705:

> Where problems in post-discharge care or discharge placement are anticipated, discharge planning should be initiated as soon as possible after admission to the short-stay hospital. Discharge planning should include both preparation of the patient for the next level of care and arrangement for placement in the appropriate care setting. Information needed for the discharge planning process includes:
> (a) Prior health care status of patient (i.e., was patient receiving care in his home or some type of long-term care facility?);
> (b) Current level of care needed;
> (c) Projected level(s) of care needed;
> (d) Projected time frame for moving patient to next level of care;
> (e) Therapy(ies) and teaching that must be accomplished prior to hospital discharge;
> (f) Available resources for post-hospital care; and
> (g) Mechanisms for facilitating transfer to other levels of care. (DHEW, 1974b)

These excerpts from the ANA statement and federal regulations provide the framework for the successful intervention of Discharge Planning.

INSTITUTIONAL FOCUS

A great deal of attention is given in the recent literature and in continuing education programs to the subject of Discharge Planning methods. Much of this information relates to discharge from hospitals without sufficient emphasis on continuity of care in the broader sense. It has been left to the institutionally based health care providers to set the pattern for Discharge Planning development within the health care system even though health care providers in several settings must be cooperating to provide continuity of care. In the American Hospital Association's Patient's Bill of Rights (1972) there is a statement that the patient has the right to expect reasonable continuity of care. This implies that Discharge Planning has become synonymous with post–hospital care arrangements for many health care providers. This is inadequate since most people in the United States are not hospitalized when they receive health care.

Discharge Planning has followed the medical model of health care delivery. The existing health care system consists of a hierarchy in which physician orders are required for nonmedical health needs to ensure acquisition of continuing health care services. Many physicians, as well as nurses, social workers, and members of various other disciplines, are questioning the need for such a requirement. Payment by third party sources for any services requires physician approval, which increases administrative costs. Since payment is arranged without direct consumer involvement, there is little motivation for consumers to question this system. Furthermore, the credibility of "less traditional" modes of health care is lowered among health care providers, especially those within acute care settings, by this dependency on physician approval for any health intervention.

In the United States the emphasis on medical care for acute and short-term illness prevails. Recovery from an episodic problem denotes success. However, the needs for many individuals, particularly older persons, often extend beyond the treatment of the crisis. Home care and adult day care services are options that can extend the range of services beyond that which is available in 24 hour care facilities for those who, with some degree of assistance, can resume independent living. There are a number of efforts currently under way to standardize the method of making this determination (O'Brien and Saletta, 1980). One example is ACCESS, a system developed by the state of New York (New York State Department of Social Services, 1978).

ACCESS is a standardized preadmission screening system used in Monroe County, New York, to assess clients prior to long-term care placement or transfer. The original purpose was to stem the flow of Medicaid funds into institutional long-term care. The findings indicate 69 per cent of Medicaid-supported clients and 58 per cent of private pay clients referred for placement remained in community settings to receive needed services as a result of the screening. Community services ranged from volunteer services and equipment modification to a range of multiprofessional services on an intermittent basis.

The appropriateness of this shift in emphasis from institutional to non-institutional care settings whenever feasible has been supported by studies citing the cost-effectiveness of the noninstitutional setting when the length of hospital stay can be decreased. For example, O'Brien and Saletta (1980) found that when clients were discharged into home care programs, 13 to 16 hospital days per client were saved as a result of earlier discharges. The economic implications are obvious considering the present daily cost of hospitalization.

The economic advantages of avoiding, delaying, or shortening institutional care are well known to lawmakers, and are becoming popular among regulatory bodies. The fact that most health care providers are not oriented to thinking about cost factors and generally have had only token exposure to educational experiences that reflect a health continuum has interfered with maximizing the health care options being made possible by legislation and funding since the mid-1960s.

Even more difficult to understand is health providers' failure to recognize the humane and therapeutic value of effective Discharge Planning. It would appear that effective discharge is currently measured by the convenience to staff, the results of medical treatments, and the idea that "more care is better care" instead of focusing on the factors that maximize the client's independence, personal resources, dignity, and long-term needs.

Discharge Planning enables nurses to prepare clients and families for maximum independence. To be effective planners, nurses must learn as much as possible about the range of resources available in a community and how to assess them, as well as anticipate problems after discharge. Observations from nursing homes and home health agencies indicate we are not doing this. Some nursing home administrators indicate the majority of persons admitted as "private pay" clients deplete their personal economic resources within 6 months and must be discharged or receive financial assistance.

A number of studies indicate that many of these persons do not require 24 hour care. For example, Elconin, Egberg, and Dunn (1964) and Greenlick, Hurtado, and Saward (1966) estimated that only 7 to 9 per cent of all discharged hospital patients need home care. Later, in a 1970 study reported by Allen and colleagues, (1974), a median of 1.5 per cent of admitted patients were referred for home care, with a range of 0.3 to 3.8 per cent among all participating hospitals. In 1980 the U.S. Department of Health, Education, and Welfare estimated that 25 per cent of disabled persons needing home care were actually receiving it (Home Health Line, 1980). Studies done by the Levinson Policy Institute of Brandeis University indicate that health professionals are in considerable disagreement about in-home care needs of individual clients (Sager, 1980). The author points out that professionals do not share goals regarding client levels of well-being, a primary factor in effective Discharge Planning. How easily this could be resolved if we determined what the clients' goals were!

Selecting the appropriate level of care to match client needs is another consideration. A report published by the Department of Health and Human Services, Health Care Financing Administration, in January 1981 (Long Term Care, 1981) reports and summarizes 14 studies of clients in skilled and intermediate care facilities in the United States and concludes that 10 to 20 per cent of those in skilled care and 20 to 40 per cent in intermediate care were receiving a higher level of care than warranted by their medical problems. The report states that "a large portion could reside at home or in sheltered housing if adequate community services were available" (Long Term Care, 1981, p. 35). We believe there is reason to question whether health professionals planning continuity of care are aware of and utilizing the sources that are readily available.

Experiences of community health agencies reflect a general trend of the client, family, or neighbor seeking nursing home care and other support services when difficulties in managing health problems are encountered at home. These experience and studies of dependency levels of clients receiving care in nursing homes and in their own homes support our position that health care providers are not approaching Discharge Planning based on the level of client needs (McClelland and Kelly, 1980). Brody, Poulshock, and Masiocchi (1978) also report a survey of chronically ill subjects either receiving care in nursing homes or served by a community home health agency. "After comparing residents by their ability to perform varying functions, such as dressing, eating and bathing, the study found that the nursing home and community population had similar impairment levels which ranged from moderately to totally impaired" (Brody et al., 1978, p. 558). The critical variable identified in this study was not the level of functioning but was related to living arrangements and the presence of a caring person (e.g., spouse, child, sibling). Numerous other studies have supported this finding, as reported in various Reports to the Congress by the U.S. General Accounting Office beginning in 1974 and available from the U.S. Government Printing Office.

Similar misuse of resources may exist in hospitals. Since the initial days in hospital are historically the most expensive it would seem appropriate to develop mechanisms for preadmission screening of all but medical emergency admissions and requiring a broader use of options that include outpatient clinics, day surgeries, physicians' offices, and in-home care. The need to immediately address the apparently arbitrary approach to providing continuing health care as evidenced in the literature is urgent if we consider the estimated percentage of the United States population having functional disabilities. In 1977, 13.5 per cent (28.6 million) of the noninstitutionalized United

States population was estimated to suffer some degree of activity limitation due to a chronic health problem. Of these, 7.7 million were unable to carry out major activities and 0.8 per cent were dependent in one or more activities of daily living (Long Term Care, 1981).

Although this last statistic is currently insignificant with respect to the total population, there are two issues to consider. First, the elderly are *20 times* more likely to be dependent in daily activities, and this segment of the population is increasing more rapidly than any other age group in our population (Long Term Care, 1981). This shift in age is probably most important to future health care delivery since it is estimated that 25 per cent of the population will be over 80 years of age by the year 2010 (Ball, 1977). Second, the estimated 7.7 million people with limitations in major activities should have guidance in planning for optimal independence.

As nurses, we have the tools and mechanisms to implement the ANA and PSRO expectations. We must remember that our efforts in resolving life-threatening problems may be lost if we do not plan to prevent or control the more subtle or insidious events that complicate an individual's health. For the past several decades, the focus of nursing has been on crisis. Because we are used to dramatic and highly technical interventions, we are not cognizant of issues as basic as food preparation, transportation, medication management, homemaking, and adaptation of the home or work situation to personal limitations. If nursing is to assume a leadership role in establishing continuity in health care delivery we must be critical of our efforts in Discharge Planning. Only by recognizing impediments to continuity of care will nursing achieve this role.

BARRIERS TO EFFECTIVE DISCHARGE PLANNING

There are specific reasons why nurses and other health care professionals have not used Discharge Planning as a means of improving health care delivery and controlling costs. In 1957 it was shown that early release of acute care patients and efficient long-term care management was possible through greater utilization of public health nursing services (Associated Hospital Service of New York, 1957). Smith (1962), in her frequently quoted publication, used this and other investigative reports to substantiate the need for improving continuity of care.

Why then, have we not done so? Developments in the health industry during the 1950s and 1960s, such as the Hill-Burton Act, have perpetuated an acute care model of care delivery that subverts the concept of Discharge Planning. In the case of the Hill-Burton Act, the fact is that hospital beds, once provided, should be kept occupied to restrict operating costs per day; thus, the economic incentive conflicts with planning care that will minimize use of the facility.

Another phenomenon inhibiting Discharge Planning based on level of client needs is Medicare legislation, in which reimbursement guidelines for inpatient hospital care are broad and nonspecific, whereas outpatient and home care coverage remain very stringent, and day care coverage is non-existent.

Approximately 10 years ago Ziegler (1974) summarized the basic problems curbing the development of positive attitudes and skills in assuring effective continuity of health care. His points were as follows:

1. The provider's view of health is limited to what is available in his agency.

2. Health providers from various disciplines and care settings do not trust each other.

3. Discharge Planning will be poorly done and the consequences—loss of valuable health information, fragmented care, and increased cost—will continue so long as more value is placed on hospital care than on its alternatives.

4. Most health providers have inadequate knowledge of available resources.

5. Resources and administrative support for doing effective Discharge Planning are lacking.

As the barriers to effective discharge planning are analyzed it is sometimes difficult to differentiate problems from symptoms or to determine the best approach to elimination of the barrier. For purposes of illustration, we have organized the barriers to Discharge Planning in two categories: intrinsic and extrinsic. Intrinsic barriers we have defined as those causes of ineffective Discharge Planning that result from actions or omissions on the part of health professionals. Ziegler's first four problems are intrinsic barriers. Extrinsic barriers are those we consider precipitated by United States society, economics, and the prevailing political climate. Ziegler's fifth problem is an extrinsic barrier. Critics of the United States health care system raise the issue that health professionals as a group may contribute in some ways to perpetuating some extrinsic barriers. If we, as individuals, are to contribute to an improvement in the continuity of care system, we must analyze these major barriers to determine specific behaviors we can modify. Tables 27–1 and 27–2 provide tools for such an analysis.

What this overview demonstrates is that it is within the capabilities of health professionals, individually and collectively, to develop a delivery system that not only supports but also is contingent on providing continuity of care based on individual client needs. This would mean optimal utilization of every health care resource for which there is a demonstrated need and which is cost-efficient. (Cost-efficiency relates to achieving desired effect for least expense, not unit costs.)

We believe nurses in every care setting are in crucial positions to make the difference in change from a haphazard approach to Discharge Planning to developing plans that respond to client needs most effectively.

INTERVENTION

For Discharge Planning to be successful, it is our belief that administratively approved, formal systems should be established within every health care setting. A review of current literature supports this position (ANA, 1975; Beatty, 1980; McKeehan, 1981; Smith, 1962).

Models

The literature describes several Discharge Planning models, including those related to the primary nurse, discharge planner, liaison nurse, bedside staff nurse, or a combination of these, and multiprofessional collaboration.

Primary nurses have as their major objectives continuity of care and accountability for client care, which promotes consistency in planning for discharge (Marran, Schlegel, and Beves, 1979). The nurse, in the practice of primary nursing, has responsibility for developing a plan of care that encompasses all aspects of the client's needs. When the implementation of the plan

Table 27–1. INTRINSIC BARRIERS TO EFFECTIVE DISCHARGE PLANNING

Barriers	Professional Contributions to Barriers		
	Education of Health Professions	Inadequate Role Models and Research	Underestimate Client, Family, and Community Resources
1. Limited concept of the health continuum	X	X	X
2. Lack of professional rapport and collaboration	X	X	
3. Lack of a discharge planning system crossing over care setting boundaries	X		X
4. Care providers lack knowledge of available resources and their potential	X	X	X

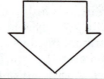

Contributing Factors

Philosophy and goals vary greatly among individuals and care settings.

Abstract concepts and management skills involved are traditionally not valued among health professions.

Overtreatment occurs in an effort to achieve quality.

Discharge Planning is equated with referral.

Literature is on hospital discharge, confuses issue of responsibilities.

Table 27–2. EXTRINSIC BARRIERS TO EFFECTIVE DISCHARGE PLANNING

Barrier	Indirect Professional Contributions to Barrier
1. Lack of Resources and Accessibility	A functional continuum of health care is not reflected in regulatory guidelines for funding (developed with health professions' input).
	Reimbursement by National Health Insurance (Medicare, Medicaid) reflect an acute care, medical model, which major professional associations have not questioned.
	The marketing within the professions and trade industries promote our societal expectations for "hi-tech" medically managed, institutionally located health care.
	Resources for nontraditional health services vary dramatically among communities, depending on the politics and power groups; health professionals more often represent their "practice group" rather than the needs of their clients when we attempt to impact these forces.
	A passive acceptance of the United States health care system and an unwillingness to test some alternative systems used in other societies.

utilizes the range of resources needed to facilitate continuity of care, the ideal situation exists. In reality this is not likely to be the usual occurrence.

The discharge planner, a specially designated nurse or other health care professional in the hospital setting, usually begins with an assessment of the anticipated post-hospital needs of a client at the time of admission to the hospital. The discharge planner, as a hospital employee, is governed by that institution's policies and procedures. This includes involvement in utilization review, orientation and in-service for hospital personnel, and reassessing client's post-hospital needs. The degree to which continuity of care is implemented is related to the discharge planner's knowledge of community resources, referral expertise, and effective coordination of communication among all participants in the clients' care.

The liaison nurse, a nurse who is based in a community agency, serves as a link between the community agency and the hospital to ensure that continuity of care occurs. As an employee of a community agency the liaison nurse is governed by its policies and procedures. The liaison nurse's role includes participation in hospital in-service and orientation programs; evaluation of clients referred for home care; consultation with other health care professionals in developing a predischarge plan for home care; facilitation of communication between hospital staff and community staff; and serving as a resource person to hospital personnel regarding community resources and home care practices. The person in the liaison role is sometimes called the Community Care Coordinator (National League for Nursing, 1979).

When continuity of care plans for an individual patient are the responsibility of many nurses, such as all the bedside staff who provide care for the client, too often inconsistency results. The Discharge Planning part of the plan may receive inadequate attention. Frequently the lack of accountability for the plans results in lack of continuity of patient care (Beatty, 1980). This could still work if Discharge Planning were done across all levels and in instances in which care providers from different levels are equal collaborators with the client in the planning process. Because this does not happen consistently, clients frequently receive higher cost care for longer periods of time, which may lead to greater dependency in clients than is therapeutic.

Multiprofessional collaboration is most useful when independent assessments are revised and synthesized, giving a more complete picture of the client's situation. Decisions regarding continuity of care should be made by the appropriate mix of health team members in close communication with the client and family. The choice of care should be made after considering all options, from the simplest to the most complex. Obviously health care providers must keep abreast of the options available to maintain the best chances that needs will be met by the care received. We are more likely to provide more care than less care because of our orientation to 24 hour care settings, but, as stated in the *Accreditation Manual for Hospitals*, "conservation in provision of medical and health services is an element of quality" (Joint Commission on Accreditation of Hospitals, 1977, p. 28). In other words, not only may resources be wasted by giving excessive care but also, if dependence is promoted and rehabilitation opportunities are missed, poor outcomes can result.

Nursing Process in Action

Effective Discharge Planning will reflect the essence of the nursing process from assessment to evaluation. Regardless of the intervention model, identi-

Table 27–3. IDENTIFICATION OF AT RISK POPULATION

At Risk Groups	Related Nursing Diagnoses*
Disabled and elderly	Impaired Physical Mobility
Terminally ill	Anticipatory Grieving
Disrupted family	Alteration in Family Processes
Chronically ill	Potential for Growth in Coping
Surgeries affecting body image or function	Disturbance in Self-Concept
Ethnic or cultural isolation	Social Isolation
Economic deprivation	Powerlessness, Anxiety
New, young parents	Potential Alterations in Parenting
Single parents	Alterations in Family Processes
Persons living alone	Social Isolation
Known substance abuse	Alterations in Thought Processes
Homebound	Social Isolation, Activity Intolerance
Sensory impairment	Sensory Perceptual Alterations

*These are examples of commonly accepted "at risk" categories and related nursing diagnoses and should not be considered all-inclusive.

fication of "at risk" groups and the need for specific services is an initial step in any care setting, which can be included within a larger assessment (see Table 27–3). It is essential that the client be oriented initially for care beyond the immediate setting. Ideally the client is involved in each stage of planning for continuity of care.

To demonstrate the application of nursing diagnosis and nursing process to Discharge Planning, a nursing process model for Discharge Planning has been developed as a basis of nursing intervention (Table 27–4).

This model represents the key concepts involved in effective Discharge Planning. The first of these concepts is "mutuality of assessment, need or problem identification and determination of objectives." Mutuality in this context refers to the pooling of data from the client and various health professionals to arrive at consensus about the client's future health care needs. This may often involve compromise on the part of each one involved to accommodate the perspectives of provider and client.

A second key concept in Discharge Planning is "client withdrawal." This refers to the third alternative in implementation when the client (or significant others) elects to reject help. In these situations, which should be limited in number, the nurse's responsibilities focus on maximizing the opportunities for the clients to learn, by role modeling, keeping communication open to reestablish Discharge Planning activities, and identifying the possible outcomes of failure to accomplish needed discharge plans. The following example will clarify this concept. If a new mother does not show any willingness to care for (or be taught to care for) her newborn baby before discharge from the hospital, refuses a post-hospital referral, and identifies no means for providing infant care within a family support system, the nurse can anticipate some serious implications for both the mother and the infant. In this instance the Discharge Planning process encounters a barrier that should be treated as a serious health hazard, based on what we know about maternal-infant bonding and child abuse research.

Finally, the concept of "evaluation" based on client and multiprofessional feedback is critical to effective use of the nursing process in Discharge Planning. The methods of this feedback vary greatly, and may be based on data from all clients or a random sample. Regardless of the sample, the criteria should be a formal part of the Discharge Planning program, should have administrative and multiprofessional acceptance, and should be convenient for respondents to provide.

Table 27-4. NURSING PROCESS MODEL FOR DISCHARGE PLANNING

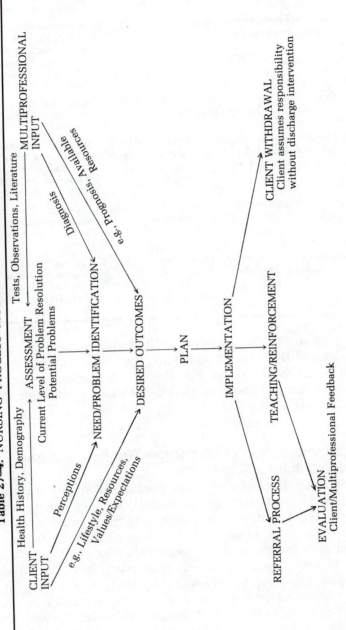

Table 27–5. EVALUATING EFFECTIVENESS OF DISCHARGE PLANNING

Client Outcomes That Would Demonstrate Effective Discharge Planning	Process for Achieving the Identified Outcomes
1. Client status is improved (comfort, cure)	1. Completion of medication and treatment regimens, facilitation of support systems (referal or family), assess status, monitor progress, and evaluate client status
2. Client has reduced hospital stay, delayed admission, or no readmission	2. Arrangement of predischarge home visit(s); on-going liaison or consultation in contact among staff in care settings. Prevention early and identification of problems. Timely reassessments and modification of treatment plans
3. Client or family expresses satisfaction with discharge planning arrangements	3. Collaboration of key health care professionals, identification of client or family wishes
4. Client or family displays independence in specified health behaviors (e.g., injections, exercises, appliances, etc.)	4. Facilitation of optimal independence in activities of daily living. Assess level of knowledge and observed level of skill. Treatment or equipment used appropriately
5. Client or family is directly involved in planning and evaluating the care provided	5. Provision of information regarding community resources. Familiarizing patient or family with expectations for specific care settings
6. Client receives services appropriate to the dependency level demonstrated	6. Referral(s) made to the appropriate provider(s) of needed services(s) (nursing home, Meals on Wheels, social worker, hospital, etc.). Timely reassessment(s) and modification of treatment plans

Table 27–5 is one example illustrating some client-related indicators of successful Discharge Planning and the process for achieving these outcomes. To ensure that Discharge Planning is indeed effective, these elements need to be reflected in criteria for staff performance evaluations and recorded audits of the care setting.

Implementation of Discharge Planning [as an Intervention]

The requirements for effective Discharge Planning are administrative recognition, sufficient staffing, documentation, and on-going evaluation. In reality, these may be artificial and exist only on paper. The concepts of Discharge Planning and continuity of care must be incorporated into staff orientation and development with the expectation for Discharge Planning included in written job descriptions. Only then can it be evaluated and rewarded. It is apparent that written policies and procedures alone are not sufficient.

Literature over the last five years has focused extensively on operationalizing various Discharge Planning models (Beatty, 1980; Steffl and Eide, 1978; Waters, 1980). Steffl and Eide (1978) describe models for Discharge Planning applicable to hospital settings, long-term care facilities, and the community agencies. Multidisciplinary involvement is identified in each instance. Other key elements include identification of discharge options for patients, provisions for patient input, and a defined problem-solving approach.

Beatty (1980) comments that the common characteristic of Discharge Planning models in several university hospital settings is "a centralized, coordinated approach to continuity of care assessment and implementation" (p. 166). Accountability is determined by identification of specific responsibilities with the major assignment delegated to either the department of nursing service or department of social services. Planning is interdisciplinary, and implementation occurs in appropriate departments. Nursing roles may range from involvement as a team member to that of primary coordinator.

Waters (1980) provides a tutorial approach in which she outlines ways for a Discharge Planning program to be developed and implemented. The practical suggestions described provide a framework for organizing discharge planning in a health care setting where none exists. McKeehan (1981) emphasizes the roles of various health professionals in the Discharge Planning process. The multiprofessional approach to Discharge Planning expands the potentials for meeting the range of clients' needs to assure that continuing care may in reality be achieved. Social workers, dietitians, physicians, physical therapists, and occupational therapists along with nurses may contribute the essential expertise needed for health care planning teams.

If it is accepted that the goal of nursing is to assist individuals and communities to attain, maintain, or regain health or move from illness to wellness, there should be no question about the need for implementation of activities to promote continuity of care. The value of nursing diagnosis in providing such care and communication among care levels is unlimited.

To demonstrate how Discharge Planning is applicable to any situation but operationalized on an individual basis the following case study is included.

CASE STUDY

The head nurse of a medical unit, Ms. R., placed high priority on reviewing all admissions occurring during her days off the unit. Recently she returned from a four day leave to find that three persons had been admitted with cardiac arrhythmias. What was especially noteworthy was that all three clients were readmissions after recent hospitalizations for the same problem. Ms. R. hypothesized that these clients had not been adequately prepared for self-care.

To explore this possibility, Ms. R. instructed the staff nurses on the unit to review each client's records, complete a current assessment, and determine nursing diagnoses for each of them. In addition to gathering data to assist her in evaluating her unit, she viewed this as an opportunity for staff nurses to analyze continuity of care needs on an organized, comparative basis. The similarity of the presenting problems should clearly demonstrate the impact individual circumstance has on Discharge Planning. When the intervention for these three cases is approached according to a medical model the individual differences could be overlooked. By developing nursing diagnoses the individuals' differences become apparent and implications for Discharge Planning take on a new meaning.

Clients A, B, and C were assessed using the departmental tool. Table 27–6 reflects the findings and interactions of staff, patient, and significant others that resulted.

Such hypothetical situations are not fantasies but represent the types of problems that can be gleaned by routinely reviewing client situations. Furthermore, they illustrate the scope of circumstances that may cause the presenting problem, with each situation requiring a totally different response following the initial assessment. This is the essence of Discharge Planning—the commitment to a comprehensive standardized assessment followed by an individualized plan reflecting the scope of problems and the continuum of care necessary for resolution, control, or prevention.

We have offered only a few examples of the strategies that will impact favorably on Discharge Planning. When health care professionals place con-

Table 27–6. PLANNING CONTINUITY OF CARE

Client	Assessment of Findings	Problem Identification	Nursing Diagnoses	Goals or Plan
A	Understood treatment regimen. Had appropriate medications available. Identified side effects and hazards of not following prescribed use of medications. Finances adequate for needs	Went on long weekend trip and forgot medication supply. Unable to obtain new supply enroute	Self-Care Deficit	Regulation and discharge with plans for maintaining a travel kit that includes medication supply
B	Understood drug effects and frequency ordered. Took one daily; sublingually	On discharge had received a prescription for "heart pills." Believed all such pills were to be placed under tongue. Did not associate pills given during previous hospitalization with this prescription.	Knowledge Deficit	Client will describe the action, schedule, and method of taking medication. Practice self-medicating prior to this discharge. Obtain materials on self-medicating and review with primary nurse
C	Medication supply available at home, but has used only one tablet since previous discharge. Takes numerous over-the-counter medications and dietary supplements	Lack of commitment to medication management. Mild electrolyte imbalance	Noncompliance Coping, Ineffective Individual	Regulate cardiovascular status. Arrange staffing and referral re: medication management, nutrition, and safety. Arrange predischarge home visit if client is receptive

certed effort on improving Discharge Planning activities (i.e., focus discharge planning on individual needs) the benefits will be felt by clients, health care professionals, employing agencies, and the general public. Clients benefit by receiving more care, often at less cost than care arranged through arbitrary referral. Health care professionals benefit through greater job satisfaction achieved by creative and efficient problem resolution through collaborative working relationships with other health professionals. For the employer, effective Discharge Planning is an important marketing tool and a means of focusing available resources at the level of greatest need. For the general public, effective Discharge Planning would achieve what United States legislators and some state legislators have sought—that is, matching the level of care to the level of need for the purpose of controlling health care costs and distributing available resources to meet a growing demand.

EDITORS' COMMENTS AND QUESTIONS

Although Discharge Planning is most frequently done in the acute care setting, the key to its successful implementation is good communication with fellow health care workers and clients. Thus, the intervention of Discharge Planning was placed in this section of the book. The authors stress that the key to successful Discharge Planning is sound planning at the institutional level as well as the individual client level.

Questions for Discussion

1. *What are the cost-effectiveness implications for this intervention? What impact do DRGs have on Discharge Planning? Can you design a study to evaluate the cost-effectiveness of Discharge Planning?*

2. *Does every hospitalized patient need this intervention?*

3. *How can the use of nursing diagnosis facilitate Discharge Planning?*

4. *What type of administrative support is necessary for Discharge Planning?*

References

Allen, D., Kuhns, P. L., Werley, H., and Peabody, S. R. Agencies' perceptions of factors affecting home care referral. *Medical Care*, 1974, 12(10), 828–844.

American Nurses' Association. *Continuity of care and discharge planning programs in institutions and community agencies*. A statement of the American Nurses' Association Division on Medical-Surgical Nursing practices and the Division on Community Health Nursing Practice. Kansas City, Mo.: American Nurses' Association (Publications Code NP-493000), November 1975, p. 2

Associated Hospital Service of New York. *Report of a study concerning the feasibility of providing nursing service following hospitalization for Blue Cross subscribers*. New York: Associated Hospital Service, 1957, pp. 61, 62.

Ball, R. United policy toward the elderly, in A. N. Exton-Smith and J. Grimley Evans (Eds.), *Care of the elderly*. New York: Grune and Stratton, 1977, pp. 20–32.

Beatty, S. *Continuity of care—the hospital and the community*. New York: Grune and Stratton, 1980.

Brody, S., Poulshock, S. W., and Masciocchi, F., The family caring unit: A major consideration in the long-term support system. *Gerontologist*, 1978, 18(6), 556–561.

Department of Health, Education, and Welfare. Medicare–Medicaid, *Federal Register*, Part III, 1974a, 39(85) (May 1), p. 15232.

Department of Health, Education and Welfare. *PSRO program manual*, Chapter 7, Section 705.29, 1974.

Elconin, A. F., Egberg, R. O., and Dunn, O. J. An organized hospital-based home care program. *American Journal of Public Health*, 1964, 54, 1106.

General Accounting Office. *Entering a nursing home*. Report to the Congress, PAD-80-82. Washington, D.C.: U.S. Government Printing Office, 1979.

General Accounting Office. *Home health—the need for a national policy to better provide for the elderly*. Report to the Congress, HRD-78-19. Washington, D.C.: U.S. Government Printing Office, 1977.

Home Health: An Industry Composite, Chicago: Arthur Young and Company, 1980.

Home Health Line. *Home health line decade report—1980*. Washington, D.C.: National Press Building, 1980.

Iowa Health Systems Agency. *Home health reference manual*. Des Moines: Iowa Health Systems Agency, 1980.

Iowa Health Systems Agency, *Long-term care in Iowa, Part I and II*. Des Moines: Iowa Health Systems Agency, 1981.

Joint Commission on Accreditation of Hospitals. *Accreditation manual for hospitals* (supplement to 1976 Edition). Chicago: Joint Commission on Accreditation of Hospitals. 1977.

LaVor, J. Long term care and home health care: A challenge to service systems. *Home Health Service Quarterly*, 1979, *1*(1), 19–73.

Long term care; background and future directions. Washington, D.C.: U.S. Department of Health and Human Services, HCFA publ. #81–20047, 1981.

Maddox, G. Community and home care: United States and United Kingdom. in A. N. Exton-Smith and J. Grimley Evans (Eds.), *Care of the elderly.* New York: Grune and Stratton, 1977, pp. 147–160.

Marran, G. M., Schlegel, E., and Beves, E. *Primary nursing* (2nd ed.). St. Louis: C. V. Mosby Company, 1979.

McClelland, E., and Kelly, K. Characteristics of clients referred for post hospital care. *Home Health Review*, 1980, *3*, 11–22.

McKeehan, K. M. (Ed.). *Continuing care—a multidisciplinary approach to discharge planning.* St. Louis: C. V. Mosby Company, 1981.

Moss, F., and Halmandaris, V. *Too old, too sick, too bad.* Germantown, Md.: Aspen Systems Corporation, 1977.

New York State Department of Social Services. Monroe County demonstration of a community-wide alternative to long-term care models. 1978, SRS Grant No. 11–P–90130. Albany: New York State Department of Social Services, 1978.

O'Brien, C. L., and Saletta, A. Home health care and adult day health care—options for serving older adults. *Nursing administration quarterly, community outreach Part I.* Germantown, Md.: Aspen Systems Corporation, 1980.

Reif, L. *Community based in home health services.* San Francisco: San Francisco Foundation, 1977.

Sager, A. *Decision-making for home care: An overview of study goals and methods.* Waltham, Mass.: Levison Policy Institutes, Brandeis University, 1980.

Smith, L. Factors influencing continuity of nursing services. New York: National League for Nursing, Publ. 62–12063, 1962.

Steffl, B. M., and Eide, I. L. *Discharge planning handbook.* Thorofare, N.J.: Charles B. Slack, 1978.

Waters, E. J. *How to do patient discharge planning.* North Miami, Fla.: Waters, 1980.

Weiler, P. Geriatric care abroad. *Forum*, 1978, *2*, 32–35.

Yura, H., and Walsh, M. *The nursing process.* New York: Appleton-Century-Crofts, 1976.

Ziegler, D. Overview of the discharge referral planning problem: What is being done locally, in *Patient discharge and referral planning—whose responsibility?* New York: National League for Nursing, Publ. 20–1515, 1974.

28

FUTURE DIRECTIONS

GLORIA M. BULECHEK
JOANNE C. McCLOSKEY

We have been nurses for approximately 20 years and have participated in the recurrent debate over the issue "Is nursing a profession?" After working for two years on the preparation of this book, it is exciting to conclude that there is a professional model of nursing. This model is characterized by direct service to clients that is based upon theory developed and modified through research. The service is delivered via the autonomous acts of diagnosis and treatment and is evaluated by peers against standards established by the profession. At present, this professional model is being implemented by only a few nurses, most of whom have graduate preparation and are working as clinical nurse specialists or nurse practitioners. The professional model of nursing is being promoted by the nursing diagnosis movement. Nurses must assume accountability for the health problems being identified through the movement. This book describes some of the interventions that nurses are currently implementing to treat nursing diagnoses. Much work remains to be done to place a professional model of nursing in the mainstream of nursing practice. We offer the following suggestions.

Continued Development and Refinement of Nursing Interventions

More clarification of the term "intervention" is necessary. There is confusion about what is a theory, what is a philosophy, and what is a treatment. For example, is Patient Advocacy a treatment to use with a specific diagnosis or is it the philosophical basis of all nursing? Is Counseling the essence of a definition of nursing or is it an intervention? We hope the discussion and description of interventions in this book helps us begin to answer these questions.

An intent of this book was to identify nursing interventions for specific nursing diagnoses. Owing to the early stage of diagnostic taxonomy development, the research on interventions is just beginning. Although some interventions have been tested in some patient populations, none have been tested in relationship to specific nursing diagnoses. In this book, the authors, drawing upon their own knowledge base and practice experience, have identified nursing diagnoses related to interventions. The next step is to test their ideas. To facilitate this we have constructed an index of related nursing diagnoses and interventions. In Table 28–1, each of the 50 diagnoses approved by the Fifth National Conference Group has been listed next to the intervention that

Table 28–1. NURSING INTERVENTIONS: TREATMENTS FOR NURSING DIAGNOSES

Nursing Diagnoses	Nursing Interventions
Activity Intolerance	Relaxation Training
Airway Clearance, Ineffective	Surveillance
Anxiety	Active Listening Assertiveness Training Culture Brokerage Discharge Planning Music Therapy Presence Relaxation Training Structured Preoperative Teaching Support Groups Truth Telling
Bowel Elimination, Alterations in: Constipation Bowel Elimination, Alterations in: Diarrhea Bowel Elimination, Alterations in: Incontinence	Exercise Program Nutritional Counseling
Breathing Patterns, Ineffective	Relaxation Training Structured Preoperative Teaching Surveillance
Cardiac Output, Alterations in: Decreased	Exercise Program Surveillance Truth Telling
Comfort, Alterations in: Pain	Relaxation Training Music Therapy Structured Preoperative Teaching
Communication, Impaired Verbal	Assertiveness Training Culture Brokerage Group Psychotherapy Music Therapy Patient Advocacy Presence
Coping, Ineffective Individual Coping, Ineffective Family: Compromised Coping, Ineffective Family: Disabling Coping, Family: Potential for Growth	Assertiveness Training Cognitive Reappraisal Counseling Crisis Intervention Culture Brokerage Discharge Planning Group Psychotherapy Music Therapy Patient Contracting Patient Teaching Preparatory Sensory Information Presence Relaxation Training Reminiscence Therapy Role Supplementation Sexual Counseling Structured Preoperative Teaching Support Groups Truth Telling

the authors in this book recommend. It must be remembered that the diagnosis list is incomplete. Indeed, our authors had additional diagnoses to suggest in relationship to certain interventions. For example, Impaired Decision Making is the critical diagnosis for Values Clarification and Depression is one of the major diagnoses for Music Therapy.

It is apparent from the index that most of the interventions in this book

Diversional Activity, Deficit	Music Therapy Reminiscence Therapy Support Groups
Family Processes, Alterations in	Counseling Discharge Planning Support Groups
Fear	Active Listening Assertiveness Training Cognitive Reappraisal Counseling Crisis Intervention Music Therapy Preparatory Sensory Information Presence Relaxation Training Reminiscence Therapy Structured Preoperative Teaching Support Groups Truth Telling
Fluid Volume, Alterations in: Excess Fluid Volume Deficit, Actual Fluid Volume Deficit, Potential	Nutritional Counseling Surveillance
Gas Exchange, Impaired	Structured Preoperative Teaching Surveillance
Grieving, Anticipatory Grieving, Dysfunctional	Counseling Crisis Intervention Discharge Planning Exercise Program Music Therapy Presence Reminiscence Therapy Role Supplementation Support Groups Truth Telling
Health Maintenance Alteration	Cognitive Reappraisal Culture Brokerage Exercise Program Self-Modification
Home Maintenance Management, Impaired	Patient Teaching
Injury, Potential for	Crisis Intervention Exercise Program Patient Teaching Presence Support Groups Surveillance
Knowledge Deficit (specify)	Counseling Culture Brokerage Patient Contracting Patient Teaching Support Groups Structured Preoperative Teaching

Table continued on next page

Table 28–1. NURSING INTERVENTIONS: TREATMENTS FOR NURSING DIAGNOSES (Continued)

Nursing Diagnoses	Nursing Interventions
Mobility, Impaired Physical	Discharge Planning Exercise Program Music Therapy Relaxation Training Truth Telling
Noncompliance (specify)	Counseling Culture Brokerage Patient Contracting Patient Teaching Support Groups
Nutrition, Alterations in: Less than Body Requirements Nutrition, Alterations in: More than Body Requirements Nutrition, Alterations in: Potential for More than Body Requirements	Culture Brokerage Exercise Program Nutritional Counseling Self-Modification Support Groups
Oral Mucous Membrane, Alterations in	No intervention
Parenting, Alterations in: Actual Parenting, Alterations in: Potential	Counseling Culture Brokerage Discharge Planning Patient Contracting Patient Teaching Role Supplementation Support Groups
Powerlessness	Cognitive Reappraisal Crisis Intervention Culture Brokerage Discharge Planning Patient Advocacy Preparatory Sensory Information Relaxation Training Support Groups Truth Telling
Rape-Trauma Syndrome	Counseling Crisis Intervention Sexual Counseling
Self-Care Deficit (specify level: Feeding, Bathing/hygiene, Dressing/grooming, Toileting)[1]	Counseling Patient Contracting Patient Teaching Reminiscence Therapy
Self-Concept, Disturbance in	Active Listening Counseling Crisis Intervention Culture Brokerage Discharge Planning Exercise Program Group Psychotherapy Music Therapy Reminiscence Therapy Role Supplementation Support Groups

[1]The primary interventions to treat this diagnosis would be interventions such as Bathing, Feeding, Positioning, Bowel Training, Bladder Training, Oral Hygiene, and Skin Care. We were not able to include these interventions in the book.

are treatments for psychosocial diagnoses. We made a purposeful decision not to include the interventions to treat the Self-Care Deficit diagnoses. Interventions such as Bathing, Feeding, Positioning, Bladder Training, Bowel Training, Skin Care, and Oral Hygiene would be the primary interventions for the diagnoses Self-Care Deficit, Oral Mucous Membrane Alteration, Impairment

Table 28–1. NURSING INTERVENTIONS: TREATMENTS FOR NURSING DIAGNOSES (*Continued*)

Nursing Diagnoses	Nursing Interventions
Sensory Perceptual Alterations	Discharge Planning Music Therapy Reminiscence Therapy Structured Preoperative Teaching
Sexual Dysfunction	Counseling Music Therapy Patient Teaching Sexual Counseling
Skin Integrity, Impairment of: Actual Skin Integrity, Impairment of: Potential	No intervention
Sleep Pattern Disturbance	Exercise Program Music Therapy Relaxation Training
Social Isolation	Active Listening Assertiveness Training Culture Brokerage Discharge Planning Music Therapy Presence Reminiscence Therapy Support Groups
Spiritual Distress	Counseling Crisis Intervention Culture Brokerage Music Therapy Presence Reminiscence Therapy Support Groups Truth Telling Values Clarification
Thought Processes, Alterations in	Cognitive Reappraisal Crisis Intervention Discharge Planning Music Therapy Reminiscence Therapy
Tissue Perfusion, Alterations in	Exercise Program Structured Preoperative Teaching
Urinary Elimination, Alterations in	No intervention
Violence, Potential for	Counseling Support Groups Surveillance Truth Telling

of Skin Integrity, Alteration of Urinary Elimination, and Alteration in Bowel Elimination. More attention needs to be directed to the testing of these interventions and the development of other interventions for biological diagnoses. This puts us in the middle of the controversy over the degree of independence a nurse has to treat pathophysiological problems. We believe that nurses do exercise a great deal of independence in the care of critically ill and long-term patients. It is also apparent from the index that some of the psychosocial diagnoses need to be refined. For example, Ineffective Coping, Fear, Anxiety, Powerlessness, and Disturbance in Self-Concept are so abstract that multiple interventions can be recommended. It is apparent that to choose an intervention, the nurse must know more about the cause (etiology). As these diagnoses are further developed, subcategories of each diagnosis will appear in the taxonomy and specific interventions will evolve.

There is a great deal of variation in the research base for the interventions described here. Sensory Preparation and Structured Preoperative Teaching have had extensive testing, and the findings are providing direction for practice. Interventions such as Presence and Patient Advocacy are still being defined. Other interventions, such as Relaxation Training and Assertiveness Training, are widely used but the outcomes have not been documented. Some interventions, such as Role Supplementation and Values Clarification, have been borrowed from other fields and as yet have had little application in nursing. Research related to the reliability and validity of nursing interventions is needed. The reliability question is, "Will two nurses doing the same intervention for the same patient get the same result?" The validity question is, "Is the intervention appropriate for the diagnosis?" Obviously, further research is needed on almost all of the interventions in this book. *Therefore, the clinician should be cautioned not to take this index as a prescription for practice.*

Tool Development for Nursing Interventions

An early step in defining, implementing, and evaluating an intervention is the development of a tool that outlines the specific nature of the intervention. For some interventions, such as Patient Teaching, several tools have been developed to assist with consistent implementation of the intervention. The current need is psychometric testing and standardization of the tools. For an intervention such as Surveillance, one comprehensive tool that may be modified depending on the nature of a specific critical care unit may need to be developed.

Tools are important because they guide the intervention and provide criteria from which to judge its effectiveness. In addition, documentation forms often control the delivery of services. While nurses complain about paperwork, they structure their care so that the required forms get filled out. If the forms reflect a philosophy of the nurse as a dependent assistant to the doctor who delivers technical care in a functional manner, this is the way the nurse will act. If the forms reflect a philosophy of the nurse as a professional member of the health team with a unique independent function, the nurse will act accordingly. In the future, with the implementation of price-per-case reimbursement vis-à-vis diagnosis-related groups, documentation will become more important than ever. Nurses must have the evaluation tools to document outcomes of interventions that have implications for cost effectiveness by keeping the client self-sufficient and out of the acute care institutions.

Organizational Changes for Delivery of Nursing Service

Attention must be given to organizational structures that will provide for a professional model of nursing. One nurse needs both the authority and the accountability to select a nursing intervention for a given client. The nurse will need the assistance of others to carry out the nursing orders associated with the intervention once the decision is made. These orders must be binding. Primary nursing is much closer to this ideal than team or functional nursing.

How can delivery of nursing service be structured to accommodate the professional model of practice and still effectively deliver the technical component? Society and employers expect nurses to continue to carry out physicians' orders. Will all RNs continue to be responsible for both technical and professional practice or do job descriptions need to separate the two? Will nurses be forced out of bureaucratic organizations in order to adopt a professional model of practice?

Increased Specialization and Advanced Education

The astute reader will have concluded by now that few of the 26 nursing interventions described in this book are currently being taught in nursing curricula. Indeed, at the present time these interventions are being implemented by nurses who practice in specialized areas. Any one nurse will be observed conducting only a few of these interventions. As the knowledge base of nursing advances, increased specialization will occur. It is our prediction that these interventions plus others that will be developed at this same conceptual level will be the foundation of professional nursing practice in the future.

Where do nurses learn how to do these interventions? What level of education is necessary for the nurse who will use these interventions? We hope that all RNs will be able to benefit from this book, and we hope that diagnosis and intervention books will eventually replace traditional medical model books at the undergraduate level. Indeed, curricula across the country are moving from the medical model to a conceptual model. This trend will continue, and the conceptual approach now utilized for assessment and diagnostic purposes will extend to the intervention portion of the nursing process. This is occurring first in graduate programs preparing clinical nurse specialists but will "trickle down" to undergraduate curricula. At the present time we believe the appropriate level of preparation for nurses who can implement these interventions is at the master's level. As several chapter authors have pointed out, the skills needed by a nurse to implement these interventions are many and complex. Once an intervention is well defined and a protocol established, the intervention is easy enough to learn—Preparatory Sensory Information is an example. However, the judgment as to when to do the intervention, the evaluation of whether it works, and the delineation of further research all require advanced preparation.

Legislative Changes

Many states have revised their nurse practice acts in recent years to accommodate an expanded role for nurses. Recent acts include provisions for the nurse to diagnose, prescribe, and treat. These efforts to give legal recognition to the expanded role of the nurse need to continue.

Specifically, more effort is needed to attain third party reimbursement for nurses. While recent gains have been made in this area for nurse midwives and other nurse practitioners in some states, there is a long way to go. Related to third party reimbursement for nurses are several questions that the profession needs to answer: Should all nurses receive third party reimbursement? If only certified nurses are to be reimbursed, what criteria will be used for certification? Should the American Nurses' Association be the certifying organization? Should master's preparation be required for certification?

In several states nurse practitioners are legally prescribing medications.

Should this become the norm for more nurses? Will the power of prescription facilitate autonomous nursing practice? Do nurses need the power of prescription to be effective in the eyes of the public?

Implementation of the Baccalaureate Degree as the Minimal Entry Level

Much has been said and written about the minimal level of entry into professional nursing practice in the past two decades. We can only add our voices to those who say that it is time for a speedy resolution of this issue. Baccalaureate preparation at a minimum is needed to implement the professional model of practice indicated in this book. The 1985 proposal is a step in the right direction; we need to take it.

In conclusion, this is an exciting time in nursing. It is a time of rapid change, which offers both individual nurses and the profession as a whole a unique opportunity to grow. In 1980 the American Nurses' Association specified the nature and scope of nursing practice in *Nursing: A Social Policy Statement*. Each individual nurse is obligated to assist the profession to fulfill the commitment spelled out in the statement and thereby assist the profession to more fully meet its responsibility to society. This book is our contribution.

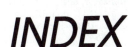

INDEX

Note: Page numbers followed by the letter t refer to tables.